MIND BODY MEDICINE

HOW TO USE YOUR MIND
FOR BETTER HEALTH

Edited by Daniel Goleman, Ph.D.,
and Joel Gurin

CONSUMER REPORTS BOOKS
A Division of Consumers Union
Yonkers, New York

Library of Congress Cataloging-in-Publication Data

Mind / body medicine: how to use your mind for better health / edited by Daniel Goleman and Joel Gurin.
        p.   cm.
    Includes index.
    ISBN 0-89043-580-4
    1. Psychosomatic medicine.   2. Mind and body.   3. Healing—Psychological
aspects.   I. Goleman, Daniel.   II. Gurin, Joel, 1953-
    RC49.M523   1993   92-35904
    613—dc20   CIP

ISBN 0-89043-840-4

Editorial production by Spectrum America
Illustrations by Harriet Greenfield
Design by Alex Jay

Fifth printing, December 1998
This book is printed on recycled paper.
Manufactured in the United States of America

The editors thank the following for permission to print adaptations of their copyrighted material:

    On page 24, "The Symptoms of Stress," from "Cognitive Behavioral Stress Management Intervention for an AIDS Risk Group" by Michael H. Antoni et al., University of Miami, 1988.
    On pages 35-38, "The Stresses of Life," from "Epidemiological Studies of Life Change and Illness," by Richard Rahe, *International Journal of Psychiatry in Medicine*, 6(1/2): 133-146, 1975. On page 71, "How Stressful Is Your Job?" from "The Political Implications of Psychosocial Work Redesign" by Robert Karasek, *International Journal of Health Services*, 19(3): 495, Baywood Publishing Co., 1989.
    On page 235, "How Metabolism Changes with the Relaxation Response"; page 238, "How the Relaxation Response Differs from Sleep"; page 243, "Physiological Changes with Different Techniques" from *The Relaxation Response* by Herbert Benson with Miriam Z. Klipper, William Morrow & Company, Inc., 1975.
    On page 240, "How to Elicit the Relaxation Response" from *Beyond the Relaxation Response* by Herbert Benson and William Proctor, Times Books, 1984.
    On page 388, "Keeping Depression in Check" from "Cognitive-Behavioral Stress Management Intervention Buffers Distress Responses and Immunological Changes Following Notification of HIV-1 Seropositivity" by Michael H. Antoni et al., *Journal of Consulting and Clinical Psychology*, 59(6): 910, American Psychological Association, 1991.

Consumer Reports Books gratefully acknowledges the cooperation and support of The John E. Fetzer Institute, Inc., of Kalamazoo, Michigan. The Fetzer Institute facilitated the planning and development of *Mind/Body Medicine*.

Mind/Body Medicine is a Consumer Reports Book published by Consumers Union, the nonprofit organization that publishes *Consumer Reports*, the monthly magazine of test reports, product Ratings, and buying guidance. Established in 1936, Consumers Union is chartered under the Not-For-Profit Corporation Law of the State of New York.

The purposes of Consumers Union, as stated in its charter, are to provide consumers with information and counsel on consumer goods and services, to give information on all matters relating to the expenditure of the family income, and to initiate and to cooperate with individual and group efforts seeking to create and maintain decent living standards.

Consumers Union derives its income solely from the sale of *Consumer Reports* and other publications. In addition, expenses of occasional public service efforts may be met, in part, by nonrestrictive, noncommercial contributions, grants, and fees. Consumers Union accepts no advertising or product samples and is not beholden in any way to any commercial interest. Its Ratings and reports are solely for the use of the readers of its publications. Neither the Ratings, nor the reports, nor any Consumers Union publication, including this book, may be used in advertising or for any commercial purpose. Consumers Union will take all steps open to it to prevent such uses of its material, its name, or the name of *Consumer Reports*.

CONTENTS

ACKNOWLEDGMENTS

This book has been a collaborative effort, and we have been fortunate to work with a remarkable group of associates. As editors, we are immensely grateful to this book's 31 contributors. They have produced comprehensive, authoritative chapters under tight deadlines and have been graciously patient with our editorial efforts to give the book a unified structure and consistent style.

Several other people have made important contributions to this book at various stages of its development. Kathleen Anderson, Harris Dienstfrey, David Eisenberg, David Grubin, and Judith Reemtsma all offered early advice on the book's structure and content. Robert Ader provided a valuable overview of current research in psychoneuroimmunology. Malcolm Schoen, one of Consumers Union's medical advisers, reviewed much of the book and raised important questions on several points. Steven Locke shared his perspective on the physiology of mind/body interactions and his knowledge of research on psychologically based interventions, which proved invaluable. We also thank the many anonymous peer reviewers who read individual chapters for us and offered insights, questions, and advice.

Numerous people played important roles in the editorial and production process. Carl Sherman and Rick Weiss worked with us in editing several chapters. Adria Pauze and Paula Tamburrino, and especially Donna Pough, coordinated the trafficking of manuscripts through many different versions. Mary Ann Larkin, with assistance from Sandra Cohen, checked and updated the Resources appendix. Dale Ramsey of Spectrum America and Meta Brophy of Consumer Reports Books ensured consistency of style and timeliness of publication.

Special thanks are due to three people who played key roles in shaping this book. Nan Silver worked closely with us, and with the contributors, to perform the initial structural and text editing on most of the chapters; the overall clarity and readability of the book are largely the result of her efforts. Marvin Lipman, Consumers Union's senior medical adviser, reviewed the entire manuscript meticulously and raised many thoughtful questions and criticisms that improved it greatly. And Ruth Turner, director of Consumer Reports Books, was a champion of this project from the very beginning. Without her strong support, the book would not have come into being; without her substantial involvement and input, it would be a lesser book.

We are especially grateful, too, to The John E. Fetzer Institute, Inc., which provided support that facilitated the planning and development of this project.

Several contributors wish to acknowledge the help they received on their chapters. An earlier, unpublished version of Chapter 5 was written under the auspices of the Institute for the Advancement of Health. The preparation of Chapter 12 was supported by funds from the Faulkner Institute for Reproductive Medicine. The authors of Chapter 6 express their appreciation to Caryn Feldman, Bruce Sorkin, Jane Gradwohl Nash, and Lorraine Turk for their comments on an earlier version of the chapter. And the authors of Chapter 18 thank several colleagues and friends who provided suggestions on an earlier draft: Jack Hartje, David Krebs, Joel Lubar, Doil Montgomery, Mike McKee, Susan Middaugh, Patricia Rollins, Richard Sherman, and Steven Wolf.

Finally, we owe a special debt of gratitude to Tara Bennett-Goleman, Carol Duchow Gurin, and two children—Alison and Joanna Gurin—for their love, patience, and support during this book's gestation.

PREFACE: ABOUT THIS BOOK— AND HOW TO USE IT

"CONTROL OF THE IMMUNE SYSTEM COMES INTO YOUR HANDS!"

"Trigger Your Body's Own Natural Immunities! For 21 Days, Absolutely Free!"

"Visions to Boost Immunity!"

Such blurbs call to us—from popular magazine articles, from ads, from brochures in our third-class mail—hailing medical miracles and touting breakthrough products. And too many of them are fraudulent, exaggerating or skewing what medical science is finding to be the actual relationship between the mind and physical health, a field now called *mind/body medicine*.

The particular examples we cite come from Robert Ader, a psychologist at the University of Rochester, who collects them because they misrepresent a field that he pioneered, psychoneuroimmunology (or PNI)—the study of the links between thoughts and emotions, the brain and nervous system, and the immune system. Ader has been joined by a growing cadre of researchers who are documenting, piece by piece, the role that the mind can—and cannot—play in disease and healing.

That scientific effort is beginning to reveal the physiological mechanisms that seem to allow mind to affect body. But as those headlines show, many of the popular claims made for the power of the mind to heal the body are distorted or inflated, going far beyond what science has established. Although the discerning medical consumer can find much of value in this new approach to medicine, there is also much to be wary of: Some reports about mind/body medicine that seem too startling to be true are simply false.

Some popular writers, for example, have taken a single case study of what seems to be a miraculous cure and presented it as proof of the mind's power to heal. Such claims go far beyond the scientific data; they amount to wishful thinking about positive thinking.

Other writers have done a disservice by claiming that people's illnesses are due to their "wishing" themselves to be sick. That unfortunate approach takes far too literally the connection between mind and body. Worse, it leaves sick people, who are already suffering, feeling guilty for their supposed role in becoming ill. No responsible advocate of mind/body medicine subscribes to that point of view.

But if some entrepreneurs and journalists have overinterpreted the meaning of mind/body medicine, others have not taken this growing field seriously enough. The media have tended to treat it as a "New Age" phenomenon more than as a serious scientific undertaking. Recent cover stories on alternative medicine in national magazines have treated relaxation, biofeedback, and hypnotherapy—mainstream mind/body approaches—together with homeopathy, aromatherapy, and crystal healing, which have nothing to do with mind/body medicine. One major magazine recently ran a sober article on hypnosis, biofeedback, and acupuncture (which is not a mind/body technique) under the headline "Wonder Cures from the Fringe."

Mind/body medicine does not offer miracle cures, any more than nutrition and exercise do. And yet, like those other "life-style" approaches, it has much of real value to offer the ill and the well alike. The best of mind/body medicine has helped bolster resistance to disease and brought relief from symptoms in thousands of patients. More and more medical centers—the nation's most prestigious among them—are offering mind/body interventions to their patients and encouraging research on this approach to healing.

To sort out the truth about mind/body medicine from the many fictions that surround it, we have brought together in this book many of the leaders in the field to report on the state of the art. We have asked them to explain what is already known in their areas of specialty and to reflect on what remains to be learned. Each chapter concludes with a brief summary, called "The Bottom Line," synopsizing the current state of that field. Reference material keyed to each chapter is given in the Resources appendix at the end of the book.

The book is divided into sections that cover the basic areas of mind/body medicine: its scientific principles, its application to specific diseases, its most widely used techniques, and its role in the hospital and the doctor's office. We have structured the book so that you can either read it from beginning to end for a thorough understanding of the field, or pick and choose the chapters you feel will be most helpful to you in your particular situation. Each chapter in the book has been written to stand on its own, without assuming the reader has read the entire book up to that point, in order to make the information in each chapter as useful and accessible as possible.

The scientific basis for mind/body medicine is emerging from recent research on the physiological mechanisms that connect the brain and nervous system with the hormonal and immune systems. Readers who want to understand these biological underpinnings of mind/body medicine—which are referred to throughout the book—will find them presented in Part I, Mind/Body Basics. This section offers a general overview of the field, a review of what science has established about the relationship between stress and disease, and a detailed look at the growing body of research connecting psychological states and physiological functions.

In Part II, The Mind's Role in Illness, we look at what science can tell us about the role of psychological states in specific medical conditions—in bringing them about, in worsening symptoms, in healing. The medical conditions covered in Part II include heart disease, cancer, headaches and other kinds of chronic pain, diabetes, skin disorders, gastrointestinal disease, arthritis, asthma, and problems in fertility and pregnancy. We also look at those instances where medical symptoms have no known biological cause but seem to be the result of psychological conditions. Many of these chapters, as well as those that follow, include descriptions of individuals the author of the chapter has treated with mind/body approaches; in those cases, names and identifying details have been changed to preserve anonymity.

Although there are many other diseases we might have included, this section covers the principal medical conditions for which sound research has begun to evaluate the effectiveness of mind/body approaches or to trace the ways psychological states affect the course of disease. We have intentionally said little about psychological problems like anxiety and depression or behavioral problems like smoking and overeating—not because they are unimportant, but because they are outside the main focus of this book.

Perhaps of greatest interest to readers who are themselves considering a mind/body approach for a medical problem are Part III, What You Can Do: Relaxation and Beyond, and Part IV, What You Can Do: Friends, Attitudes, and Coping. In these sections our experts write about the interventions that have produced the best results, as research and clinical experience have shown.

These clinically tested interventions include meditation, hypnosis, imagery, biofeedback, exercise, and support groups—as well as methods like psychotherapy, attitude change, and stress management—which can alter how we react to life's large and small challenges. For each of these methods, the experts tell us what to expect, the medical problems for which research has shown the approach may be most effective, what its limitations are, and what warnings to keep in mind.

Finally, should you want to apply some of the principles of mind/body medicine to your dealings with the medical system, consult Part V, Becoming an Active Patient. Mind/body medicine demands that patients become active partners in their own medical care. Rather than passively waiting for a doctor to cure you, you need to take an active role in caring for yourself.

That active participation is a part of mind/body medicine for two reasons: It enables you to deal with psychological reactions to medical treatment that could impede your recovery; and it gives you a sense of being in control of your treatment, which to some degree can be therapeutic in itself. Part of being an active patient is to prepare yourself psychologically for stressful medical procedures—whether a diagnostic test with a high-tech MRI machine, which has been likened to spending an hour inside a clanging metal can, or the often terrifying prospect of surgery. Another crucial part of being an active patient, discussed in the book's final chapter, is to find the best ways to communicate with your physician to make yourself your doctor's close ally in your own medical care. Ultimately, one of the most appropriate roles for mind/body medicine is to add a humane dimension to conventional medical treatment.

DANIEL GOLEMAN, PH.D., AND JOEL GURIN

I

MIND/BODY BASICS

1

WHAT IS MIND/BODY MEDICINE?

BY DANIEL GOLEMAN, PH.D., AND JOEL GURIN

- AT THE UNIVERSITY OF MASSACHUSETTS MEDICAL CENTER, 30 patients with diverse medical conditions—including heart disease, cancer, diabetes, chronic back pain, and colitis—sit meditating with eyes closed, focusing in utter stillness on the feeling of their breath moving in and out of their bodies. Most people who make this simple practice a part of their daily routine report a lessening of their distress and even relief from many medical symptoms.

- At the Ohio State University College of Medicine, second-year students undergoing the stress of final exams are taught a relaxation technique. Blood tests of immune function show that the stress of exams weakens the students' resistance to viruses. But those who practice the relaxation method most diligently show the least impairment of resistance.

- At a hospital in Cleveland, children with chronic, intractable pain from cancer are being taught to escape it by visualizing themselves in a relaxed, happy place.

Such studies are producing an ever-growing body of evidence that portends a sea change in the way health-care professionals and patients are viewing the role of the mind in the treatment of illness. Relaxation, hypnosis, and other mind/body approaches have been used in Western medicine for decades, even centuries, and very possibly for millennia by traditional healers.

DANIEL GOLEMAN, PH.D., writes for *The New York Times* on health and human behavior. JOEL GURIN is the science editor of *Consumer Reports*.

Two things are different today. First, the use of these approaches is becoming more widespread and they are gaining more respect and interest from researchers in major medical institutions. And second, evidence is mounting that mind/body techniques may not only improve the quality of life—particularly for someone dealing with a serious illness—but actually affect the course of disease itself.

The most compelling study to date was done at Stanford University by David Spiegel, a psychiatrist who never anticipated that his work would show that the mind has an impact on physical health. In the mid-1970s, Spiegel had led support groups for women being treated for advanced breast cancer that had spread throughout the body—a pattern that carries the grimmest of prognoses. His intent was to show that women placed at random into these groups, which allowed them to talk over their day-to-day troubles in a supportive setting, would suffer less from the emotional distress that accompanies cancer than other women in the same medical situation. The experiment was a success: The data soon showed that the groups did improve the women's quality of life.

The surprise came a decade later, when Spiegel went back to the women's records to see how long they had survived after the groups disbanded. As he recalls in Chapter 20, his original intention was to *disprove* the notion, spread by some popular books in the mid-1980s, that mental and emotional factors could influence the course of cancer. Instead, he was surprised to find that the women in the support groups had survived twice as long as the others. The added months of life—18 months, on average—were more than even cancer medications could have been expected to provide at that point in the women's disease. When Spiegel published these findings in the journal *The Lancet* late in 1989, they stunned the medical community and inspired many investigators to look more closely at the possible clinical effects of mind/body treatments. At least half a dozen research teams are now in the process of repeating his study to see if his results can be replicated.

Other scientists, laboring to unravel the physiology of the mind/body connection, have begun to outline plausible ways in which the mind and emotions could affect physical health. They have deepened our understanding of the effects of stress on the body and are accumulating convincing evidence that the immune system, along with other organs and systems in the body, can be influenced by the mind.

Taken together, these research efforts and clinical experiments suggest that the split between mind and body, long taken for granted in Western philosophy, is illusory indeed. The studies are also part of a new synthesis in medical science. They are part of *mind/body medicine*: an approach that sees the mind—our thoughts and emotions—as having a central impact on the body's health.

For patients, this new synthesis has a very practical significance. It means that by paying attention to and exerting some control over emotional and mental states—your worries, hostility, habitual reactions, pessimism, and depression—you may help yourself stay healthy or recover more rapidly from being sick.

From the perspective of doctors, nurses, and other health-care professionals, this new way of seeing things suggests there is much to be gained if they go beyond attending to physical disease and attend as well to the overall experience of illness—the way the disease affects a patient's spirits and the emotional reactions it calls forth.

In short, one basic tenet of mind/body medicine is that it is best to treat the whole person: Treating emotional distress should be an essential complement to standard medical care. Another tenet is that people can be active participants in their own health care and may be able to prevent disease or shorten its course by taking steps to manage their own psychological states.

Of course, these principles must be tempered with a realistic view of the many other factors at work in health and illness. No one is promising that people can cure themselves of disease just by thinking happy thoughts. That simplistic idea ignores the complexities of biology and the wired-in destiny of our genes. Worse, it can leave people feeling guilty about being sick at all. That is not the message of mind/body medicine.

But the evidence *is* growing stronger that states of mind can affect physical health. And while that effect may not be as dramatic as, say, the power of penicillin to fight a strep throat, it can be meaningful nonetheless. Mind/body approaches can certainly reduce the severity and frequency of medical symptoms. For example, they can make chronic headaches less frequent, reduce the nausea that accompanies chemotherapy, speed recovery from surgery, and help people with arthritis feel less restricted by their pain. Moreover, the same approaches may help strengthen the body's resistance to disease.

THE QUIET BEGINNINGS

The research that laid the basic scientific foundation for modern mind/body medicine began with an accidental discovery that attracted little attention at first. That discovery was made one day in 1974, in a laboratory at the University of Rochester School of Medicine and Dentistry. It led to research that would redraw biology's map of the body.

On that day, psychologist Robert Ader analyzed data from an experiment showing that the immune systems of white rats had learned a specific conditioned reaction. The results were startling because the prevailing wisdom held that the immune system should not have been capable of "learning" anything. Learning was something done only by the brain and central nervous system—certainly not by the immune system, the body's disease-fighting network of cells.

The discovery was serendipitous. Ader had been conducting a classic Pavlovian conditioning experiment, trying to teach the rats to respond with aversion to saccharin-flavored water. His study had a simple design. The rats were given a drink of saccharin-laced water and then received an injection of the drug cyclophosphamide, which Ader gave them to produce nausea. One shot should have been enough to condition them to associate saccharin water with nausea and avoid it.

But there was a problem. For some reason, many of the rats—though young and healthy—were getting sick and dying. Looking into the problem, Ader realized that the drug he was using to nauseate the rats also suppressed their immune systems. In particular, it lowered the number of T-cells, immune system cells that fight viruses and infections as they circulate through the body (see Chapter 3).

It seemed to Ader that giving the rats the saccharin water alone, *without* the immunosuppressive medication, was decreasing the number of T-cells in the rats' bloodstreams. Classical conditioning had triggered a learned association between the taste of the saccharin and the suppression of T-cells, so that later—when the rats tasted the flavored water alone—their immune systems reacted as though they were exposed to the drug itself. And that, in turn, made them more susceptible to disease.

But that just should not have happened, according to what was then the best scientific understanding of how the brain and immune system function.

Immune system cells travel the entire body, contacting virtually every other cell. Those cells they recognize, they leave alone; those they do not recognize, they attack—defending the body against tumors and virus-infected cells.

Until Ader's experiment, anatomists, physicians, and biologists all believed that the brain and the immune system were separate entities, neither one able to influence the functioning of the other. They were not aware of any pathway that connected the brain centers monitoring what the rats tasted with the areas of bone marrow that manufacture T-cells.

Ader himself could not quite believe his findings. To test the possibility of a connection, he teamed up with Nicholas Cohen, an immunologist at Rochester. In an elegant series of studies, they demonstrated that aspects of the immune system can, in fact, be conditioned, just as Pavlov had shown that dogs can be conditioned to salivate at the sound of a bell after food had been paired with the sound.

Ader's experiments have now been repeated successfully, and his discovery has opened the way to identifying the links between the immune system and the central nervous system. As a result, science is finding that there are many physiological connections between these two systems. These findings have generated the field of medical science known as *psychoneuroimmunology*, or PNI: *psycho* for mind, *neuro* for the neuroendocrine system (the nervous and hormonal systems), and *immunology* for the immune system.

While no one is yet quite sure just how the connections among these areas function, few medical researchers now doubt that such connections exist. Ader likes to quote a basic immunology textbook, published in 1991, that teaches that research studies in PNI now "confirm the long-standing belief that the immune system does not function completely autonomously." In the last decade, he says, the reaction of the scientific community to PNI "has gone from, 'It's impossible,' to, 'We knew it all along.'"

An explosion of interest in PNI has brought about renewed research on a whole range of physiological mechanisms, some of them known for decades, by which the mind and emotions may affect physical well-being. As scientists learn more about the hormones and neurotransmitters that brain cells use to communicate with each other and with the rest of the body, they are developing a deeper understanding of the stress response. They are learning more precisely how the physiological changes that occur under stress—or with emotional distress—may, for example, raise the risk of heart disease, make diabetes more difficult to control, or make it harder for some women to conceive.

Research is now revealing a range of likely avenues through which our mental states may influence our health. Although it will take years of work to piece together the precise biological mechanisms involved, the research done so far provides the beginnings of a sound scientific basis for mind/body medicine.

THREE LINES OF EVIDENCE

The scientific evidence for the mind's influence on the body now comes from three converging areas of research:

- Physiological research, which investigates the biological and biochemical connections between the brain and the body's systems.
- Epidemiological research, which shows correlations between certain psychological factors and certain illnesses in the population at large.
- Clinical research, which tests the effectiveness of mind/body approaches in preventing, alleviating, or treating specific diseases.

Each of these areas, taken alone, is incomplete; each has produced promising findings, but also raised unanswered questions. Taken together, however, the different kinds of research in mind/body medicine are beginning to show a coherent picture—like a jigsaw puzzle that still has many pieces missing, but that is starting to form a recognizable image.

Physiological research in mind/body medicine (described in detail in Chapters 2 and 3) dates back to Walter B. Cannon, who discovered the "fight-or-flight response" to stress during World War I. But the modern study of mind/body physiology began in the 1940s, when the pioneer researcher Hans Selye investigated the physical effects of psychological stress. This avenue of investigation was a precursor of current physiological research, which ranges from studying the intricacies of PNI to examining the ways in which emotions like anger may lead to biological changes that raise heart attack risk.

The key question for physiological researchers is whether the biological changes that stem from psychological factors actually make a difference to health. For example, even if stress or depression does lower the effectiveness of the immune system, is the drop great enough to increase the risk of illness?

In addition, because many physiological studies are done on experimental animals, their relevance to humans may be uncertain.

Epidemiological studies in this field look for relationships between psychosocial factors and patterns of illness in large populations. They date back to the early 1960s, when a study done for the U.S. Navy showed that men who had gone through serious life changes—a divorce, move, job loss, or the like—had an increased chance of becoming seriously ill within the months following those upsets. A more recent, and very significant, series of studies covering thousands of people has shown that men and women with few social ties are significantly more likely to become ill and die than people with a rich network of family, friends, and other social involvements.

The provocative findings of studies like these often suggest avenues for both physiological and clinical research. For instance, some researchers are now trying to unravel the reasons why upsetting experiences may be associated with illness and why strong social networks are linked to better health.

Clinical research provides the third major line of evidence, one that is now getting increased attention. David Spiegel's work with support groups for women with breast cancer is a paradigm of the new research in this area. The main shortcomings here are that such studies, while promising, must be seen as preliminary until they can be repeated by other, independent scientific investigators. And even then, without carefully designed follow-up studies of the people treated, it is by no means clear how and why such interventions may work. For instance, support groups for patients may work because they encourage patients to comply better with what their physicians tell them to do, or because the emotional changes the groups produce help boost immunity directly—or for both reasons.

The issues become even more complex when social support and relaxation training are combined with changes in diet and exercise, as they were in one of the most impressive clinical studies in this field. Internist Dean Ornish, director of the Preventive Medicine Research Institute at the University of California, San Francisco, conducted a study with patients who had severe coronary heart disease. He placed them in groups and led them through several significant life-style changes, combining mind/body approaches with a very-low-fat diet (one in which fat accounted for less than 10 percent of total calories). After one year in the groups, patients showed actual reversal of their severe atherosclerosis, something that had never previously been accomplished without the use of medication. Ornish's further research is showing that, in general, an even greater degree of reversal occurs in people who stay on the program over several years.

But the success of Ornish's patients cannot be attributed to any single, isolated part of the program, even though each part of the program was correlated independently with reversal of heart disease. The patients made full use of several mind/body approaches: They met weekly to share their emotional concerns and offer each other support; they changed their life-styles to lead less stressful, more fulfilling lives; and they practiced yoga and meditation. They also began to exercise several hours a week—a change that, in itself, can have significant effects on mood and the mind.

A large number of new clinical studies are now under way at leading U.S. medical institutions to measure the effects of mind/body techniques and to explore the physiological basis for those effects. Here are just a few examples of those studies (all related to work described in later chapters of this book):

- At Harvard Medical School, a series of ongoing studies suggests that a simple technique for eliciting the body's "relaxation response" can help patients with diseases ranging from hypertension to migraine headaches to irritable bowel syndrome.
- At Duke University, men and women with cardiovascular disease participate in groups that help them control their feelings of hostility and anger. (Earlier studies at Duke and elsewhere had shown that hostility is a risk factor for heart disease.) The researchers will follow the patients over time to see whether these emotional changes directly help their hearts.
- At the University of California, Los Angeles, a prospective study has been designed to follow up on David Spiegel's groundbreaking findings. Support groups for cancer patients at UCLA have already been found to strengthen key elements of the immune system. These patients are now being studied further to see whether the immunological changes are correlated with better clinical results, such as longer survival.
- At the University of Miami, the focus is on AIDS. There, in a comprehensive stress management program, men with HIV infection meet on Monday and Thursday nights to talk over the stresses of the week, to practice relaxation methods, and to help each other find ways to improve how they handle the range of life's demands. Again, early results are promising: heightened emotional resilience, positive effects on the

immune system, and a delay in the onset of the more serious symptoms that signal AIDS.

Mind/body medicine is still far from being an exact science, and many perplexing questions remain. But the areas of uncertainty are no greater than one would expect in a complex, evolving field. And the volume of well-designed research now under way or just beginning attests to the scientific excitement the field has generated in a fairly short period of time.

For most people, the question is not whether mind/body medicine is a legitimate field for research (it is), or whether its potential has been fully defined and proven (not yet). The immediate, practical question is whether mind/body medicine as it now stands can be of value to people dealing with a range of serious illnesses and to healthy people who want to stay that way.

We believe that it can. Although mind/body medicine is still evolving, enough is now known to make it worth trying in a number of situations. It may do a great deal to improve patients' quality of life, and possibly to improve their physical health, with very little risk.

A key reason is that mind/body medicine is not so much an "alternative" approach as a complementary one. It is perfectly compatible with standard medical treatment and can be a powerful way of augmenting it, not challenging it or replacing it. In fact, the mind/body approach harkens back to some of the best traditions of Western medicine—although some of those traditions have been ignored in the expanding, high-tech era of modern health care.

BEYOND THE PLACEBO

Long before research in PNI began, the mind's power to affect the body was well known in medicine. In the centuries before antibiotics and other "miracle drugs," caring physicians hoped that a reassuring bedside manner would mobilize hidden resources within their patients to fight their illness, and they consciously used the power of the mind to help heal the body. This approach was essential in the days when physicians had relatively few effective medications or procedures to offer; indeed, a motto of medicine until a century ago was, "Comfort always, cure seldom."

But the tradition drew on a deeper wisdom that can be traced back to Hippocrates: the understanding that the physician's manner is as potent as many a medicine. For centuries, wise doctors tried to capitalize on the *placebo effect*, the power for healing that can stem simply from a patient's belief that a treatment will be effective.

Offering patients hope and reassurances may seem quaint in a day when, finally, the doctor's bag contains medications that are truly effective and the tools of medicine daily grow more technologically dazzling. Yet the power of the placebo is still very real. In fact, it is implicitly acknowledged by every major medical journal in the world, as well as the U.S. Food and Drug Administration. The scientific method now requires that every new drug must be tested against a placebo, a dummy medication given to patients as if it were a real drug.

The optimum study is prospective, randomized, and double-blind. Patients are divided at random into two groups: One receives the real drug, the other receives a look-alike placebo, and neither the patient nor the physician knows which is which (a necessary precaution because that knowledge itself could affect the outcome). If the placebo effect were not a powerful one—powerful enough to derail an otherwise careful medical experiment—such elaborate precautions would be unnecessary.

The placebo effect has long puzzled medical researchers, who were at a loss to explain it but unable to dismiss it. Study after study showed that, for virtually any disease, a substantial portion of symptoms—roughly one-third, by most estimates—would improve when patients were given a placebo treatment with no pharmacological activity. Patients simply believed that the treatment would help them, and somehow, it did.

Although some medical researchers may think of the placebo effect as the experimental "static" that can interfere with an otherwise clean study, it is a striking demonstration of the mind's effect on health. In many ways, mind/body medicine is an attempt to harness the same forces that are behind the placebo effect, but in ways that enable patients to become active partners with their physicians in helping to heal themselves.

REHUMANIZING MEDICINE

Unfortunately, the development of modern medicine has made that kind of partnership more difficult to achieve. Over the last few decades, medicine has become more centered on high technology, physicians have become ever more specialized into narrow niches, and economics has forced doctors to spend less time with each patient. Physicians are not reimbursed as well for talking and listening to their patients as they are for performing tests and administering treatments. Although many physicians and nurses still offer their patients sensitive care, too many lack both the time and the training to help patients deal with their anxieties and other emotions—even though a patient's emotional state can be closely related to his or her physical health and can influence the course of treatment and recovery.

There is now a growing movement within medical schools and medical specialty organizations to improve the doctor/patient relationship. That movement has been fueled largely by evidence that many people find their physicians insensitive to their needs: Surveys show considerable dissatisfaction with conventional medical care, and the growing interest in "alternative" practices like chiropractic, acupuncture, and homeopathy certainly reflects it. There is also increasing evidence (described in Chapter 25) showing that good communication between doctor and patient can have a direct, beneficial effect on physical health.

Because the doctor/patient relationship has long been considered a major part of medical care, many physicians should welcome this return to traditional values. But effective, caring communication is only part of mind/body medicine, although an important part. Mind/body medicine also includes a number of specific self-help techniques—such as relaxation training, meditation, hypnosis, and biofeedback—that physicians may be unfamiliar with and may view with suspicion. In general, these approaches are barely covered in medical school, if they're mentioned at all.

Physicians are also likely to be unaware of the research that has made mind/body medicine a more credible field within the last decade. Older physicians may have received some exposure to "psychosomatic" medicine during their training. But many psychosomatic theories of disease—such as the notion that specific personality types predispose people to different kinds of illness—have not held up over time. Younger physicians may have learned something about the concepts of psychoneuroimmunology, but only if they were recent medical school graduates—and only if they had the interest to pursue those concepts.

Even physicians who follow the medical literature faithfully could have missed the development of mind/body medicine. Much of the research in this field has been published in journals of psychiatry or psychology or in journals that cover individual medical specialties. Relatively few research papers have been published in the most widely read journals, such as *The Lancet* and *The*

New England Journal of Medicine, although some recent key papers in those journals have brought mind/body medicine to more general attention. As the quality of mind/body research continues to improve—and it has improved dramatically in the last few years—the number of reports in major main-stream journals should also increase.

Ultimately, many physicians may be hesitant to use mind/body approaches for a fundamental reason: The new field of mind/body medicine is still in search of a comprehensive, unifying theory. Psychoneuroimmunology, which comes closest, is still incomplete from a scientific point of view. The working hypothesis for much PNI research is that psychological distress can suppress the immune system; that this effect can be great enough to increase the risk of physical illness; and that people who learn relaxation, stress management, or other mind/body approaches can increase their immunological resistance to disease. But although that hypothesis is consistent with a growing body of evidence, it is still far from proven.

THE CERTAIN BENEFITS

If research in PNI were the only justification for using mind/body approaches, it would certainly be premature to use them widely. But because there is other strong evidence supporting their use, we believe that physicians, psychologists, and other health-care professionals should be using these approaches more extensively than they are doing now, for several reasons:

- Many of the links between mind and body have little or nothing to do with the immune system. As later chapters in this book show, psychological stress can also affect the endocrine (hormonal) system and the circulatory system in ways that can create or worsen medical problems. Mind/body approaches can be useful in managing a number of illnesses related to those systems, from migraine headaches to diabetes.
- There is abundant evidence that psychological factors affect the way people *experience* medical symptoms, even when the mind does not affect the underlying disease process. Two people with chronic pain, for example, may have precisely the same underlying physical problem, and yet, for psychological reasons, one may function reasonably well while the other is incapacitated (see Chapter 6). The same can be said of people with arthritis or irritable bowel syndrome. In some cases (see

Chapter 13), psychological problems can lead to debilitating physical symptoms in people who have no diagnosable medical illness at all. Psychotherapy, stress management, and other mind/body approaches can do a great deal to help these people reduce their symptoms—and their medical bills.

- It is now indisputable that mind/body approaches can greatly improve the quality of life for people with physical illnesses. This is especially clear for people with cancer, a terrifying disease and one whose primary treatments, radiation and chemotherapy, have extremely unpleasant side effects. Relaxation methods, hypnosis, psychotherapy, and support groups like David Spiegel's have all been shown to help cancer patients deal effectively with their fears and anxieties about the disease and the treatments they must take. Even if these mind/body approaches did not extend the life of a single cancer patient, their emotional benefits would make them a valuable part of every cancer patient's care.

- Finally, the physical and emotional risks of mind/body techniques are virtually nonexistent. Even if some of their benefits are still hypothetical, no one is likely to be harmed by giving these approaches a try—as long as they're not used in place of conventional medicine.

WHAT DOES IT COST?

Mind/body approaches are generally inexpensive; some are even free. It costs next to nothing, for example, to learn the "relaxation response" (Chapter 14)—a basic method of meditation that is now used to treat a range of physical problems. Participation in groups that teach other forms of meditation, such as "mindfulness" meditation (Chapter 15), generally costs little or nothing. If you want to use relaxation or meditation to help you deal with a medical problem, however, you should discuss your specific program with your doctor, at the cost of a medical consultation.

Self-help groups for people with different medical problems offer social support, now recognized as a major psychological aid—and these, too, cost little or nothing to join. Some groups offer specific education in dealing with a disease, which can have both practical value and the psychological value of helping you feel a greater sense of control. A model for this approach, the Arthritis Self-Help Course, is now offered at hundreds of locations by the Arthritis Foundation, at an average cost of about $20 (see Chapter 10).

Hospital-based stress management courses can be considerably more expensive. One well-respected program costs just over $500 for eight weekly group sessions plus two individual sessions. Other programs may cost twice as much, or more.

At the high end of the scale are the individualized approaches: hypnosis, biofeedback, and psychotherapy. Costs for these treatments can range from around $50 a session to over $100. Biofeedback and hypnosis, however, are designed to help you learn to regulate your mind and body on your own; you will need only a limited number of sessions with a professional. And many physical problems that can be helped with psychotherapy require only a few months or less of weekly sessions.

Anyone thinking of trying a fee-based approach will naturally want to know how much of the cost is covered by medical insurance. There is no clear answer. In fact, the level of insurance reimbursement can vary from nearly complete to nothing at all. It depends on such factors as the policies of the insurance carrier, the nature of the mind/body approach, the setting in which the treatment is given (such as a hospital or a private office), and the reason for the treatment. For example, someone who learns biofeedback to help control Raynaud's disease—a circulatory problem for which biofeedback is a well-recognized treatment—will be more likely to be reimbursed than someone who enters psychotherapy to deal with more general emotional problems (even though those problems may affect physical health).

Overall, mind/body approaches are generally not reimbursed at the same rate as conventional medical treatments. Most insurance companies, for instance, pay only 50 percent of the cost of psychotherapy (as opposed to 80 percent for other procedures). In addition, they set low limits for the allowable cost per session and for the total amount that will be reimbursed for therapy over the life of the policy.

Such limits are unfortunate, because there is increasing evidence that psychological interventions can not only alleviate suffering but also reduce the overall cost of treatment. A number of studies, described in Chapters 13 and 22, have shown that people with medical problems who undergo psychotherapy lower their medical bills enough to pay for their therapy, and more. Similarly, certain kinds of psychological preparation for surgery can speed a patient's recovery enough to save many dollars in hospital costs—$1,000 or more, according to studies of some procedures (see Chapter 24). Although these studies are not definitive, the evidence so far suggests that mind/body approaches may be highly cost-effective.

On top of that, no one has even begun to estimate the potential savings, both in illness and in dollars, of using mind/body approaches to *prevent* disease as well as treat it. Preventive care in general has gotten short shrift from our medical institutions and third-party payers, which largely follow a disease management model, one that focuses on the treatment of symptoms and diseases only after they emerge. As a society, however, we are being forced to confront the economic costs of slighting disease prevention. In 1992, health-care costs in the United States exceeded $800 billion. By the year 2000, at the present rate of increase, that figure would more than double, and make up roughly 20 percent of the projected gross national product.

Something has to change. And one reasonable alternative, among many, is to emphasize disease prevention by encouraging a healthy life-style—including mind/body methods—particularly for groups of people at risk for specific diseases. To the degree that emotional turmoil and stress speed the disease process, mind/body interventions might well save money as well as protect health. Although these benefits are not yet proven, the possibility is already leading forward-looking insurance companies, health-care organizations, and corporations to examine mind/body methods as one way to decrease the cost of medical care.

THE BOTTOM LINE

Mind/body medicine includes a variety of treatments and approaches, ranging from meditation and relaxation training to social support groups, that are designed to enlist the mind in improving emotional well-being and physical health. A growing body of research now supports the use of these techniques. Nevertheless, they are probably being used by only a fraction of the people who could benefit from them.

Although many questions about mind/body medicine remain to be answered, we believe mind/body approaches can and should become much more widely used as a regular part of medical care, for several reasons:

- Mind/body approaches have shown great potential for improving the quality of life and reducing the pain and difficulty of symptoms for people with various chronic diseases.
- They may help control or reverse certain underlying disease processes.
- By reducing the effects of stress, they may help to prevent disease from developing.

- The physical and emotional risk of using these techniques is minimal, while their potential benefit is high.
- The economic cost of most mind/body approaches is low; many can be taught by paraprofessionals and involve no high-tech interventions.
- These techniques can easily be applied in the context of conventional medicine, rather than standing in opposition to it. They can and should be used along with standard medical care.

Despite encouraging trends, both physicians and insurance companies are lagging behind the needs of ordinary patients. More and more people are looking for medical care that takes into account their thoughts and emotions as well as their overt medical problems—in short, mind/body medicine. Informed consumers who want to try a mind/body approach often want answers to a number of questions that their doctors may not be able to help them with: What actually works? What is known about these methods and their strengths and limitations? And how do you find a reliable practitioner?

This book is designed to answer such crucial questions, as fully as current scientific knowledge allows.

2

Between Mind and Body: Stress, Emotions, and Health

by Kenneth R. Pelletier, Ph.D.

Asthmatics sneeze at plastic flowers. People with a terminal illness stay alive until after a significant event, apparently willing themselves to live until a graduation ceremony, a birthday milestone, or a religious holiday. A bout of rage precipitates a sudden, fatal heart attack. Specially trained people can voluntarily control such "involuntary" bodily functions as the electrical activity of the brain, heart rate, pain, bleeding, and even the body's response to infection.

Mind and body are inextricably linked, and their second-by-second interaction exerts a profound influence upon health and illness, life and death. Attitudes, beliefs, and emotional states ranging from love and compassion to fear and anger can trigger chain reactions that affect blood chemistry, heart rate, and the activity of every cell and organ system in the body—from the stomach and gastrointestinal tract to the immune system.

All of that is now indisputable fact. However, there is still great debate over the extent to which the mind can influence the body and the precise nature of the linkage. There is even greater debate over whether, and how, the mind/body connection can be harnessed to help people stay well or recover from illness.

Yet despite the uncertainties, effective and responsible mind/body ap-

KENNETH R. PELLETIER, Ph.D., M.D. (hon.), is a senior clinical fellow at the Stanford Center for Research in Disease Prevention and director of the Stanford Corporate Health Program at the Stanford University School of Medicine.

proaches are beginning to be used widely—in university and private clinics, in hospitals, and as an integral part of health promotion programs offered by such Fortune 500 corporate giants as AT&T, Johnson & Johnson, IBM, and General Motors. These programs are gaining support because they empower individuals, teaching them skills for self-management and giving them the knowledge to make informed choices that can promote better health.

Today, the medical research community is also taking mind/body interactions more seriously. One sign of the shift in attitudes was a recent report by the Institute of Medicine, a branch of the National Academy of Sciences, which conducted an inquiry into behavioral influences on the relationship between hormones and immunity. The report's conclusion: "Scientific data generally support the idea that the nervous system directly or through neuroendocrine mechanisms [the effects of the nervous system on hormones] can affect the immune system." Similarly, a 1992 review of stress and disease from two physicians, researchers at the National Institutes of Health, noted the role of stress in a wide array of psychiatric disorders, autoimmune diseases, coronary heart disease, functional disorders of the intestinal tract, chronic pain, and a range of other medical and psychological disorders.

As one who has investigated and worked with mind/body approaches for more than 20 years, as both a researcher and a clinician, I have seen a dramatic shift in the medical acceptance of these concepts in the last decade. The point was brought home to me recently when a new patient walked into my office at the Stanford University School of Medicine.

Actually, this patient was a former colleague of mine, a cardiologist who had been at the University of California School of Medicine in San Francisco (UCSF) when I was a faculty member there during the 1970s and 1980s. I remembered him particularly from a story that one of my patients at UCSF had told me a decade ago. On the day she arrived for her first visit with me, she told me that she had ended up on the wrong floor and asked a cardiologist—this cardiologist—how to find our Behavioral Medicine offices in the Department of Medicine. "Oh, the bones-and-rattles types!" he said sarcastically. "They're right upstairs."

Now, almost ten years later to the day, the cardiologist had referred himself to me for treatment. He had developed a severe heart arrhythmia, which was not adequately controlled by medication. As he stated it, his "last resort" was to determine whether stress was playing a part.

During the course of treatment, he realized that the times when his arrhythmia became most severe were related to tensions he and his wife were experiencing over physical intimacy. Specifically, he found that when he wanted his wife to touch him, he would have episodes of arrhythmia, which allowed him to be touched and cared for without having to be sexual. When, in the course of his therapy, he and his wife talked the issues over and found more ways to be physically intimate, his arrhythmia cleared up and he needed no further medication. For both of us, the experience confirmed the observation that what goes on in the mind of the patient is at least as important as what goes on inside the body—or, as the eminent physician Sir William Osler once observed, "The care of tuberculosis depends more on what the patient has in his head than what he has in his chest."

Mind/body medicine has attracted increasing interest from physicians, psychologists, nurses, numerous researchers in immunology and endocrinology, and other health-care professionals as the science behind it has become better established. Surely, the most important recent development has been the explosion of research in the new field of psychoneuroimmunology (PNI). As described in Chapter 1, the field attempts to encompass the domains of the mind and emotions, the brain and central nervous system, and the immune system, which defends the body against both internal cancerous cells and external invaders, such as bacteria or viruses.

There is now a great deal of evidence for direct connections between the central nervous system and the immune system—parts of the body that had long been thought to be independent. Nerve endings have been found in the organs and systems of the immune system—the thymus, lymph nodes, spleen, and bone marrow—and immune system cells respond directly to chemical signals produced by the nervous system and released into the bloodstream.

Although PNI research is still at an early stage, it is already offering strong support for the observation that there is an intimate interaction between mind and body at the heart of health and disease. That idea, however, is hardly new. Since the early part of this century, clinicians have known that psychological conflicts and difficult life events—what we generally think of as stress—could affect the body's hormones and cardiovascular system and could increase the risk of illness. More recent discoveries in PNI have brought a higher level of precision to the research process, suggested more sophisticated possible explanations for the mind's role in certain diseases, and raised a host of new and provocative questions.

Now the challenge is to understand the intricate relationships between mind, body, stress, and the psychosocial and physical environment, at every level. There are two broad, basic questions: What are the psychological events that have the greatest effects on health, and how, precisely, do they affect the body physiologically?

"FIGHT-OR-FLIGHT" AND BEYOND

Actually, the mind's influence on health has been recognized by medicine since its beginnings. Although it may have been underestimated or poorly understood at times, it has never been ignored. In the fourth century B.C., Hippocrates—the founder of Western medicine who originated the Hippocratic Oath—equated health to a harmonious balance of mind, body, and the environment. By contrast, disease was due to a disharmony of these elements. Hippocrates' dictum that "nature is the healer of disease" remains a mainstay of medicine to this day. Later, in the second century A.D., the Greek physician Galen observed that "melancholic" women appeared to be especially susceptible to breast cancer.

During the Renaissance, Thomas Sydenham extended Hippocrates' observations about the "healing power of nature," proposing that a person's internal adaptation to external forces was a major factor in disease and health. In the mid-1800s, the eminent French physiologist Claude Bernard, who defined the role of the pancreas in digestion, also emphasized the role of the *milieu intérieur*, or inner state, as essential to understanding health and disease. Then, at the beginning of this century, that idea was given a scientific basis by Harvard physiologist Walter B. Cannon, who first described the *fight-or-flight response*: the internal adaptive response of the body to a threat.

In this response, the body secretes *catecholamines*, "stress hormones" that immediately arouse key organs, preparing a person or animal under threat to fight or run. Best known of these hormones is epinephrine, also called adrenaline, which is produced by the adrenal glands (located just on top of each kidney).

This fight-or-flight response was essential to survival in a time when human beings faced physical threats, such as wild animals, that caused acute stress and could be dealt with effectively by either fighting or running away. By contrast, the stresses we face in modern life are much more likely to be psychological and interpersonal and not able to be handled by fighting or fleeing. Unfortunately—as Hans Selye, a pioneering stress researcher at McGill

University, demonstrated in the 1950s—the body reacts to today's stresses as though it were still facing a real physical threat.

Two forms of stress—short-term or acute, and long-term or chronic—have different consequences for health. (The biology of both forms of stress and the appropriate clinical interventions are detailed in my book, *Mind as Healer, Mind as Slayer*.)

If you are under chronic stress—for example, if you're under constant deadline pressure, or having major difficulties with your spouse—your body reacts with the same physical changes that would be appropriate if you were under acute stress (for example, a near-miss on the freeway or the reaction to a sudden loud noise). Catecholamines trigger a cascade of physiological changes that marshal the body to readiness: Heart rate, blood pressure, and muscle tension all rise sharply; the stomach and intestines become less active; and the blood level of glucose, or blood sugar, rises for quick energy. This physical turmoil generally goes along with a psychological response: You may experience racing thoughts, anxiety, and even panic. (See "The Symptoms of Stress.")

Under conditions of chronic, long-term stress, the perfectly normal responses that occur under short-term stress are abnormally protracted and can lead to chronic disease or contribute to the development of disease. With chronic stress, the immune system tends to be suppressed or become less active, the blood-cholesterol level rises, and calcium is lost from the bones. When protracted over time, the normal short-term increases in blood pressure can become hypertension, increased muscle tension can lead to headaches or aggravate pain, unusual changes in the activity of the intestinal tract can lead to diarrhea or spasms, increases in heart rate can raise the risk of an arrhythmia. In addition, depressed immunity may make an individual susceptible to colds and the flu or possibly to more serious diseases.

If psychological stress suppresses immunity, as recent research suggests, why would this mechanism have persisted throughout evolution? There are at least three possible explanations: First, these changes are an unfortunate side effect of the fight-or-flight response but are outweighed by its benefits for survival; second, perhaps evolution has not kept pace with modern forms of stress, and we may be evolving a more adaptive response; or third, perhaps these changes in immunity are within normal limits and are usually benign, so that natural selection would not have worked against them.

Reactions to stress are governed largely by the *autonomic nervous system*, a part of the nervous system over which we have virtually no direct voluntary

THE SYMPTOMS OF STRESS

(The following list was compiled by University of Miami psychologist Michael Antoni and colleagues.)

Cognitive symptoms
Anxious thoughts, fearful anticipation, poor concentration, difficulty with memory.

Emotional symptoms
Feelings of tension, irritability, restlessness, worries, inability to relax, depression.

Behavioral symptoms
Avoidance of tasks; sleep problems; difficulty in completing work assignments; fidgeting; tremors; strained face; clenching fists; crying; changes in drinking, eating, or smoking behaviors.

Physiological symptoms
Stiff or tense muscles, grinding teeth, sweating, tension headaches, faint feelings, choking feeling, difficulty in swallowing, stomachache, nausea, vomiting, loosening of bowels, constipation, frequency and urgency of urination, loss of interest in sex, tiredness, shakiness or tremors, weight loss or gain, awareness of heart beat.

Social symptoms
Some people in stressful times tend to seek out others to be with. Other people withdraw under stress. Also, the *quality* of relationships can change when a person is under stress.

control. It has two branches: the *sympathetic nervous system*, which regulates the kind of arousal described above, and the *parasympathetic nervous system*, which controls a countervailing set of responses. Generally, the parasympathetic nervous system induces relaxation and helps the body compensate for periods of high arousal—for example, by lowering heart rate, blood pressure, and muscle tension. These relaxing responses are a biologically regenerative state, helping the body to recuperate. However, the parasympathetic nervous system is not "better" because of its role in relaxation nor is it always benign. Experimental studies of bereavement, in which animals are stressed by separating them from close family members, show that this form of stress actually produces a form of depression characterized by increased parasympathetic activity.

All stress management techniques, from meditation to biofeedback, aim to induce a positive parasympathetic state. One name for this response is the *relaxation response*, a term coined by Herbert Benson of the Harvard Medical School (see Chapter 14). Overall, the goal of stress management is not only to help people withstand short-lived stressful events, but to defuse the effects of chronic stress—a more serious threat because chronic stress may not give the body the respite it needs to recover.

Some early ideas about the link between stress and illness are now being fleshed out. Research has suggested that chronic stress may impair the function of the immune system, although, in general, immunity is temporarily enhanced under short-term stress, such as physical trauma or injury. Researchers have found many pathways through which stress may influence immunity; for example, under certain conditions, adrenaline, cortisol, and related hormones can affect the activity of immune system cells.

There is also growing evidence that stress hormones may play a role in a wide variety of illnesses, from hormonal diseases like diabetes and thyroid conditions to psychiatric diseases, including anorexia nervosa, panic attacks, and obsessive-compulsive disorder. In addition, there is renewed interest in the 1936 discovery that the proliferation of certain immune system cells (eosinophilia) is associated with severe heart failure. If the eosinophilia is influenced by psychological factors, that would provide an intriguing link between the nervous, immune, and cardiovascular systems. Current research is making it clear, however, that the link between stress and disease operates through many different pathways, not just a handful of hormones or a finite net of neurons.

Take the case of heart disease. There is now good evidence from animal and human studies that stress and strong emotions—particularly hostility and anger—can contribute to long-term damage to the heart and blood vessels and can precipitate sudden heart attacks (see Chapter 4). Bouts of anger seem to trigger ischemia, or a deficiency in blood flow to the heart, to a small but significant degree in healthy individuals—and to a greater degree in people with heart disease. Their blood-flow decreases are greater during anger than during exercise.

Recent research has shown that the precise ways in which stress works on the heart are both varied and complex. Numerous studies have been conducted with both animals and humans with the following findings confirmed in human studies. Changes triggered by stress may injure the heart in a number of ways:

- Various stressors, ranging from mental arithmetic to physical discomfort, induce elevated blood pressure in both healthy individuals and people with borderline high blood pressure. Increases are greater and more prolonged for those individuals with borderline or preexisting hypertension.
- Mental stress, such as doing complex math (a standard experimental stressor), can induce a spasm or sudden constriction of the coronary arteries for people with preexisting heart disease.
- Stress hormones may indirectly increase the blood's tendency to clot, raise the blood-cholesterol level, or induce a sudden constriction of the coronary arteries—which can block the supply of blood to the heart muscle and lead to a heart attack.
- Under extreme stress or exertion, the brain's control over heart rate may be disrupted, leading to fibrillation and sudden death.

Future research and clinical studies will not only clarify these mind/body connections, but lead to more effective programs in the prevention and reversal of coronary heart disease.

WHO IS UNDER STRESS, AND WHY?

Just as the physiological consequences of stress vary widely, so do its causes. The mind's reaction to stress is as complex as the body's. In recent years, research on the psychological roots of the stress response has given us a much better chance of learning to control that response.

Although we all know what stress is when we experience it, coming to grips with it scientifically has been a major challenge. One problem is that the very definition of *stress* has been vague and inconsistent, sometimes referring to an outside force, sometimes to the body's reaction to it. Early in 1986, several private foundations funded a major conference in Tucson, Arizona, of psychologists, immunologists, and physicians. They met to define a common ground in terminology, research procedures, and measurement in the area of psychoneuroimmunology. Ironically, the first stumbling block was an attempt to define stress, which led to the unanimous conclusion that any absolute definition was literally impossible. It was agreed, however, that stress is not what happens to someone—those outside forces are the *stressors*—but how a person *reacts* to what happens.

That distinction comes at the end of a long evolution in our understanding of stress. In a great deal of early work, stress was thought of largely as a universal force acting on the passive body. It was assumed that all people would react in more or less the same way to major disruptions—the death of a loved one, a divorce, a fight with the boss—and that such "stresses" were likely to be hazardous to health.

Our modern study of these stressors was really moved forward by psychiatrists Thomas Holmes and Richard Rahe, at the University of Washington School of Medicine, who found ways to quantify the effects of stressful events. In the late 1950s and early 1960s, based on tests of more than 5,000 people, Holmes and Rahe developed the classic, systematized method of correlating the events in people's lives with their illnesses. They showed that the more stress a person had experienced, the more likely it was that he or she would become sick over the next several months.

Events that were linked to illness covered a wide emotional range, including divorce, a death in the family, changing jobs, pregnancy, and obtaining a large mortgage. Holmes and Rahe found that even occasions for joy and celebration, like marriage or retirement, can take their toll, if only from the sheer amount of change that they demand we cope with. When life brings many such changes at once, a prolonged, intense, and potentially dangerous stress reaction is more likely. (See "The Stresses of Life" at the end of this chapter.)

These studies by Holmes and Rahe were ground-breaking and highly influential, but they needed to be more fully developed. Although many studies have now found links between stressful life events and disease—one recent study, for example, found a relationship between the amount of stress in a person's life and the risk of catching cold (see Chapter 3)—other studies have failed to find such connections. In many studies, in fact, the correlation between such stressors and subsequent illness is markedly low.

There is no simple, direct connection between life stress and illness: Subjected to the same stressors, some people will get sick and others will not. This is an observation confirmed and supported by Holmes's and Rahe's more recent research. A number of theories have been developed to try to explain the differences.

DISEASE AND PERSONALITY

One set of theories, which began to gain currency in the 1950s, held that people with "disease-prone personalities" were especially likely to develop specific illnesses. Rheumatoid arthritis, for example, was thought to be correlated with perfectionism, compliance, subservience, nervousness, restlessness, reserve, and anger. Cancer was allegedly linked with nonassertiveness, an inability to express emotion, and hopelessness. Other personality types were thought to be especially prone to asthma, or ulcers, or migraines.

One aspect of this research still seems promising: Coronary heart disease does seem to be especially common in people with a specific hostile and angry personality type and in those who are "hot reactors"—people who react excessively to moderate stressors (see Chapter 4). With that exception, the notion that specific personality types are linked to specific illnesses—including asthma, ulcerative colitis, and rheumatoid arthritis—has not been proven. In particular, the purported cancer-prone personality has not been supported by persuasive evidence (see Chapter 5).

Nevertheless, there may be such a thing as a *general* disease-prone personality type, one that gives the individual a higher risk overall of becoming ill. Several years ago, Howard Friedman and Stephanie Booth-Kewley, psychologists at the University of California, Riverside, analyzed the results of more than 200 studies purporting to link specific personality types to asthma, arthritis, ulcers, headaches, or coronary heart disease. Although they found little evidence for such specific linkages, they did find suggestive evidence for "a generic 'disease-prone' personality that involves depression, anger/hostility, anxiety, and possibly other aspects of personality." These character traits, they found, seemed to raise the overall risk of disease. Precisely what disease an individual develops may depend largely on his or her specific vulnerabilities, determined by family history, health-related habits (smoking, drinking, and diet), environmental exposures, socioeconomic status, racial and ethnic background, as well as medical care.

Neuroscientist Candace Pert, formerly of the National Institute of Mental

Health, has suggested that anxiety, hostility, and other emotional states may affect the immune system directly—a hypothesis that would help explain their connection to illness. Support for Pert's hypothesis comes from the study of receptors: molecular structures on the surface of cells that enable those cells to respond to other molecules, such as hormones and brain chemicals. Cells in the limbic system—the part of the brain that controls emotional behavior—have an unusually large number of receptors for neuropeptides, a special class of chemicals that modulate the way in which nerve cells respond to signals from other nerve cells. Best known of the neuropeptides are the endorphins (substances produced in the body that are similar to morphine), which Pert helped discover with neuroscientist Solomon Snyder nearly two decades ago.

This concentration of receptors in the limbic system suggests that neuropeptides may play a role in the emotions. As Pert and other researchers point out, the same chemicals may also influence the immune system. This hypothesis is supported by the recent discovery that immune system cells contain receptors for endorphins and other neuropeptides.

COPING: A CRITICAL FACTOR

Individual differences in the way people cope with stressful events may be at least as important as the stressors themselves in determining health or illness. A variety of psychological factors—including mood, personality characteristics, coping style, suppressed anger, a sense of hopelessness, psychological vulnerability, and defensiveness—can all affect the way a person deals with stress and thus can potentially modulate the impact that stress will have on the immune system.

If negative psychological traits can intensify the effects of stressors, positive ways of coping may buffer the body from stress. Psychologist Suzanne Kobasa, at the City University of New York, has identified and measured a style of psychological coping she terms *hardiness*, which can modify the relationship between stress and illness. People high in hardiness, she has found, are more resistant to illness than low scorers.

While at the University of Chicago, Kobasa studied a group of business executives over eight years as they faced the normal crises and turmoil of running a corporation. She found that certain personality traits marked those who stayed healthiest while steering their companies. One trait was seeing life's demands as a *challenge* rather than a threat, responding with excitement and energy to change. Another was having a *commitment* to something they felt was meaningful—their work, the community, their family. A third trait—a critical one—was a sense of being in *control*: having the right information and being able to make decisions that can make a crucial difference.

Animal experiments also suggest that a sense of control may be especially important in avoiding illness. In experimental animals, a variety of stressors—including overcrowding, electric shock, high-intensity sound, and exposure to predators—can decrease the functioning of immune system cells. But the immune system is especially disrupted by stressors that an animal can do nothing to escape—as opposed, say, to an electric shock that a cat can jump away from.

One of many studies of this effect was conducted at the University of Pennsylvania by psychologist Martin E. P. Seligman—who formulated the concept of *learned helplessness* (see Chapter 21)—and his colleague Madelon Visitainer. In their research, laboratory mice were subjected to inescapable shock, escapable shock, or no shock at all one day after being injected with a solution that could lead to the growth of tumors. Fully 73 percent of the mice who received shocks they could not escape developed at least some tumors. By contrast, only 37 percent of the mice who *could* escape suffered from tumor growth.

Numerous animal studies like this one, and a growing number of studies in human beings, have shown that having a sense of control—or of lacking control—over the sources of stress in life can have a profound effect on health. For example, researcher Robert A. Karasek, when he was at the Cornell University Medical College, found that a high rate of heart disease was linked to the "job strain" of certain jobs: those where people felt highly pressured but had little or no control over how they met the job's demands. One of these hazardous occupations, for instance, was bus driving: The driver had to keep to the schedule in the face of impossible-to-control traffic conditions. People in such jobs, including air traffic controllers and secretaries, were especially likely to have elevated blood pressure and enlargement of the left ventricular area of the heart, a danger sign for heart attack (see Chapter 4).

Your ability to cope with stress is not just a matter of personal control or personal attitude; it may also reflect the strength of your social networks. Evidence is accumulating that support from family, friends, community members, and even from having a pet, is important to a person's health. According to one theory, social contacts may serve as buffers that help filter and moderate the way we interpret stressful events and may thus provide a means of coping with stress (see Chapter 20).

People with supportive social networks have been shown to have better overall health, lower rates of cancer and heart disease, less coronary blockage (as measured by angiograms), shorter hospital stays when they do get sick, and better resistance to infection than those whose social bonds are not strong. In contrast, people who are particularly isolated have a higher death rate in general and higher-than-average rates of a variety of illnesses, including arthritis, hypertension, coronary heart disease, and colds, tuberculosis, and other infections.

By the same token, although married people are generally healthier than singles, difficulties in the marriage can have negative effects on health. Marital conflict has been shown to disrupt immune system function (see Chapter 3). Loss of a spouse due to death or divorce also increases the risk of fatal heart attack, and men who have lost their wives have a higher-than-average death rate from all causes.

PSYCHONEUROIMMUNOLOGY: SORTING OUT THE VARIABLES

Because so many factors can affect a person's response to stress, it is difficult to determine the precise impact of such stressors. In addition to the social and psychological factors described above, a person's age, race, sex, and genetic makeup as well as the nature and duration of the stress may all affect the ultimate health outcome. To make things simpler, many recent studies have focused on one type of physiological response to stress—changes in the immune system—in a limited number of specific situations.

Much of the research in psychoneuroimmunology has focused on standard behavioral or psychosocial stressors, particularly examinations, bereavement, and sleep deprivation. Several studies have now shown that the academic pressure of examinations is related to immunological changes. For example, Janice Kiecolt-Glaser and Ronald Glaser at the Ohio State University College of Medicine have characterized changes that occur in immune system cells when medical students take final exams (see Chapter 3). Studies have shown that the experience of bereavement, too, may impair immune function, decreasing the ability of certain white blood cells, called lymphocytes, to grow and multiply. There is also some evidence that experimental sleep deprivation can decrease the functioning of immune system cells as well.

These findings all suggest that the immune system becomes less effective under protracted stress. However, it is not yet clear whether the changes seen in studies like these actually lead to physical illness or interfere with healing. Although many studies have yielded results that are statistically significant, that only means that they are unlikely to have occurred by chance; a larger question is whether they are *clinically* significant. Because numbers of immune system cells generally remain in the normal range even under stress, the medical impact of these changes still needs to be investigated, as described in Chapter 3.

TOWARD PREVENTION AND TREATMENT

Ultimately, the most significant challenge faced by PNI researchers is to find ways to maximize the functioning of the immune system to enhance health. The research is likely to lead to two types of treatment: new uses of behavioral approaches and new drugs used with or without behavioral interventions.

Meditation, visualization, hypnosis, biofeedback, and numerous relaxation techniques already show promise in helping prevent and treat a variety of illnesses, including coronary heart disease, autoimmune disorders, chronic lung disease, headaches, and gastrointestinal problems, as well as panic attacks, depression, and other psychological disorders. Researchers are now trying to demonstrate that such mind/body approaches can also directly affect the immune system, with some encouraging results. In one study conducted by Janice Kiecolt-Glaser and her colleagues, geriatric nursing home residents who were taught relaxation and guided imagery showed both increased activity of certain immune system cells and improved physiological control over latent herpes virus infections. Other studies have suggested that humor, positive emotions, and hypnotic suggestion may affect the immune response. Under hypnosis, some individuals are able to increase the number of lymphocytes in their bloodstream. Although these studies are still not definitive, they suggest it may be possible to control and perhaps optimize the activity of the immune system through the mind.

Group psychotherapy may also have an impact on immune response and physical health. Psychiatrist Fawzy I. Fawzy and his colleagues at the University of California, Los Angeles Neuropsychiatric Institute have treated 40 malignant melanoma patients with group therapy in addition to standard medical treatment. Another group of similar patients received medical treatment only. Compared to the control group, the patients who received group therapy showed a significant improvement in the number and activity of tumor-fighting immune system cells, as well as a greater psychological ability to cope with stressful events. These results complement the earlier, ground-breaking study by Stanford University psychiatrist David Spiegel, who reported in 1989 that women with breast cancer who received supportive group therapy survived twice as long as those who did not. (See Chapter 20.)

Most recently, psychologist James W. Pennebaker and graduate student Martha E. Francis of Southern Methodist University in Dallas concluded an intriguing study of an innovative clinical intervention. Forty-one university employees were divided into two groups. For 20 minutes, once a week for four consecutive weeks, people were asked to write about a traumatic event in one group and a general topic in the other group. Specific substances related to immunity, as well as 23 other biochemical markers, were measured before and after. Although these specific immune measures did not show a difference between the two groups, there were positive changes in measures of liver function and a reduction in absenteeism for those who wrote about a personal traumatic event, presumably because that experience provided psychological relief. A similar study conducted by Pennebaker, Janice Kiecolt-Glaser, and Ronald Glaser, using 50 undergraduate students, did show a positive influence on immunity; 25 students who wrote about "traumatic" events for 20 minutes a day over four consecutive days showed greater immune cell activity in standard laboratory tests than those who did not write about traumas (see Chapter 3). Such innovative studies need to be replicated with other measures of immunity, because they show that a simple, clear intervention appears to have a positive impact on health.

More studies are needed to clarify the range of effects that mind/body approaches can have—the precise psychological, immunological, and hormonal changes, as well as the overall effects on physical health. Perhaps the ultimate challenges are to find the best techniques to use for specific physical and psychological ailments and to couple those techniques with other behavioral changes (such as diet and exercise), overall health care, and pharmaceuticals.

Studies are also needed to probe the limits of mind/body approaches and to find out just how great an effect they can have under optimal conditions. In this regard, researchers can gain much by using as experimental subjects people who are already expert in using mind/body techniques, rather than relying on large numbers of inexperienced subjects. If you wanted to study the physiology of piano playing, you would learn more from concert pianists than from randomly selected novices who were still learning their finger exercises. Similarly, researchers could learn a great deal by studying the small number of individuals who can alter their neuropsychological and immunological functions at will. By understanding what these exceptional people do, scientists could learn how to teach such skills to a wider range of people and help them use these methods to enhance their health.

In one innovative study, reported in the *Archives of Internal Medicine*, researchers at the University of Arkansas College of Medicine worked with a 39-year-old woman who was an experienced meditator. After her normal immunological responses were measured, the woman was able voluntarily to reduce her immunological reaction to a skin test, for a period of three weeks. At the request of the researchers, she was then able to bring it back up to her normal level voluntarily. Although other similar volunteers failed to produce this effect, this innovative study shows that it is possible, in principle, for a practiced individual to voluntarily regulate a specific immune response through meditation and visualization. This study is similar to a series of studies I conducted with researchers Joe Kamiya and Erik Peper at UCSF in the early 1970s. We found clear evidence that experienced meditators could control pain, bleeding, electrical activity in the brain, muscle tension, and infection.

Researchers are now planning further studies to see whether other adept meditators and individuals who rate high on hypnotic susceptibility can change their immune responses at will, under controlled conditions. If such direct mental control over immunity can be demonstrated, a logical step would be to teach mind/body strategies to patients with immune or autoimmune diseases to see if they could consciously improve their medical condition.

THE BOTTOM LINE

Despite the sometimes conflicting findings of current research, there is increasingly compelling scientific evidence that mind and body are inextricably linked. General effects of stress on the body have been known for decades in research and observed for centuries in clinical situations. Now a new body of research is showing that stress can also have an impact on the immune system. Furthermore, psychological factors play a role in determining whether people subjected to stressful events will get sick or not. A growing number of studies indicate that mind/body approaches could help prevent or treat many diseases related to life-style.

Given the current crisis in medical care, greater attention to health promotion and disease prevention, including the role of psychological factors and mind/body interventions, would serve us well. Many psychological and behavioral approaches have earned a place in mainstream clinical practice. One major direction is the combination of behavioral and pharmacological approaches in treating heart disease, arthritis, smoking, and chemical dependencies. More research will help clarify the value of these approaches and the best ways to maximize their effectiveness.

Research is also needed to clarify the role of such hard-to-measure factors as beliefs, positive emotions, and even spiritual values. Although these subjects might seem to be grist for idle philosophical speculation, they are crucial to psychological well-being, physical health, and the future development of a truly effective health-care system.

THE STRESSES OF LIFE

This table from Richard Rahe, a leading stress researcher, shows estimates of the relative amounts of stress associated with different events. These estimates are derived from questionnaires in which people were asked which events they had experienced recently and then asked to gauge the degree of adjustment each event required. The estimates, given in "life change units" (LCUs), range from 25, for a change in political beliefs or a minor illness, to 105, for the death of a child or spouse.

HEALTH	LCU
An injury or illness that:	
kept you in bed a week or more or sent you to the hospital	42
was less serious than described above	25

Major dental work	40
Major change in eating habits	29
Major change in sleeping habits	31
Major change in usual type or amount of recreation	30

WORK

Change to a new type of work	38
Change in work hours and conditions	33
Change in responsibilities at work:	
more responsibilities	31
fewer responsibilities	29
promotion	31
demotion	57
transfer	38
Troubles at work:	
with your boss	39
with coworkers	35
with persons under your supervision	30
other work troubles	31
Major business adjustment	38
Retirement	49
Loss of job:	
laid off work	57
fired from work	64
Taking a correspondence course	29

HOME AND FAMILY

Major change in living conditions	39
Change in residence:	
move within the same town or city	28
move to a different town, city, or state	38
Change in family get-togethers	26
Major change in health or behavior of family member	52
Marriage	50

Pregnancy	60
Miscarriage or abortion	53
Gain of a new family member:	
birth of a child	49
adoption of a child	45
a relative moving in with you	57
Spouse beginning or ending work outside the home	37
Child leaving home:	
to attend college	28
to marry	30
for other reasons	29
Change in arguments with spouse	34
In-law problems	29
Change in the marital status of your parents:	
divorce	38
remarriage	33
Separation from spouse:	
due to work	49
due to marital problems	56
Marital reconciliation	42
Divorce	62
Birth of grandchild	31
Death of spouse	105
Death of other family member:	
child	105
brother or sister	64
parent	66

PERSONAL AND SOCIAL

Change in personal habits	31
Beginning or ending school or college	32
Change of school or college	28
Change in political beliefs	25

Change in religious beliefs	29
Change in social activities	28
Vacation	29
New, close, personal relationship	32
Engagement to marry	39
"Girlfriend" or "boyfriend" problems	30
Sexual difficulties	49
"Falling out" of a close personal relationship	35
An accident	44
Minor violation of the law	32
Being held in jail	57
Death of a close friend	46
Major decision regarding the immediate future	45
Major personal achievement	33

FINANCIAL

Major change in finances:	
increased income	27
decreased income	60
investment and/or credit difficulties	43
Loss or damage of personal property	40
Moderate purchase	26
Major purchase	39
Foreclosure on a mortgage or loan	57

3

MIND AND IMMUNITY

BY JANICE K. KIECOLT-GLASER, PH.D., AND RONALD GLASER, PH.D.

IN JUNE 1985, THE *NEW ENGLAND JOURNAL OF MEDICINE* PUBLISHED A study about the effects of social and psychological factors on the course of cancer. The investigators had examined whether a range of psychological factors affected the medical outcome of patients with advanced tumors, and they had found no correlation. The study was later criticized on a number of counts. At the time, however, an accompanying editorial by an editor of the *New England Journal* took the opportunity to question the entire notion that the mind could have a demonstrable effect on health. The much-quoted editorial stated that "Most reports of such a connection are anecdotal," and concluded, "It is time to acknowledge that our belief in disease as a direct reflection of mental state is largely folklore."

Six years later, in the fall of 1991, the *New England Journal* published a watershed report showing a direct link between mental state and disease. That study demonstrated a striking correlation between levels of psychological stress and susceptibility to infection by a common-cold virus. The publication of such a study in the world's most respected medical journal marked a turning point in medical acceptance of the mind/body connection and, in particular, of the notion that stress and psychological factors could affect the function of the immune system.

Although the 1991 study didn't identify the physiological mechanisms

JANICE K. KIECOLT-GLASER, PH.D., is a professor of psychiatry and psychology at the Ohio State University College of Medicine, where RONALD GLASER, PH.D., is professor and chairman of the Department of Medical Microbiology and Immunology.

responsible for the findings, other scientists (we were among them) had already begun to accumulate convincing evidence that the immune system might provide a major link between the brain and physical health. The medical literature has long included informal observations in which severely stressful life events appeared to be linked to the sudden onset or worsening of illnesses that involve a disruption of the immune system, such as cancer, autoimmune disease, and allergies. But the field had always suffered from a lack of reliable clinical studies and the absence of any known mechanism to explain such a link between the brain and the immune system.

The conceptual wall between the brain and the immune system began to break down in the mid-1970s, when psychologist Robert Ader and immunologist Nicholas Cohen performed a breakthrough experiment. Their study, described in Chapter 1, involved giving rats an immunosuppressant drug in conjunction with saccharin-flavored water. The immune system of the rats became conditioned to the taste of the saccharin; eventually, giving the harmless saccharin water alone led to immune suppression, sickness, and death.

By showing that the immune system could "learn" such associations, Ader and Cohen provided persuasive evidence that the brain could directly influence immunity. Their study, published in 1975, reopened a long-standing debate as to whether stress and other psychological states might affect immune function and health. It triggered an explosion of research.

Researchers have since found a number of physiological connections between the brain and the immune system (see "The Evidence for PNI—An Overview"). They have shown that immune system cells can respond to chemicals once thought to affect only the nervous system and that nerve cells respond to chemical messengers secreted by the immune system, which provides a plausible means by which the two systems might communicate with each other. Changes in levels of stress hormones can also modulate immune function, as described in Chapter 2. And nerve cells connect the brain to the spleen and other organs directly involved in producing immune system cells.

These physiological discoveries, along with several clinical studies of illnesses ranging from the common cold to AIDS, have given rise to the rapidly growing field of psychoneuroimmunology (PNI). In many respects, PNI is a natural outgrowth of more than half a century of research on the physiology of stress, described in Chapter 2. But because the immune system is central to so many basic disease processes, PNI has also become a major field of investigation in its own right.

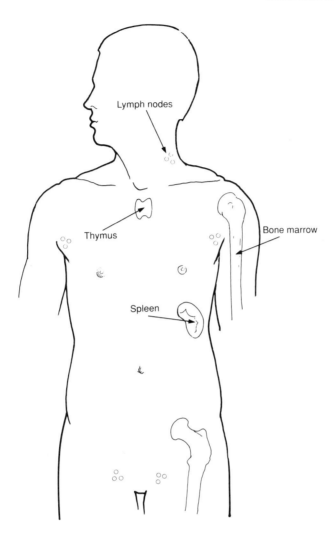

ANATOMY OF THE IMMUNE SYSTEM

The organs of the immune system are also known as the lymphoid organs, *because they produce* lymphocytes—*the white blood cells that mediate the immune response. Lymphocytes are initially produced in the* bone marrow. *One set of lymphocytes, the T-cells, spend time early in their development in the* thymus; *there they mature and develop the ability to distinguish self from nonself. While lymphocytes travel throughout the body, small armies of these cells are kept at alert in the* lymph nodes *and the* spleen, *which have specialized compartments for different kinds of immune system cells. All of these immunological organs have now been shown to contain networks of nerve cells, which provide a pathway for the brain and central nervous system to influence immunity.*

A WHO'S WHO OF THE IMMUNE SYSTEM

The cells of the immune system form a multifaceted and powerful army. The key ones are the *lymphocytes*—small white blood cells that attack threats to the body in a number of ways.

B-lymphocytes, or *B-cells*—so named because they were first discovered, in chickens, in a gland called the *bursa*—are the cells that produce circulating antibodies. *Antibodies,* in turn, are tiny proteins—members of the family of proteins called *immunoglobulins*—that attack bacteria, viruses, and other foreign invaders (called *antigens*). Antibodies "fit" the molecules of the antigens they attack, much as a key fits a lock. Each antibody will attack only a single kind of antigen—one will go after a common-cold virus, for example, while another will attack a bacterium that causes pneumonia—and each B-lymphocyte produces only one kind of antibody.

T-lymphocytes, or *T-cells,* don't produce antibodies. Instead, these cells themselves attack foreign invaders or work with other cells that do. (The *T* comes from the *thymus* gland, where these cells undergo much of their development.)

The several different groups of T-cells have different functions. *Cytotoxic (cell-killing) T-cells*, along with other blood cells called *natural killer (NK) cells*, constantly patrol the body, searching for dangerous rogue cells. Once they find them, these T-cells attach themselves to the invading cells and release microscopic packets of toxic chemicals that destroy them. Each cytotoxic T-cell, like each antibody, is "designed" to attack only a very specific target: Some attack cells that have been infected by viruses, some attack cancer cells, and some attack transplanted tissues and organs (to the frustration of transplant surgeons and their patients). Each NK cell, in contrast, has a broad range of targets and can attack both tumor cells and a wide variety of infectious microbes.

Two other classes of T-cells, called *"helper"* and *"suppressor" T-cells*, are especially important because of their overarching regulatory effects on immunity. Helper T-cells stimulate B-lymphocytes to produce antibodies, while suppressor T-cells shut off the helper

T-cells when enough antibodies have been produced. These cells communicate with each other by producing *interferons, interleukins,* and other chemical messengers that govern the activity of immune system cells.

For optimal health, the *helper/suppressor cell ratio* should be in balance. People with AIDS and other immunodeficiency diseases have low ratios (too few helper cells); people with autoimmune diseases, characterized by an overactive immune system, often have high ratios.

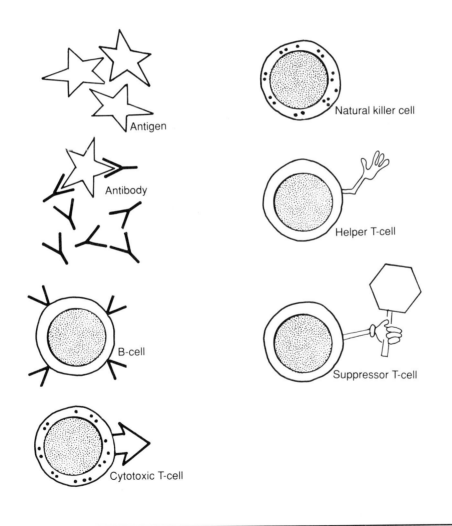

Antigen

Antibody

B-cell

Cytotoxic T-cell

Natural killer cell

Helper T-cell

Suppressor T-cell

SOME BACKGROUND: THE IMMUNOLOGICAL BASICS

The immune system is the body's means of defense against infectious disease and cancer. It has two primary tasks: to distinguish between "self" and "nonself," and then to destroy, inactivate, or eliminate foreign substances that are identified as nonself—not naturally part of the body.

The two major arms of this protective complex are the humoral and the cellular immune systems. In the former, white blood cells called *B-lymphocytes* produce *antibodies*, proteins that are key to the body's defense against bacteria and viruses in body fluids. In contrast, the cellular immune response defends against cancer cells and viruses that have taken up residence inside the body's cells. (It's also the branch of the immune system that attacks transplanted tissue, and that has to be controlled to keep organ transplants from being rejected.)

The cellular immune response is not carried out by antibodies, but by various immune system cells. Among them are *T-lymphocytes*, which help organize the overall immune response; *macrophages*, which engulf and dissolve invading organisms; and *natural killer (NK) cells*, which defend against virus-infected cells and cancer.

Most recently, the AIDS epidemic has highlighted the importance of the immune system in maintaining health. The AIDS virus invades and destroys critical immune system cells, leaving the infected person open to a host of diseases that would be rebuffed by a normal immune system. But less severe immunological problems can also have an impact on health: A person with an underactive immune system will be especially susceptible to infections. Someone with an overactive immune system, one that cannot accurately distinguish between self and nonself, is at risk for allergies or autoimmune disease. And many experts believe that immune dysfunction can contribute to the development and spread of cancer.

DO SMALL STRESSES REALLY MATTER?

When PNI researchers first turned from rats to human beings, they began by examining the effects of very intense events on the immune response. For example, they found altered immune function in astronauts at the end of their mission; in Swedish volunteers who endured 77 hours of noise and sleep deprivation; and in people whose spouses had recently died. (All these studies showed decreases in the response of immune system cells to stimulation in the test tube.)

While the physical response to such extreme events is interesting, it's not immediately relevant to everyday life; fortunately, no one loses a spouse or goes for three days without sleep very often. But a decade ago, only a handful of PNI researchers had used human subjects—the vast majority of studies were still being done on rodents—and virtually all the human studies looked at the effects of extreme stress.

It was at that point that we began our research, which has been aimed at studying the connection between stress and immunity under more natural circumstances. Although we were married, we had never thought about working together. One of us (Janice Kiecolt-Glaser) was a psychologist whose research had focused on assertiveness training, while the other (Ronald Glaser) was an immunologist studying the possible role of Epstein-Barr virus in a form of nasal cancer. While our relationship was based on many things, the prospect of professional collaboration was not one of them.

But as we began to become aware of the growing body of research in PNI—which we each saw through the lens of our respective backgrounds—we realized that we had a unique opportunity to pool our disciplines and make a contribution together. In 1982, we began clinical studies at Ohio State University to try to synthesize the tantalizing but scattered findings on stress and immunity and to investigate their relevance to human health.

We reasoned that if stress was indeed an important risk factor for infectious disease (and perhaps for cancer as well), then immunological changes should be associated with ordinary stressful events as well as intense ones. To find out, we began conducting annual studies of medical students. Every year since 1982, we have collected immunological and psychological data from the students throughout the academic year, including the three-day period in which they take their examinations. We have found that the simple stress of exams adversely affects a very wide range of immunological functions.

For example, we found that exams brought about a decline in the activity of natural killer cells—the cells that fight tumors and viral infections. The body's production of an immune system chemical called *gamma interferon,* which stimulates the growth and activity of NK cells, decreased by as much as 90 percent during examinations. The medical students' T-cells also showed a poorer response to test-tube stimulation during examinations.

THE ANTIBODY RESPONSE: HOW IT WORKS

The diagram on the next page shows how the immune system mounts an antibody response against an invader, as well as the roles that various cells play in the process.

Billions of B-cells are on guard in the body at all times, each one geared to recognize a single specific kind of invader, or antigen. When an antigen appears in the bloodstream, it is "caught" by a receptor on the surface of the appropriate B-cell. Like the antibodies the B-cell will produce, this receptor has a molecular shape that fits only this specific antigen.

Next, the B-cell engulfs the antigen and exposes part of the antigen on its surface, where it can be recognized by a helper T-cell. When a helper T-cell recognizes the signal, it attaches itself to the B-cell and releases *interleukins*—chemicals that stimulate the B-cell to become an antibody factory called a *plasma cell*. The plasma cell then multiplies, and the cells it produces pump out millions of identical antibodies into the bloodstream, where they hunt down the invading antigen.

Antibodies can render invaders harmless in a number of ways. For example, they can latch onto toxic substances produced by bacteria, inactivating the toxins. The antibodies may coat the bacteria themselves, a process that attracts other immune system proteins or cells that then destroy the invader. Or they can latch onto a virus, making it impossible for that virus to infect the body's cells.

In one of our recent medical-student studies, we placed catheters in students' arms for 24 hours during a low-stress academic period, and then again during exams, so we could draw hourly blood samples to measure changes in stress hormones (which can affect immunological activity). Nurses waited outside the students' classrooms during the day in order to get their hourly samples, and students slept in the university hospital's research unit at night. William Malarkey, the endocrinologist who conducted the hormone studies, found that levels of adrenaline and noradrenaline increased significantly at

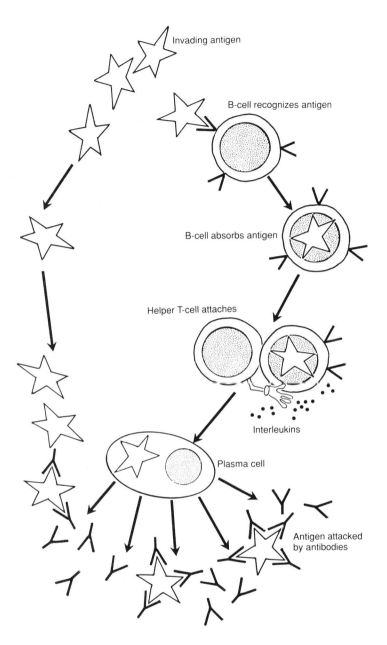

exam time, during both waking *and* sleeping hours. These changes could have led to some of the immunological changes we have observed.

All these findings are especially meaningful when you consider that medical students are experienced at taking examinations; the simple fact that they have been admitted to medical school shows that they have repeatedly done

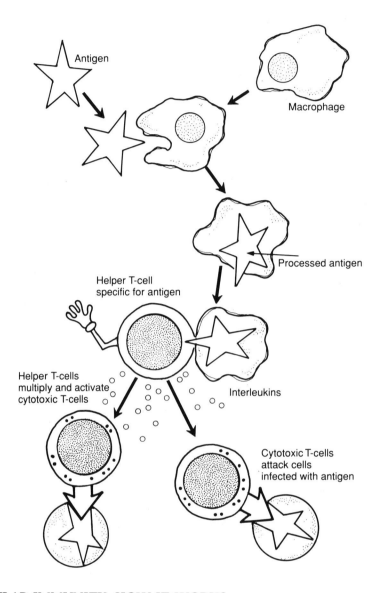

Antigen

Macrophage

Processed antigen

Helper T-cell
specific for antigen

Helper T-cells
multiply and activate
cytotoxic T-cells

Interleukins

Cytotoxic T-cells
attack cells
infected with antigen

CELLULAR IMMUNITY: HOW IT WORKS

When an antigen such as a virus enters the bloodstream, it can trigger a cellular immune response in various ways. Any cell that has been infected by a virus can "present" the antigen to helper T-cells that are specially geared to recognize it. Specialized cells, called macrophages, *also engulf invading antigens and present them to helper T-cells. Once the helper cells recognize the presence of an antigen, they mature and multiply rapidly, in order to enable the body to fight the invader. One way they do this is by helping to activate cytotoxic T-cells, which then find and destroy cells infected with the virus. (Helper T-cells also help carry out the antibody response.)*

well on college exams. Yet despite their relative competence in this stressful situation, it consistently regulates their immunological function to a lower level.

Are these studies relevant to those of us who no longer take exams? We think so. The stress of examinations should actually provide a good model for understanding people's responses to other commonplace stressors—events that people experience on a fairly routine basis but that still cause stress. For example, the several days before you go on a vacation or a business trip are often filled with frenzied activities at work and at home. Your emotional response to the pressures of those periods may be quite similar to the medical students' feelings of stress and anxiety as they cram for exams. Similarly, you may feel tension or strain if you have to spend several days in the company of your least favorite relatives. If the stress you experience in these common situations is similar to our medical students' responses to academic pressures, your immune system, too, may show the effects.

By learning how to relax, however, you may be able to affect your immune system's functioning. In one study, we took 34 medical students before exam time and randomly assigned half of them to a group where they were given hypnosis and relaxation training. During exams, we compared the immune function of students in the training group with that of the other students, who received no such training. We saw no difference at first: Students in the relaxation group showed the same average downward alterations in immune function as the others. But a closer look showed that the students trained in relaxation varied tremendously in how often they practiced their relaxation techniques. And those who took their relaxation seriously, who practiced the techniques often, showed significantly better immune function during exams than did those who practiced less frequently or not at all.

IS STRESS REALLY HARMFUL TO HEALTH?

Although the immunological changes we and others have measured are reasonably clear and consistent, they don't necessarily demonstrate that everyday stress is a health hazard. In fact, no one really knows whether relatively small immunological changes can actually affect the incidence, severity, or duration of infectious disease or cancer. Equally little is known about the clinical value of psychological approaches that lead to small improvements in immune measures. The health effect probably depends on the type of approach, its intensity, the degree of immunological change, and prior health status.

Moreover, it is difficult to demonstrate clearly that stress has helped cause an infectious illness or that stress reduction has helped stave one off. Infections such as strep throat or the flu are relatively infrequent—most adults don't experience many such episodes each year—so changes in their frequency are extremely difficult to detect. This is a special problem because PNI studies can use only relatively small groups of human subjects, due to the time and expense of doing such studies.

Finally, any effort to find connections between emotions, immunity, and health will be complicated by the fact that people under stress are likely to have lifestyles that put them at greater risk of disease. They're more prone to alcohol and drug abuse, poor sleep habits, poor nutrition, and inactivity—all of which can affect immunity.

The 1991 *New England Journal of Medicine* study of stress and the common cold, mentioned above, is one of the most persuasive demonstrations that emotional factors can indeed have a measurable affect on health. In that study, psychologist Sheldon Cohen at Carnegie Mellon University and his colleagues inoculated volunteers with measured doses of a cold virus—five different viruses were tested—or a placebo, a noninfectious "dummy" shot. As expected, some of the volunteers came down with colds and some did not. But among the volunteers injected with any of the five viruses, the chance of getting a cold or respiratory infection was directly proportional to the amount of stress the volunteers said they had experienced during the past year. The study was the first well-controlled demonstration that stress can increase the risk of infection.

Those results notwithstanding, stress is only one factor in determining your risk of infectious disease. The frequency with which you are exposed to viruses or bacteria, of course, has a major effect. So does the overall status of your immune system. That's particularly important for older adults because the immune system declines with age.

Our best understanding at this point is that the people most likely to become ill in response to stress are probably those whose immune systems are already compromised to some extent, either by a disease like AIDS or by a natural process like aging. These people start out with poorer immunological defenses, so that small changes associated with stress could have more important consequences. But even young, generally healthy people may find themselves getting sick more often if they are subject to severe or ongoing, long-term stress.

WHEN STRESS BECOMES A CHRONIC PROBLEM

What happens when people are faced with a stressful situation that lasts months or years, such as caring for a family member with Alzheimer's disease? The weight of the evidence to date suggests that the immune system does not adapt to the situation, but stays active at a lower level.

Caring for a spouse or a parent with Alzheimer's disease or another progressive form of dementia is a major hardship. There is no treatment for Alzheimer's disease, the course of the illness is uncontrollable and unpredictable, and the only certainty is the patient's eventual death. Since survival time sometimes extends to more than 20 years after the onset of the disease, caregivers have described the process as a kind of living bereavement, in which they watch the personality and intellect of their loved one slowly disintegrate. For five years, we have been studying people who are caregivers for a loved one with Alzheimer's to see how the long-term stress affects their immunological responses.

Joe, a retired lawyer in his mid-sixties, is typical of the caregivers in our study. He began taking care of his wife full-time about five years ago. The first time we saw him, he told us how his wife's symptoms had worsened over the prior year. Joe and his wife used to spend time at their summer home, located on an island in the middle of a lake. When he helped his wife into the boat the previous summer, she became very upset and confused; and when they reached the island, she jumped out, yelling to bystanders that her husband was a thug who was attacking her.

Fortunately, the local people knew Joe and his wife, and they helped calm her down and bring her back to him. Now, however, he feels that he can no longer take her out in public because he is afraid that the same thing might happen again around strangers. But he also can't leave her home alone because she might injure herself accidentally or wander away. Joe's story is typical of many we hear. It's not surprising that caregivers for people with Alzheimer's disease have high rates of clinical depression, much higher than their counterparts in the general population.

In our study, published in 1991, we measured certain aspects of immune function in 69 people who were caregivers for a spouse with dementia and in

69 people from our community who were the same gender, roughly the same age, and had the same income level. (The caregivers had been providing care for an average of five years when we first saw them.) During the 13-month interval between the beginning of the study and the follow-up, caregivers showed decreases in three measures of cellular immunity, relative to the non-caregivers, and were ill for more days with respiratory tract infections. This study provides the first good evidence that chronic stress leads to chronically lower immune system activity—which in turn may lead to a higher rate of illness.

Although these findings are provocative, they don't mean that everyone subjected to chronic stress will react in the same way. We found that the caregivers who were most distressed by their spouse's erratic behavior were most likely to show large negative immunological changes. The same was true of caregivers who were dissatisfied with their close personal relationships at the start of the study. Conversely, other studies have shown that friends and family can help caregovers deal with this kind of stress; in one study of women whose husbands were being treated for urologic cancer, those who had higher levels of social support had better immune function than those who reported less support.

THE IMPORTANCE OF RELATIONSHIPS

Some of the strongest evidence in the area of PNI now shows that poor personal relationships and social support can adversely affect the immune system. Sociologist James House and his colleagues reviewed data from large, well-controlled epidemiological studies and concluded that stressful social relationships rivaled smoking, high blood pressure, high blood cholesterol, obesity, and physical inactivity as a risk factor for illness and early death (see Chapter 20). The immune system may be part of the connection that explains this link.

Studies of several diverse groups of research subjects have found that people who are lonely, as measured by psychological tests, tend to have poorer immune function. In one of our earlier studies, we found that the loneliest medical students had the lowest levels of NK cell activity. Similar links between loneliness and suppressed immunity have been found in groups of psychiatric patients and adolescents.

Looking at the flip side of loneliness, psychologist Sandra Levy and her colleagues at the University of Pittsburgh found a connection between supportive personal relationships and improved immune function in women with breast cancer. The researchers measured NK cell activity and gave the women psychological tests just after they had undergone their initial surgery to remove a tumor, and then again three months later, after they had begun radiation or chemotherapy treatments. Several psychological aspects of support were linked to higher NK cell activity, including support from their husbands or other intimate relationships, support from their physicians, and efforts by the patients to actively seek support as a way of coping with stress.

A good deal of our own research is now designed to measure the impact of relationships on the immune system. We have found, for example, that divorced people who have the most negative feelings about the separation or the most difficulty "letting go" of a former spouse tend to show the greatest downward regulation of the immune system (see Chapter 20).

Our studies also suggest that sharing your feelings about issues that trouble you can have a positive effect on immunity. In collaboration with psychologist James Pennebaker at Southern Methodist University, we studied students who agreed to keep journals in which they wrote their feelings about disturbing, traumatic events—an analogy for the process that takes place in the intimate relationship of psychotherapy. Students who went through this process, we found, had better immune system function and fewer visits to the university's health clinic.

In our study with Pennebaker, 50 healthy undergraduates were asked to write either about personal and traumatic events or about trivial topics for 20 minutes a day during four consecutive days. The 25 students randomly assigned to the "trauma" writing group took the assignment seriously; the topics they discussed were personal and quite traumatic, ranging from problems with homesickness after coming to college, loneliness, and relationship conflicts, to parental problems such as divorce, family quarrels and family violence, and the death of a loved one. The "trivial" group had an assigned topic each day, such as descriptions of the shoes they were wearing or of a recent social event.

Although there were no immunological differences between the two groups before they began the writing assignment, differences emerged by the end of the study. Immune system cells from students who wrote about traumatic events showed greater activity in standard laboratory tests than did cells

HOW IMMUNE FUNCTION IS TESTED

Because it is difficult to measure the functioning of the immune system within the body itself, researchers have devised various laboratory methods to do so indirectly. Such studies are typically performed by taking a sample of white blood cells from the person being tested and exposing the cells to certain compounds, called *mitogens,* that essentially mimic an attack by a foreign substance. Healthy white blood cells will respond by secreting other compounds and by proliferating when stimulated by a mitogen. By comparing the activity of stimulated to unstimulated cells, and by tracking the mitogen response when a person is under varying degrees of stress, it is possible to see how stress affects this kind of immunological activity in that person.

There are many different kinds of immunological lab tests, but they can be roughly divided into two classes: qualitative and quantitative tests. The qualitative tests provide information about the relative activity levels of particular cells under particular conditions—a kind of "performance" measure. In contrast, quantitative tests show the actual numbers or percentages of different cell types relative to each other. In general, psychological stress appears to affect qualitative aspects of immunity—the activity of different cells—more than it affects quantitative aspects.

taken from the blood of the other students, suggesting improved immune responsiveness.

With the students' permission, we then looked at their health center records. We compared the average rate of visits for illness during the five months prior to the study with the rate over a six-week period beginning at the time of the study. Students who wrote about traumatic events showed a drop in clinic visits, relative to those who wrote about trivial events.

STRESS AND SPECIFIC CONDITIONS

In addition to studying immune system changes in experiments like these, a number of researchers (including ourselves) have looked at conditions and diseases that involve the immune system to see if psychological factors might alter their course.

HERPES VIRUSES

Several recent studies have provided strong evidence that stress increases both the initial risk of developing a herpes infection and the risk that symptoms will recur.

Unlike other common viruses, which are usually eliminated from the body by the immune system, herpes remains in the body for life and may flare up unpredictably. Different kinds of herpes viruses cause genital herpes, cold sores, mononucleosis, cytomegalovirus infection, and chicken pox and shingles.

Several studies have now shown that stress can disrupt the body's immune response to these viruses. One study followed West Point cadets for the four years after they entered the military academy. Those cadets who had three risk factors for stress—a high level of motivation for a military career, poor academic performance, and fathers who were "overachievers"—were more likely to develop infectious mononucleosis and were hospitalized longer in the infirmary. (None of the cadets in this study were infected with Epstein-Barr virus, the cause of mononucleosis, when they entered the academy.) Other studies have shown that nursing students who tend to be unhappy (as measured by psychological testing) are more likely to have recurrent cold sores, and that unhappy people in general have higher rates of recurrent genital herpes.

Some studies have used blood samples to measure the body's response to herpes viruses under stress. The cellular arm of the immune system is responsible for controlling both the initial herpes virus infection and later recurrences. When cellular immunity fails to do its job, the body may try to fight off the virus by producing antibodies to it. Paradoxically, then, high blood levels of antibodies to herpes virus mean the immune system is *not* controlling the virus effectively; in other words, high antibodies to herpes are a sign of low immune function. For example, medical students have higher levels of antibodies to certain herpes viruses during final examinations and lower levels after summer vacation.

People under various kinds of stress tend to have high levels of antibodies to herpes viruses, even if they don't develop symptoms of infection. In the West Point study, for example, even cadets who did not get sick were more likely to have high antibodies to Epstein-Barr virus (EBV) if they were in the high-stress group. In another study, separated and divorced men and women had higher EBV antibody levels than a group of married volunteers of the same age and education. (The separated and divorced men also had high levels of antibodies to HSV-1, the herpes virus that causes cold sores.) Caregivers for family members with Alzheimer's disease have higher EBV antibodies than similar people in the community, and psychiatric inpatients have higher HSV-1 antibody levels than people with no psychiatric disorders. Taken together, all these studies provide consistent and convincing evidence that stress can affect the body's control over herpes virus infections.

ALLERGIES

Allergies are triggered when the immune system becomes oversensitized to something in the environment—such as pollen grains or a particular food— and overreacts with an intense inflammatory response whenever the allergen is present. In the case of hay fever, for example, exposure to pollen grains sets off the production of massive amounts of antibodies, which in turn signals a class of white blood cells, called *mast cells,* to spring into action. The mast cells then produce a chemical called *histamine,* which in turn inflames the nasal passages and causes sneezing, itching, and tearing eyes.

While it is not clear whether stress can trigger or worsen allergies, there is good evidence that the mind can affect the allergic response in other ways. Animal experiments have shown that allergies can be learned as a conditioned response. In one study, guinea pigs were sensitized to a specific chemical—in essence, made allergic to it—and then repeatedly exposed to that chemical at the same time that they were made to smell an innocuous, unrelated odor. After a few weeks, the odor alone would trigger the release of histamine in these animals, just as if they had been exposed to the allergen.

A few studies have suggested, too, that people can modulate the allergic response under hypnosis. Some of the better studies have used the "double-arm" technique: Both arms are injected with substances that produce an allergic response, but the subject is told under hypnosis that only one arm will show the redness, itching, burning, and swelling that characterize an allergy. In most of these experiments, though not all, one arm is indeed more affected than the other. However, the difference may be due simply to circulatory changes in the skin rather than to a difference in the underlying immune response.

AUTOIMMUNE DISEASE

Autoimmune diseases, like allergies, stem from excessive immune system activity. In these diseases—which include rheumatoid arthritis, systemic lupus erythematosus, and Type I diabetes—the immune system becomes overactive or imprecise in its duties. Antibodies or immune system cells mistakenly identify the body's healthy cells as foreign invaders and attack them. The results are chronic inflammation and, in some cases, life-threatening organ damage.

The possibility that stress is linked to autoimmune disease is intriguing but still speculative. It is not immediately clear how stress could precipitate these illnesses; chronic stress is typically associated with immune *suppression,* although acute stress can activate the immune system. But a number of anecdotal reports suggest that there could be a link—perhaps operating through an immunological pathway that has not yet been discovered—and several researchers are beginning to study that possibility.

CANCER AND AIDS

These two diseases, perhaps the most feared of all modern illnesses, are generally modulated by the immune system. According to one widely held theory, cancer cells arise in the body all the time, but they are normally held in check by immune cells that recognize them as invaders and destroy them; it is only when these cells are ineffective that cancer spreads. And AIDS, the ultimate immunological disaster, results from the wholesale destruction of the cellular immune system, caused by a virus that invades and kills key "helper" T-cells.

One area of great interest is the possibility of using mind/body techniques to influence cancer and AIDS by improving the immune response. Although a number of clinicians have advocated the use of such techniques as guided imagery for cancer patients, there is no good evidence that this has a direct physiological benefit for people with cancer. However, a few recent studies—described in detail in Chapters 5 and 20—now suggest that group therapy, oriented toward relaxation training and psychological support, may improve certain components of the immune response and possibly survival for people with certain kinds of cancer. Similarly, early studies show that stress management groups and exercise can help maintain immune function in men infected with HIV, the virus that causes AIDS (see Chapters 19 and 23).

THE EVIDENCE FOR PNI—AN OVERVIEW

Robert Ader, a psychologist at the University of Rochester School of Medicine and Dentistry, performed the key experiments in the mid-1970s that ushered in the field of psychoneuroimmunology (PNI). Today, he is coeditor of the major reference work in the field, *Psychoneuroimmunology*, and editor-in-chief of its primary journal, *Brain, Behavior, and Immunity*, as well as an active researcher. In a recent interview with the editors of this book, he summarized the essential evidence that has been found to date for connections between the mind, the immune system, and the nervous system, as follows:

Nerve endings have been found in the tissues of the immune system. The central nervous system is linked both to the bone marrow and thymus, where immune system cells are produced and developed, and to the spleen and lymph nodes, where those cells are stored.

Changes in the central nervous system (the brain and spinal cord) alter immune responses, and triggering an immune response alters central nervous system activity. Animal experiments dating back to the 1960s show that damage to different parts of the brain's hypothalamus can either suppress or enhance the allergic-type response. More recently, researchers have found that inducing an immune response causes nerve cells in the hypothalamus to become more active and that this brain cell activity peaks at precisely the same time that levels of antibodies are at their highest. Apparently, the brain monitors immunological changes closely.

Changes in hormone and neurotransmitter levels alter immune responses, and vice versa. As this chapter and the previous one have shown, the "stress hormones" generally suppress immune responses. But other hormones, such as growth hormone, also seem to affect immunity. Conversely, when experimental animals are immunized, they show changes in various hormone levels.

Lymphocytes are chemically responsive to hormones and neurotransmitters. Immune system cells have receptors—molecular structures on the surface of their cells—that are responsive to endorphins, stress hormones, and a very wide range of other hormones as well.

Lymphocytes can produce hormones and neurotransmitters. When an animal is infected with a virus, lymphocytes produce minuscule amounts of many of the same substances produced by the pituitary gland.

Activated lymphocytes—cells actively involved in an immune response—produce substances that can be perceived by the central nervous system. The interleukins and interferons—chemicals that immune system cells use to "talk" to each other—can also trigger receptors on cells in the brain, more evidence that the immune system and the nervous system speak the same chemical language.

Psychosocial factors may alter the susceptibility to, or the progression of, autoimmune disease, infectious disease, and cancer. Evidence for these connections comes from many researchers (and is cited in this chapter and others in this book).

Immunologic reactivity may be influenced by "stress." Chronic or intense stress, in particular, generally makes immune system cells less responsive to a challenge.

Immunologic reactivity can be influenced by hypnosis. In a typical study of this type, both of a subject's arms are exposed to a chemical that normally causes an allergic reaction. But the subject is told, under hypnosis, that only one arm will show the response—and that, in fact, is often what happens.

Immunologic reactivity can be modified by classical conditioning. As Ader's own key experiments showed, the immune system can "learn" to react in certain ways as a conditioned response.

Psychoactive drugs and drugs of abuse influence immune function. A range of drugs that affect the nervous system—including alcohol, marijuana, cocaine, heroin, and nicotine—have all been shown to affect the immune response, generally suppressing it. Some psychiatric drugs, such as lithium (prescribed for manic depression), also modulate the immune system.

VACCINATION

Vaccines help protect us from disease by providing the immune system with a "sneak preview" of a disease-causing bacterium or virus, thus priming the system for a quick attack if that organism later makes a real assault on the body. Because stress can clearly affect immune function, might it also affect the response to a vaccine?

A recent study from our laboratory shows that it can. We gave each of three vaccinations against hepatitis B to 48 medical students on the last day of a stressful examination period. As expected, a few students made antibodies to the hepatitis virus after the first injection—the sign of a stronger immune response. Others made antibodies only after a booster shot, and some required all three shots before responding. Our research showed that the small number of students who produced antibodies after the first injection—25 percent of the total group—were less stressed and less anxious than those who required two or three shots to trigger antibody production. These data suggest that the response to a vaccine can be affected by a relatively mild stressor in young, healthy adults—a finding that may have important public-health implications.

THE BOTTOM LINE

Taken together, the evidence from human and animal studies clearly shows that stress can suppress immune function. For most stressors, these immune system changes may be quite small and probably will not have any severe consequences, particularly if you are otherwise healthy. But if you have recently experienced a major disruption in your life, like a divorce or a move, then your health may indeed be affected, especially if age or a medical condition has already weakened your immune system.

Relaxation, group support, and other forms of stress management may well enhance immunity. One caveat, however: If your immune system is already functioning well, it may not be possible to "enhance" it above normal levels.

The evidence suggests that there are things you can do to improve your chances of staying healthy—beyond following such basic preventive advice as getting flu shots, eating sensibly, exercising, and getting enough sleep. If you feel you are under serious stress, you may want to try one of the many stress reduction programs now available. In addition, it may be helpful to talk about your feelings with people close to you or with a therapist; supportive personal relationships appear to help maintain the immune response and physical health.

What if you have a serious illness like cancer or are infected with the AIDS virus? First and foremost, continue with standard medical treatments recommended by your physician. No form of relaxation, support, or imagery can substitute for the well-documented benefits of standard medical care, though they may complement it. As an adjunct to your medical treatment, you may want to consider joining a group for people who have cancer or who are HIV-positive or meet with a mental health professional accustomed to dealing with medically ill patients.

Finally, whatever you do, don't blame yourself for any negative changes in your health. Although the results of PNI research are promising and are beginning to suggest ways that we can affect the balance between health and disease, remember that we still know little about the extent to which these approaches can actually be used to improve health. Rather than leading you to blame yourself for your illness, this research should motivate you to do whatever possible to stay healthy.

II

THE MIND'S ROLE
IN ILLNESS

4

HOSTILITY AND THE HEART

BY REDFORD B. WILLIAMS, M.D.

"How is it that you have contrived this deed in your heart? You have not lied to men but to God." When Ananias heard these words, he fell down and died.

—Acts of the Apostles, Chapter 5, Verses 4–5

TWO THOUSAND YEARS AGO, WHEN PETER AND THE APOSTLES WERE establishing the Christian church, many believers sold their houses and lands and laid the proceeds at the apostles' feet to help support the mission. Among the contributors were Ananias and his wife, Sapphira. However, Peter discovered that the couple had secretly withheld some of the profits. He called Ananias to his presence and chastised him so severely for the deception that, according to the passage from Acts quoted above, Ananias "fell down and died."

About three hours later, when Sapphira came to see Peter, he confronted her as well, saying, "How is it that you have agreed together to tempt the Spirit of the Lord? Hark, the feet of those that have buried your husband are at the door, and they will carry you out." According to the biblical account, she, too, died instantly.

Today we would describe the fate of Ananias and Sapphira as examples of "sudden cardiac death brought on by acute, massive stress." To my knowledge, theirs are the earliest recorded examples of the profound effect that state of mind can have on the heart.

REDFORD B. WILLIAMS, M.D., is director of the Behavioral Medicine Research Center and head of the Division of Behavioral Medicine at Duke University Medical Center.

There are now many reports in the medical literature of sudden death precipitated by intense emotional stress. At Harvard Medical School, physiologist Richard Verrier and his colleagues have shown that acute stress can cause dangerous heart rhythm abnormalities in people who already have coronary heart disease, a progressive blockage of the arteries that supply blood to nourish the heart muscle.

Coronary heart disease is America's number-one killer. In its major manifestation, heart attack, it accounts for nearly half of all deaths in the United States every year—over twice as many as are caused by all forms of cancer. And in addition to triggering sudden cardiac death, which is a relatively rare occurrence, stress seems to play a more subtle, long-term role in the development of coronary heart disease overall.

Many people are well aware of the established physical risk factors for coronary heart disease: high blood pressure, smoking, and elevated blood cholesterol. Now epidemiologic research has identified specific psychosocial risk factors—hostility, lack of social support, and job strain—that can also set the stage for the disease to develop and, once it has been diagnosed, contribute to a poor prognosis. At the same time, laboratory investigators have begun to identify the biological factors that could explain why hostile people are at high risk for coronary heart disease, as well as other serious ailments.

There is also growing evidence that learning to become less hostile and angry and developing stronger networks for social support can improve the prognosis for many people with coronary disease. So there is good reason to hope that similar approaches may help prevent the disease from developing in the first place.

The Behavioral Medicine Research Center at the Duke University Medical Center is one of about ten centers nationwide investigating the role of psychological and social issues in cardiovascular disorders. For the past two decades, our research team of physicians and psychologists has worked to define the aspects of personality that place people at high risk for heart disease, as well as the biological mechanisms through which the damage is done. Although some of our conclusions are still tentative, we can now provide a great deal of useful information for people hoping to protect or improve their health.

THE TYPE A HYPOTHESIS

Although anecdotal reports of a mind/body connection in heart disease date back to the days of Ananias and Sapphira, it was only in the 1960s that solid scientific evidence of the link began to emerge. The pioneers were San Francisco cardiologists Meyer Friedman and Ray Rosenman, who identified a cluster of behavioral characteristics—constant hurriedness, free-floating hostility, and intense competitiveness—that seemed to be present in most of their patients with coronary disease. They coined the term *Type A* to describe this behavior pattern; *Type B* describes people who do not display these qualities.

Friedman and Rosenman undertook a prospective study to demonstrate that Type A behavior is a risk factor for coronary heart disease—much as a famous long-term study in Framingham, Massachusetts, had shown that *physical* factors, like high blood pressure, elevated cholesterol levels, and smoking, put people in greater danger of developing the illness. Using a specially designed interview to assess Type A traits, the two cardiologists categorized the personalities of more than 3,000 healthy middle-aged men.

Over an eight-and-a-half-year follow-up period, the men who had scored as Type A developed coronary disease twice as often as those who were initially Type B. The study also confirmed the impact of the physical risk factors uncovered by the Framingham study. However, Friedman and Rosenman found that Type A behavior put the men at high risk even if they had none of those physical attributes.

Although these results were encouraging to those of us researching the mind's role in cardiovascular disease, it became clear by the late 1970s and early 1980s that the Type A hypothesis was not the whole story. Following Friedman's and Rosenman's results, several researchers studied patients undergoing coronary angiography—an X-ray procedure for visualizing the coronary arteries—to see whether those arteries were more severely blocked in Type A patients than in Type Bs. While some studies did find such a physiological connection, several more did not. In addition, Richard Shekelle, an epidemiologist now at the University of Texas Health Sciences Center in Houston, conducted a major study on the same scale as Friedman and Rosenman's and found no difference between Type As and Type Bs in the rate of coronary heart disease over a seven-year period.

Like others working on the Type A hypothesis at this time, I began to suspect that the negative findings might mean that the three aspects of Type A behavior—hurriedness, competitiveness, and hostility—are not equally harmful to the heart. They certainly don't have equal effects on one's everyday life. Being competitive and getting things done quickly can have benefits, such as helping accomplish your goals. Hostility and anger, on the other hand, have little redeeming social or psychological value.

What's more, from a medical standpoint, bottled-up anger has long been suspect as a cause of illness. It may increase the levels of stress hormones circulating in the blood, which can have a number of long-term effects on the cardiovascular system.

THE HAZARDS OF HOSTILITY

At Duke, our research team decided to focus on the hostility factor. In 1980, we published a paper showing that patients who scored high on a 50-item questionnaire designed to assess hostility were more afflicted with severe coronary artery blockages than other patients. Specifically, we found that more than 70 percent of patients with high scores had severe blockages. In contrast, fewer than 50 percent of those with low hostility scores had a marked blockage of any coronary artery.

The items in our questionnaire were culled from an extensive test called the Minnesota Multiphasic Personality Inventory (MMPI), which is widely used in psychological research. After our results were announced, other researchers took a second look at people with high hostility scores in previous MMPI studies to see if they, too, had a higher risk of developing cardiovascular disease. For example, Shekelle reviewed the scores of 1,877 middle-aged men he had enrolled in a study of Western Electric Company employees in the 1950s. He found that high hostility did predict an increased risk of suffering a heart attack or some other manifestation of coronary disease, as well as an increased risk of dying from *all* causes. These effects of hostility remained significant when other risk factors were controlled for.

My colleague at Duke, the psychologist John Barefoot, has done similar studies of doctors and lawyers who had taken the MMPI while in medical or law school at the University of North Carolina during the 1950s. The results confirmed the Western Electric findings. Over the 25-year follow-up period, Barefoot found that doctors with high hostility scores were four to five times more likely to develop coronary disease than were those with low scores. Even more dramatic, 14 percent of the doctors and 20 percent of the lawyers with high hostility scores at age 25 were dead by age 50. In marked contrast, only 2 percent of doctors and 4 percent of lawyers with low scores had died by that age.

Further study of the lawyers pinpointed the specific aspects of hostility that predicted higher death rates. These were a cynical mistrust of people in general, the frequent experience of anger, and the overt expression of aggressive behavior. Questions that pointed to other personality traits that one might think would be risk factors—including generalized anxiety, paranoid ideas, and a tendency to avoid people (introversion)—did not predict a higher death rate.

Various studies using methods other than the MMPI scale have also linked hostility to future coronary risk. The most persuasive was completed by psychologist Ted Dembroski of the University of Maryland, utilizing data from Shekelle's seven-year study (which had already failed to confirm the original Type A hypothesis). When Dembroski assessed hostility levels using a technique he had developed to score interview material, he found that hostility *did* predict increased coronary risk, even though Type A measures from the same interviews had not.

In addition to increasing the risk of developing heart disease in the first place, anger is also bad for the heart once coronary disease is present. In a study of heart patients at Stanford University, psychiatrist Gail Ironson found that recalling an incident that had made them angry led to a deterioration in the heart's pumping efficiency—a deterioration in function signifying reduced blood supply that could lead to sudden death.

As more researchers have looked for a link between scores on the MMPI hostility scale and either coronary risk or overall death rate, the results have been conflicting. Several have found no connection at all. Some of these studies, however, have had serious methodological flaws. For example, in one study medical school applicants were given the MMPI while visiting the school for admission interviews. As a group, their hostility scores were very low—not surprising, because the students were undoubtedly trying to present themselves in the best possible light. As you would expect, these scores did not predict anything because they were not true measures of hostility in these students.

There are other, better designed studies that have still failed to find a link between hostility and coronary disease or death, though they are smaller in number than the studies that do show a connection. Although the negative findings don't disprove the hostility hypothesis, they do suggest that research in this area needs further development. We need better ways to measure hostility than that provided by the MMPI scale. And we also need to consider the other psychosocial factors that influence heart-disease risk.

SOCIAL SUPPORT AND JOB STRESS

Research has also shown that inadequate social support or a high level of job stress can hurt your cardiovascular system. People who suffer from these factors in addition to hostility may have an especially high risk of illness.

Social support is defined not only by the number of social contacts you have—such as family, friends, and colleagues—but also by how well those people meet your needs. In numerous studies, healthy people have given researchers information about their social support networks and have then been monitored for a number of years. These studies have uniformly found that people with poor social support have a high risk of developing coronary disease and have higher-than-average death rates from all causes combined (see Chapter 20). This connection holds even when possible differences in pre-existing illness and physical risk factors are taken into account.

Once coronary disease has developed, people with low levels of social support also are more likely than others to succumb to the disease. My colleagues and I studied more than 1,350 patients diagnosed at Duke in the late 1970s as having severe coronary disease. Those who were unmarried and said there was no one with whom they could share their innermost concerns were three times more likely to die in the next five years than patients who had someone—a spouse or close friend—to confide in. This dramatic difference in five-year mortality rates—a 50 percent death rate for socially isolated patients, versus only 17 percent for those with someone to talk to—could not be attributed to any initial difference in degree of heart disease between the two groups. Similarly, researchers at three hospitals in New York State found that heart attack patients who lived alone were twice as likely to have another attack within six months as were patients who lived with a spouse or companion.

While these findings don't minimize the importance of high-technology treatments like angioplasty and bypass surgery, they strongly suggest that providing increased social support would further benefit heart patients. A friend and confidant can be powerful medicine in treating coronary heart disease.

Social support may affect health in a number of different ways. People with poor support may not take care of themselves as well as those who have someone to remind them to take their blood pressure pills, stop smoking, go to the doctor when they feel sick, and the like. But social support may have a direct physiological effect as well: People without good support may experience more stress than those with more social ties. In a study of people living

HOW STRESSFUL IS YOUR JOB?

A tension-filled workplace is a significant factor in cardiovascular disease. What really makes a job hard on the body as well as the mind is the combination of high psychological demands, such as pressure to meet deadlines, and a low level of control over work circumstances—what researchers call *decision latitude*. Psychologist Robert Karasek has dubbed this situation "high job strain." This chart, based on a survey of almost 4,500 working men and women, shows where different jobs fall, on average, on this scale. For example, stressful occupations include keypuncher and garment stitcher; among the least stressful are natural scientist and architect.

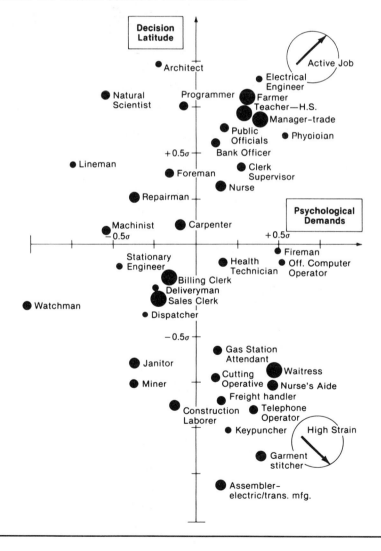

near the Three Mile Island nuclear plant after the near-meltdown, for example, psychologist Andrew Baum found that people with strong social support produced less adrenaline (as measured in their urine) than those with poor support.

A high level of job stress also raises the risk of cardiovascular disease. As defined by psychologist Robert Karasek at the University of Massachusetts in Lowell, high job strain comes from a combination of two factors: a strong demand for productivity and little freedom to determine how that demand will be met.

Karasek, along with colleagues in Scandinavia, has shown that people working at jobs characterized by high strain have an increased risk of developing cardiovascular disease and have a higher death rate overall. (See "How Stressful Is Your Job?") The connection between high job strain and high blood pressure is part of the explanation. In a study of workers in several New York firms, internist Peter Schnall and his colleagues found that those with higher blood pressures were more likely to be in high-strain jobs. Similarly, a study of a large group of Swedish military recruits, whose blood pressure was measured at induction physical exams at age 18, showed that those who went on to work at stressful jobs had the largest increases in blood pressure by age 20.

Other psychosocial factors—including depression, pessimism, and stressful life events—have been postulated at one time or another to play a role in causing or worsening cardiovascular disease. However, there is no good evidence that these factors contribute significantly to cardiovascular risk.

One remaining question is whether hostility, poor social support, and job strain affect women's hearts in the same way as men's. Most of the research I have described has focused on men, simply because much of the research in this area, like studies on heart disease in general, has used only males as subjects. Cardiovascular researchers have generally focused on men at least partly because they have a much higher rate of coronary disease than women—before women reach the age of menopause. After menopause, however, the coronary rate in women begins to increase; by age 65 or 70, there is no difference in risk between the sexes.

Though less extensive, the available evidence shows that psychosocial risk factors for heart disease do have just as great an impact on women as on men. Tests of hostility, for example, predict coronary artery blockages in women just as accurately as they do in men. So the adverse impact of psychosocial factors is not less important in women; it's just delayed. Recently, several research organizations, including the National Institutes of Health, have begun to focus new attention on women and heart disease. That effort is long overdue and should include research on the ways that psychosocial factors affect women's hearts as well.

THE BIOLOGICAL PATH TO HEART DISEASE

When Ananias and Sapphira dropped dead at Peter's feet, an immense surge of the stress hormone adrenaline was probably the immediate cause. Most likely, a jump in adrenaline precipitated a massive disturbance of the heart's rhythm known as ventricular fibrillation, which throws the heart's normally well-organized contractions into quivering chaos. Enormous surges of adrenaline and related stress hormones can also work heart muscle cells to such exhaustion that they curdle into a hypercontracted state.

In contrast to these immediately fatal effects of massive acute stress, hostility acts slowly over the years to damage the cardiovascular system. The precise physiological connections between hostility and long-term heart damage are still unknown.

It seems likely, however, that increased levels of stress hormones in hostile people play a key role. (These hormones are probably responsible for the damage caused by low social support and high job strain as well, although there is less direct evidence for this.) In recent laboratory studies at Duke by psychologist Edward Suarez, men and women with high hostility scores were harassed while trying to perform a mental task. They showed larger increases in blood pressure and stress hormones like adrenaline and cortisol than did people with low hostility scores who were subjected to the same provocation.

Adrenaline is known to raise blood pressure, make the blood clot more rapidly, and accelerate a host of other physiological processes that are likely to speed the growth of atherosclerotic plaques—deposits within the blood vessels that clog the coronary arteries. For example, adrenaline triggers the movement of fat from the body's fat stores into the bloodstream. That raises blood levels of cholesterol, which then accumulates in plaques.

The stress hormone adrenaline surges higher in hostile people in real life as well as in the lab. The amount of adrenaline excreted in the urine during the daytime is greater in men with high hostility scores, even though their

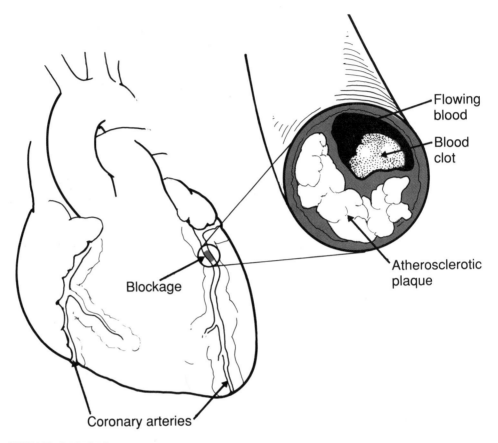

Flowing blood

Blood clot

Atherosclerotic plaque

Blockage

Coronary arteries

WHAT CAUSES HEART ATTACKS?

The coronary arteries—so named because they encircle the heart like a crown—supply heart muscle with the blood it needs to function. Over time, cholesterol and other substances can accumulate to form a plaque, a deposit in the wall of the artery. This process, known as atherosclerosis, leaves only a narrow area for blood to flow through. If a blood clot then blocks that passageway, it can choke off the blood supply to the heart muscle and cause a heart attack.

nighttime excretion of the hormone is normal—suggesting that hostile men produce more adrenaline in reaction to daily events, rather than for some innate physiological reason.

The fact that hostile people have higher-than-normal increases in blood pressure and stress hormones when they are annoyed or angry shows that they have a low threshold for triggering the sympathetic nervous system's "fight-or-flight" stress response (see Chapter 2). In addition, hostile people are slower than others to activate the parasympathetic nervous system, the part that can protect the body from the onslaught of stress hormones.

To make matters worse, hostile people who also have a biological tendency to high blood cholesterol suffer from a synergistic effect. A high level of blood cholesterol is a major risk factor for heart disease: As it deposits in plaques in the coronary arteries, it interferes with the supply of blood to the heart muscle. The higher cholesterol levels found in hostile people may result in part from the frequent surges of adrenaline they experience. In addition, the excess adrenaline is clearly more dangerous if high cholesterol levels have already contributed to coronary artery disease. The interconnections between hostility and high cholesterol levels are complex, but the important message is that the two risk factors combined are far more toxic for the cardiovascular system than either one alone.

As if the biological effects of hostility were not enough, recent research indicates that hostile people are also more likely to engage in behaviors that harm their health. At Duke, psychologist Ilene Siegler is studying nearly 5,000 University of North Carolina graduates who took the MMPI in the 1960s as first-year students. Compared to their less hostile classmates, those who had high hostility scores in college now weigh more relative to their height, are more likely to be smokers, consume more alcohol, and have higher levels of the "bad" form of cholesterol (LDL) and lower levels of the "good" cholesterol (HDL). Another large-scale study found that people with high hostility scores consume an average of 600 more calories per day than those with lower scores.

HOSTILITY AND THE BRAIN

While the precise link between hostility and these harmful characteristics remains to be identified, one speculative possibility is that they might all be part of a "syndrome" that stems from a single biological deficit: too little of a brain neurotransmitter called serotonin. Neurotransmitters are chemicals that are released by one nerve to trigger a reaction in other nerves. Every one of the characteristics making up the "hostility syndrome"—increased anger and irritability; strong sympathetic and weak parasympathetic nervous system responses; increased eating, drinking, and smoking—has been found in diverse lines of research to be a potential consequence of low brain levels of serotonin.

If the hostility syndrome is eventually traced to a brain serotonin deficiency, it would raise the possibility that drugs could help protect the cardiovascular system by raising brain serotonin levels. Such drugs could even be used preventively, much as we already use pills to control blood pressure and lower cholesterol. Although such a pharmacologic "magic bullet" to protect us from the damaging effects of hostility is far in the future, basic research into the hostility syndrome may one day make such a pill possible. Meantime, there are behavioral approaches that do help curb hostility. They will remain important even if a drug for hostility control is eventually developed, just as behavioral measures are still central to cholesterol and blood pressure control.

STEPS TOWARD SELF-PROTECTION

What specific steps can you take to guard yourself from the effects of hostility, low social support, and high job strain? First of all, be sure you are getting good medical care, with regular, preferably annual, checks of your blood pressure, cholesterol level, and other risk factors. If you have any physical warning signs of future heart disease, you should follow your doctor's advice about ways to reduce their impact on your health. Also, if you already have cardiovascular disease, there are effective medical and surgical interventions that can increase the quality and length of your life.

Along with these important steps, however, there is good reason to believe that reducing your hostility, dealing more effectively with a stressful job, and increasing your sources of social support can help prevent or alleviate cardiovascular disease.

REDUCING HOSTILITY

In the early 1980s, Type A trailblazer Meyer Friedman conducted a study in which men who had suffered a heart attack were given either routine care or routine care plus instruction in reducing their Type A behavior, with considerable emphasis on limiting hostility and anger. The result: The men who were trained to curb their hostility suffered fewer deaths or second heart attacks over a four-year follow-up period than those who received only routine medical care.

While Friedman studied only men who already had heart disease, these results raise the question of whether lowering hostility and anger might also diminish a person's risk of having a first heart attack. As yet, there is no hard evidence that it will. But people with other risk factors for heart disease—say,

---

LOW CHOLESTEROL, HIGH HOSTILITY?

Some recent research has raised a troubling question about the standard dietary advice to eat a low-fat, low-cholesterol diet. Scientists at Bowman Gray University in North Carolina have discovered that monkeys fed a low-fat diet act more aggressively than those given more fatty foods. That fits with some recent evidence that people on cholesterol-lowering regimens have a higher-than-average risk of violent death (although their risk of heart disease is low).

While it's not clear why a low-fat diet would increase hostility, further research by the Bowman Gray team suggests one explanation: Monkeys on a low-fat and low-cholesterol diet also had lower functional levels of the brain chemical serotonin. Previous research in animals and humans has already shown a link between reduced serotonin function and increased aggressive behavior.

Do these findings mean that people at risk for heart disease should now try to *avoid* a low-fat diet, because hostility increases their risk? Absolutely not. First, it will take much more research to prove that an association between this eating pattern and hostility really does exist. Even if such a connection is confirmed, it will probably be found only in a certain group of people—namely, those who already have a low serotonin level and are susceptible to hostility anyway. And even for these people, the physiological benefit of reducing fat and cholesterol may well outweigh the added psychological risk. (There will probably be drugs available someday to help these people rebalance their brain chemistry.)

Meantime, we know that a low-fat, low-cholesterol diet decreases the risk of coronary heart disease in *most* people. To prevent heart disease, your best bet is to follow your doctor's advice, stick to a low-fat diet, and consider the behavioral changes discussed in this chapter.

---

a family history of the disease and a high blood cholesterol level—might reasonably consider rethinking their style of dealing with stress as part of an overall heart disease prevention plan.

Unfortunately, finding out whether your hostility level is too high is less straightforward than checking your cholesterol or blood pressure. You can't go to the doctor or a clinic for a routine test; there is no standard measure of hostility. However, you can gain a sense of your risk by answering the questions in "Test Your Hostility Level," at right. This test assesses the three aspects of hostility that appear particularly damaging to health: cynical mistrust, frequent anger, and overt aggressive behavior.

There is not enough space here to give you a complete course in hostility control. But as a first step, consider the "17 Tips for Becoming Less Hostile" on page 80; they have been helpful for many people. For more details, you might want to consult one of the books listed in Resources or consider professional psychological help. Most hospitals with cardiac rehabilitation programs also have "wellness" programs that include training in stress management and reducing hostility and anger.

I cannot guarantee that these steps will help you avoid or postpone cardiovascular disease, but I am confident that they are not likely to cause you any harm. And whatever the benefits to your health, the consequences for your interpersonal relationships are almost sure to be positive.

SOCIAL SUPPORT

In a groundbreaking study, psychiatrist David Spiegel showed that women with widespread breast cancer who joined a support group for cancer patients survived significantly longer than similar women who received routine care (see Chapter 20). Now the same appears to be true for heart patients.

At McGill University in Montreal, psychologist Nancy Frasure-Smith tracked the fate of heart attack survivors who were randomly assigned to receive either regular care or regular care plus a social support system. (The support entailed a nurse phoning once a month and visiting if the call revealed any problems.) The patients who received the added support experienced a 30 to 50 percent lower mortality rate over a four-year follow-up than those receiving standard care.

Another important, ongoing research project (which has attracted a great deal of attention from the media) is the work of cardiologist Dean Ornish at the University of California, San Francisco. In Ornish's studies, patients with severe coronary artery disease were randomly assigned either to the usual care or to a comprehensive program designed to actually *reverse* their disease. The program involved marked dietary fat restriction, exercise, yoga training, and group support sessions.

TEST YOUR HOSTILITY LEVEL

To gain a general impression of how hostile you tend to be, answer the following questions in each of the three areas that our research has shown to be critical: cynicism, anger, and aggression. This questionnaire is not a scientifically validated test, but it will give you some sense of how you measure in these three domains.

Cynicism

- [ ] When in the express checkout line at the supermarket, do you often count the items in the baskets of the people ahead of you to be sure they aren't over the limit?
- [ ] When an elevator doesn't come as quickly as you think it should, do your thoughts quickly focus on the inconsiderate behavior of the person on another floor who's holding it up?
- [ ] Do you frequently check up on family members or coworkers to make sure they haven't made a mistake in some task?

Anger

- [ ] When you are held up in a slow line in traffic, at the bank or supermarket, etc., do you quickly sense your heart pounding and your breath quickening?
- [ ] When little things go wrong, do you often feel like lashing out at the world?
- [ ] When someone criticizes you, do you quickly begin to feel annoyed?

Aggression

- [ ] If an elevator stops too long on a floor above you, are you likely to pound on the door?
- [ ] If people mistreat you, do you look for an opportunity to pay them back, just for the principle of the thing?
- [ ] Do you frequently find yourself muttering at the television during a news broadcast?

If you answered yes to at least one question in each area or to four or more questions overall, your hostility level is probably high.

17 TIPS FOR BECOMING LESS HOSTILE

1. Admit to a friend that your hostility level is too high and let her or him know you are trying to reduce it.
2. When cynical thoughts come into your head, yell "Stop!" (silently, if you are in public).
3. Try to talk yourself out of being angry. Reason with yourself.
4. Distract yourself when you're getting angry. For example, pick up a magazine from the rack if you're kept waiting in a supermarket checkout line.
5. Force yourself to be quiet and listen when other people are talking.
6. Learn how to meditate, and use this skill whenever you become aware of cynical thoughts or angry feelings.
7. Try to become more empathetic to the plight of others.
8. When someone is truly mistreating you, learn how to be effectively assertive, rather than aggressively lashing out.
9. Take steps to increase your connectedness to others, thereby countering the tendency of hostile people to ward off social support.
10. When people do you wrong, forgive them.
11. Cultivate friends at work or in your religious group.
12. Volunteer to help others less fortunate than yourself.
13. Learn to laugh at your hostile tendencies.
14. Engage in regular exercise.
15. Get a pet. People who have pets seem to live longer and be healthier, perhaps because animals, especially dogs, are so affectionate and undemanding. Unlike many people, pets give much more than they get.
16. Learn more about the core teachings of your chosen religion: A central principle of the major world religions is to treat others as we would have them treat us.
17. Pretend that this day is your last. Your hostile tendencies will come into perspective.

Most of the patients assigned to the reversal program showed actual shrinkage of their coronary artery blockages, as documented by X-ray—an improvement that had never been achieved before in a lifestyle-oriented treatment program without the use of drugs or surgery. By contrast, most of those receiving usual care showed *enlarged* blockages. While it isn't yet possible to identify which components of the program were responsible for the partial clearing of the arteries, Ornish has suggested that the social support provided by many group activities may have been a key ingredient.

How do you increase your social support? Some of the "17 Tips for Becoming Less Hostile" also apply here. Indeed, hostile people tend to have poor social support because they often ignore or even drive off other people.

You can also work consciously to improve your social support network, just as you can work to change your own attitudes. You can find new groups to become active in—a club, a sports team, or a church or synagogue, for example. You may choose to cultivate a friend who can be a confidant and join you in playing sports, watching movies, traveling, or doing whatever other activities you enjoy. And if you are married or in a committed relationship, you can rededicate yourself to your spouse or partner and resolve to improve the quality of your interactions.

JOB STRESS

Unfortunately, most of us cannot afford the most direct solution to high job stress: quitting the job for another. I am not aware of any mind/body approaches that have been specifically designed to help individuals reduce their stress on the job. The interventions that have been proposed focus more on efforts to change the work environment, often to give workers a greater say in how job demands are met. If you see ways that you could reduce your stress level by changing aspects of your job, by all means try to persuade your boss or supervisor to let you make the changes.

Because job stress can raise your blood pressure, you might also try to lower it using one of the relaxation methods described in this book. As Herbert Benson and others have found, various forms of the "relaxation response" can bring blood pressure down in many people with hypertension (see Chapter 14).

Although this approach has not been scientifically tested, I would also suggest that you use your leisure time as an antidote to a stressful job. Don't place high demands on yourself to "produce" off the job if your work requires high output. If your job gives you little latitude in meeting its demands, be sure to engage in leisure activities that give you maximum control.

Finally, any steps you can take to reduce hostility and increase social support may help protect you against the harmful effects of a high-stress job—just as they can help protect you from other sources of stress.

A PERSONAL NOTE

It isn't a simple matter to change one's personality: I've learned this from my own experience. As a "recovering hostile guy," I have struggled to curb my cynical thoughts, angry feelings, and aggressive tendencies. Despite my progress, the short fuse is still there. Unless I watch out, my ire quickly surges when the car ahead dawdles too much, the elevator lags, my son doesn't clean his room.

But I have improved over the years. I do "watch out" more now than in the past, and often I am able to abort hostile episodes that earlier in my life would have flared into full-fledged fight-or-flight responses. I have also learned how a strong connection with other people can help you become less hostile: My wife, Virginia, has been a major influence on my own hostility control program.

I've also come to believe this: If you do only one thing to protect yourself against your own hostility and anger, it should be to strive always to treat others as you would like them to treat you. On this both modern science and our religious traditions agree.

THE BOTTOM LINE

Extensive research has shown that hostility, lack of social support, and high job stress increase the likelihood of developing cardiovascular disease and dying from it prematurely. All three factors increase the body's levels of stress hormones, which can raise blood cholesterol levels and cause other changes that lead to blockages in the arteries that nourish the heart. Hostile people are also more likely than others to have poor health habits, such as overeating, smoking, and drinking alcohol to excess—problems that may also be more common in socially isolated people.

Fortunately, there are ways to diminish the negative health effects of hostility, low social support, and job stress. Hostility can be countered with a commitment to change, to learn to control your reactions and behavior. Research also shows that support groups can improve the prognosis for heart patients, and it's reasonable to believe that strong social support could help healthy people *prevent* heart disease as well.

5

EMOTIONS AND CANCER: WHAT DO WE REALLY KNOW?

BY JIMMIE C. HOLLAND, M.D., AND SHELDON LEWIS

BARBARA BOGGS SIGMUND, THE MAYOR OF PRINCETON, NEW JERSEY, WAS furious. It had been bad enough to learn that her eye cancer—ocular melanoma—was spreading. But then the self-help books started pouring in, filled with advice on how she could heal herself and overcome the disease. Behind the upbeat suggestions to picture white blood cells "as so many little men of war against the cancer cells" or to "redirect your life" in order to save it, Sigmund detected a far darker message. As she described these books in a *New York Times* Op-Ed piece, they presumed that "I had caused my own cancer"—through "a lack of self-love," a "need to be ill," or a "wish to die"—and, therefore, "it was up to me to cure it." Facing a poor prognosis, Sigmund wasn't willing to buy the notion that "cancer cells are internalized anger gone on a field trip all over our bodies" or that "rah-rah-sis-boom-bah, I can beat the odds if I only learn to love myself enough."

Sigmund, who died soon after her essay was published late in 1989, was reacting to a trend that every cancer patient today is almost certain to encounter. A cottage industry of books, tapes, lectures, and self-help groups has emerged during the past two decades, based on the belief that patients can indeed help heal themselves by putting their heart and soul into recovery. Advocates of this approach, including the physicians Bernie Siegel and

JIMMIE C. HOLLAND, M.D., is chief of the Psychiatry Service at Memorial Sloan-Kettering Cancer Center in New York City. SHELDON LEWIS is a journalist specializing in health.

O. Carl Simonton and psychologist Lawrence LeShan, have become house-hold names among those who hope to engage the mind and spirit in fighting their disease.

Many cancer patients have been grateful for the encouragement to use their mental and emotional powers to fight the illness. Physicians, too, are increasingly accepting the value of stress reduction, counseling, self-help groups, and other approaches to the emotional side of cancer treatment, with the philosophy that they can't hurt and quite possibly could help.

But many patients, physicians, and researchers are deeply troubled by the notion—spread by some proponents of mind/body approaches to cancer—that the illness is brought on by guilt, repressed emotions, or a spiritual defi-ciency. Unlike the well-tested theories that have linked personality and behav-ior to heart disease, these formulations of the emotional roots of cancer are still too speculative to be applied with the assurance some practitioners of these approaches claim today. In fact, telling cancer patients that they made themselves sick—asking them, "Why did you need this cancer?" as some self-help approaches do—may only add to the burden of dealing with the disease.

It's become more important than ever to bring a scientific perspective to the popular mythology on cancer and the mind. To that end, a growing num-ber of medical and psychological researchers are working to answer some key questions. Is there a "cancer personality"? Can your thoughts, emotions, or stress make you sick? And if so, can you "think" yourself well?

At this point, there is no convincing evidence that thoughts, feelings, per-sonality characteristics, or any mental or emotional states play a direct role in causing cancer. However, psychological factors that alter behavior can and do lead to cancer indirectly by affecting a person's health habits—for example, if someone starts smoking as a way to cope with stress.

There is better evidence, though it is still preliminary, that providing a person with supportive social circumstances may increase the odds of recov-ery or lengthen survival time in some people with cancer. Support groups, in particular, have shown a surprisingly strong physiological benefit in some studies.

Perhaps most important, there is now excellent evidence that social and psychological approaches can help people with cancer cope with the stress of having the disease and the stresses of treatment. Even if they do nothing to slow the progress of the disease, mind/body approaches—including support groups; counseling; and control of anxiety, depression, and pain—can have a tremendous impact on a cancer patient's quality of life.

CAUSING CANCER: CAN YOUR MIND MAKE YOU ILL?

When people ponder whether psychological factors can lead to tumors, they rarely focus on the most obvious pathways: Stress, beliefs, and emotions can affect life-style choices and health-related behavior. It's quite clear that those actions have a major impact on your health.

For example, people who smoke cigarettes are at increased risk, not only for lung cancer, but for developing malignancies of the lip, larynx, esophagus, and bladder, as well as heart disease. Alcohol consumption raises the risk of cancers of the mouth, larynx, pharynx, and esophagus, as well as the liver. People who smoke *and* drink are more than doubling their danger: The physiological effect of both habits together is more deleterious than the sum of their individual effects.

Other life-style decisions also influence your vulnerability to the disease. Much attention has been focused lately on the cancer-preventing power of a healthful diet, one that is low in saturated fats and high in fiber, vitamins A, C, and E, and cruciferous vegetables (such as broccoli, cabbage, and cauliflower). Conversely, a high-fat diet leading to obesity is believed to be a factor in about one-third of all cases of cancer, particularly those of the breast, colon, prostate, and stomach.

The evidence is conclusive that an unhealthy life-style—which may be the result of a reaction to stress—can increase your cancer risk. What is less clear and needs further research is whether your social environment, emotions, and attitudes can directly increase your risk as well.

The idea that psychological factors cause cancer goes back several centuries. The same idea was applied to tuberculosis, until a cure was found. However, it's become more credible with the development of the new field of psychoneuroimmunology, or PNI (see Chapter 3). Research in PNI explores the relationship between the mind, the brain, and the immune and endocrine (hormonal) systems. It has uncovered some intriguing evidence that stress and other emotions may have a bearing on the immune system's effectiveness in fighting illness.

According to a widely accepted theory of cancer, called the immune surveillance hypothesis, the immune system plays a constant, ongoing role in preventing cancer from developing. This theory holds that cancer cells are always developing spontaneously in the body, but the immune system's ability to recognize them as abnormal and destroy them generally prevents them from developing into tumors. Natural killer cells, described in Chapter 3, are thought to play a key role in attacking cancer. It is only when the number of cancer cells becomes too great to be destroyed—or when the natural killer cells are suppressed or inactive—that cancer develops.

If this theory is true, and if emotional stress can weaken the immune system considerably, then a link between the mind and cancer causation would be theoretically plausible. Plausibility, however, is far from proof, and studies of the mind's role in causing cancer have been inconsistent and inconclusive.

For example, some researchers have studied the possibility that certain personality types are especially cancer-prone. While at the University of California, San Francisco, psychologist Lydia Temoshok and Andrew Kneier, then a graduate student, compared the responses of patients with malignant melanoma and those with cardiovascular disease to receiving mild electrical shocks. Although the melanoma patients had a stronger physical reaction than the heart patients to the test, they tended to downplay how emotionally upset they were about it when they talked to the researchers afterward. Temoshok and Kneier concluded that the cancer patients restrained their "negative" feelings.

This study and other observations of patients with cancer have led Temoshok to coin the term *Type C personality*. She hypothesizes that cancer patients are likely to be uncomplaining, cooperative, and resistant to expressing emotions, particularly anger and hostility. This fits with a decades-old notion, based on clinical observations, that cancer patients tend to be "nice people." However, others believe that Type C characteristics do not cause cancer but may be the *result* of having a frightening disease. At this point, Temoshok's conclusion is still hypothetical.

Modern folklore has it that depression makes you especially vulnerable to cancer. However, careful studies have shown no link between risk of cancer and depression. One group of researchers studied 6,400 individuals who represented a cross-section of the U.S. population. Using psychological rating scales, the researchers identified those individuals who had depressive symptoms or actually suffered from major depression. After ten years, the researchers followed up on the causes of death of those who had died. No greater incidence of cancer or deaths from cancer had occurred among those who had been depressed ten years earlier. Two studies of bereaved individuals who had lost a spouse or a child found similar results over a ten-year follow-up—despite the common belief that many people develop cancer after such a great loss.

In a widely quoted 1989 editorial in the *Journal of the American Medical Association*, Bernard H. Fox, an epidemiologist highly respected for his work on the psychosocial aspects of cancer, concluded that the data overall do not suggest an association between depressive symptoms and cancer. At most, he granted the possibility of a weak relationship, too weak to make depression a true risk factor for the illness.

Despite these findings, some scientists still believe depression may lead to cancer, based on research with animals, which can be more easily controlled than human studies. Animal experiments have examined the phenomenon of helplessness—induced by giving animals repeated shocks that cannot be avoided—which is thought to be analogous to depression (see Chapter 21). These experiments have shown a relationship between helplessness, stress, the immune system's response, and the rate of tumor growth.

One interesting set of experiments, done by psychologist Martin Seligman and his colleagues at the University of Pennsylvania, subjected two groups of mice to stress in the form of electric shocks, but the researchers allowed only the first group to escape the shocks. Mice in the second group, which could do nothing to lessen the number of shocks they received, experienced "learned helplessness." Both groups of mice had previously been injected with tumor cells. In the wake of the electric shocks, the second, "helpless," group of mice grew tumors more readily than those in the first group. Related research by Vernon Riley, working at the Pacific Northwest Research Foundation in the 1970s, showed that mice stressed in different ways had higher levels of the stress hormone cortisol and experienced immune suppression, suggesting a mechanism in animals to be explored.

This animal research is suggestive, but not definitive. In fact, other investigators using different tumors and applying stress at different times have found tumor growth to be *slower* in stressed animals. Because the tumors transplanted into the mice were different from those that develop and grow in people, neither set of animal experiments may be directly relevant to human cancer.

CAN YOUR MIND HELP YOU SURVIVE CANCER?

Whether or not psychological and social factors can cause cancer, they may affect the course of the disease once it strikes. We know, for example, that death rates for people with cancer (as well as for people with other diseases) are affected by social factors: They are significantly higher among the poor, probably because of inadequate nutrition and limited access to health care, which often means the illness is further advanced by the time the poor receive treatment. And patients who use early-detection measures (such as mammograms, Pap smears, stool tests, and skin cancer screenings) have a better prognosis than those who avoid taking these steps.

More controversial is the idea that people's social support system, attitude, or emotional state may govern their odds of survival, and the hope that mind/body therapies can give patients an edge in fighting the disease. Recently, however, these possibilities have sparked new research interest.

SOCIAL SUPPORT

Could support groups for cancer patients increase the length of their lives? More than 20 well-designed studies have shown that individual or group counseling enhances the quality of life for patients. Most interventions have not been controlled well enough to study the effect of counseling on survival. One study, however, has examined the effect on survival a decade later, with dramatic results.

In the 1970s, psychiatrist David Spiegel and his colleagues at Stanford University combined group therapy with hypnosis and relaxation, in weekly sessions over a year, for a group of women with advanced breast cancer (see Chapter 20). An equal number, who were randomly assigned to a control group, received the same medical care but did not participate in group therapy.

The goal of the group was simply to help the women cope with the stress of a painful, terminal illness, and it succeeded in that. But a decade later, when popular books began to promote the value of psychological treatments for cancer patients, Spiegel was skeptical. He went back to see whether the women in his support groups had survived longer than other women with similarly advanced disease, expecting that he would find no difference and would thus disprove the popular notions.

What Spiegel found—much to his surprise, as he later recalled—was that the women in the support groups lived an average of 18 months longer. After circulating his findings to a number of colleagues, who could find no fault with them, Spiegel published his results in the British journal *The Lancet* in late 1989.

The report has sparked a great deal of interest from other researchers, who are now trying to replicate Spiegel's results.

One of us (Jimmie Holland) is now planning a similar study with advanced colon cancer patients being treated by an identical chemotherapy regimen. In a clinical trial conducted in more than 30 cancer centers, patients will be divided into a group that receives education about the disease only and a group that receives weekly telephone interviews by a skilled therapist over four weeks, to offer them both information and support in adjusting to the illness and its treatment. In previous research, we found that telephone interventions are extraordinarily helpful for the well-being of homebound patients with advanced disease. In this study of hundreds of patients, the team will assess both the quality of life *and* survival for these patients, compared with those who receive identical medical treatment but no telephone support. Studies like this are necessary because they control for confounding medical variables of treatment.

Spiegel's results fit with earlier epidemiological research on the relationship between social support and health. Researchers have found that people who lack social support have a higher death rate from *all* diseases, including cancer, than others of the same age. A long-term study in Alameda County, California, by researchers at the California Department of Health Sciences, found that older people who were socially isolated were more likely to get cancer than others and had a higher death rate from cancer. Several other investigators have confirmed this finding.

Although many theories have been proposed, we still don't know the precise ways in which social support may lengthen survival. Obviously, people who have close friends or relatives to watch out for them are more likely to see a doctor soon after having symptoms, to eat nutritiously, and to stick with their treatments. But the negative emotions associated with social isolation may also worsen the disease directly, by suppressing the immune system—while increasing social support could reverse that effect.

There is now some evidence, described in Chapter 3, that emotional distress—including the stress linked to loneliness—weakens the immune system cells that normally attack cancer cells. In one widely noted study, psychologist Sandra Levy and her colleagues at the National Cancer Institute and the University of Pittsburgh looked for interconnections among degree of social support, psychological state, and immune function (including activity of natural killer, or NK, cells) in a group of women with breast cancer. The women were studied just after they underwent mastectomy and again three months later.

Women who were found to have cancer cells in the lymph nodes under their arms at the time of surgery also had lower NK cell activity than the women who did not. However, poor social support and symptoms of depression and fatigue were also linked to low NK cell activity. This research suffered from certain flaws in design, and it did not find differences large enough to suggest that loneliness had a *major* impact on the immune system. But it does suggest that a possible link between loneliness and immune system suppression in cancer patients is worth further study.

Conversely, enhancing a patient's social support system might work by strengthening the ability to fight cancer by "tuning up" the immune system. A study by psychiatrist Fawzy I. Fawzy at the University of California, Los Angeles, looked for immune system changes after short-term (six-week) support group therapy for patients who had undergone surgery for malignant melanoma and who had no current signs of cancer. The support consisted of psychological counseling, education about melanoma, and training in stress management (including relaxation techniques) and coping skills. Not only did these patients have less distress than similar patients who were not in the support group, but they also showed higher levels of NK cells and certain other immune system cells. Whether these changes will be reflected in lower recurrence rates and longer survival is not yet known.

ATTITUDE AND EMOTIONS

Does a positive attitude—a willingness to express emotions combined with a fighting spirit—improve a patient's chance of survival? Since 1975, about ten scientific studies have looked at this question. A few found a correlation between the patient's attitude and cancer survival, but the studies suffered from inadequate controls in their design.

In one, for example, researchers in England did a study of 35 women with breast cancer over ten years. Soon after the women were diagnosed, the researchers evaluated their psychological state. Five and ten years later, they discovered that women who initially showed a fighting spirit or who denied the seriousness of their situation lived significantly longer than those who felt helpless or hopeless or accepted the illness stoically. But the spread of cancer cells to lymph nodes under the arm—known to be the greatest predictor of recurrence—was not studied. Whether those women with a positive attitude also happened to have fewer cancerous lymph nodes is not known.

Any study of psychological factors in cancer must take such biological aspects of the illness into account. (For one thing, cancer may have a biological effect on mood, because some tumors stimulate the production of hormones that can have a depressive effect.) At New York's Memorial Sloan-Kettering Cancer Center, we led a large multicenter study of nearly 350 women undergoing chemotherapy for breast cancer to look for links between psychological factors and survival. We assessed such biological factors as the number of lymph nodes under the arm that had microscopic cancer cells and the number of tumor hormone receptors, which are known to influence survival. The result: Although biological factors did correlate with survival eight years later, psychological factors did not.

Even if more rigorous studies do eventually prove that attitude counts in cancer survival, a major reason may simply be that people with a fighting spirit adhere to medical treatment more faithfully—an advantage in fighting any illness. Clearly, there are some ways of coping that work better than others, and the role of counseling and support is to help patients deal effectively with illness.

One final note: Because popular reports have exaggerated the evidence that a positive attitude helps people fight cancer, many patients are afraid that the depression they feel during treatment will make their tumors grow faster. There is no evidence that this is so. In fact, feeling positive all the time is impossible when you are ill. Particularly for someone facing a biologically aggressive tumor and a poor prognosis, feeling like a failure for "giving in" to the tumor is an unnecessary added burden in an already painful situation.

MIND/BODY THERAPY

Despite a lack of scientific evidence for its physical benefits, active or guided imagery has become a popular way to put the mind to work to battle cancer. It clearly helps some patients psychologically to gain a sense of control and to be "doing something." In this approach—which was developed by radiation oncologist O. Carl Simonton and psychologist Stephanie Simonton—patients envision their immune system winning a battle against tumor cells. For example, some picture the immune system's cells as a legion of white knights on horseback vanquishing small, slow-moving creatures (the cancer cells). This self-help therapy is based on the theory that mental imagery can enhance the immune system's actual response.

Although such imagery may reduce the patient's sense of helplessness—a benefit that in itself can enhance health—no adequately controlled studies have yet found that this exercise helps promote the regression of tumors. Some clinicians who use the approach claim it has cured patients. The problem with these treatments comes when patients whose health does not improve believe they have failed and become depressed because they feel they are not strong enough mentally to cure or control their cancer. Eventually, through carefully controlled trials, we may be able to tell definitively whether the immune system really does benefit from imagery exercises. It is an intriguing area of inquiry.

HOPE AND SPIRITUAL VALUES

For many people, spiritual, philosophical, or religious beliefs are central to coping with cancer and help them find meaning in having the disease. Usually, these beliefs include the existence of a higher power or a conviction that life has order and meaning beyond our rational everyday perceptions. Calling on a higher power for help can bring great solace during illness, but no one yet knows whether spiritual beliefs have an impact on survival. One study of cancer patients treated in Vermont, done by oncologist Jerome Yates, found better pain control and sense of well-being, but no difference in survival, associated with spiritual beliefs.

Research in this area is just beginning. Psychiatrist Peter Silberfarb at Dartmouth headed a multicenter study in which patients were asked whether religion was important to them in coping with cancer. Ninety percent of patients reported that religion was moderately or very important to them during their illness.

Now researchers at Memorial Sloan-Kettering and the Hadassah Medical Center in Jerusalem are joining forces to study the aspects of spiritual and religious beliefs that influence the quality of a patient's life and immune function. Prayer, existential perceptions, belief in a supreme being, and being part of a close social community are all different components of spirituality. One aspect may be more critical in coping than another. Social support of a religious community, for example, might be a major factor in producing the positive effect of spirituality on coping.

COPING WITH CANCER

Although the mind's role in the development of cancer remains speculative, emotions have an undeniable effect on the *quality* of a cancer patient's life.

Cancer has shared with blindness, mental illness, and AIDS the dubious distinction of being among the world's most feared diseases. One consequence is that people who suspect they have the disease are afraid to be tested. Most often, a suspicious symptom turns out not to be a sign of cancer. But if cancer *is* present, seeing a doctor promptly may make early diagnosis possible and increase the chances of cure. The assumption that "cancer equals death" is less true now than ever; there is hope for successful treatment of an increasing number of cancers, and cure of several.

If cancer is detected, most people respond as they would to hearing any catastrophic news. At first, they have difficulty accepting the diagnosis. They may think: "There must be a mistake in the tests. Cancer can't happen to *me!*" If this denial is extreme and prolonged, it can be dangerous: It may prevent the patient from having necessary exams or life-saving early treatment.

Usually, as denial fades within a few days, the individual begins to feel restless, anxious, and, at times, hopeless. During this phase, many people eat and sleep poorly and have trouble concentrating because they're plagued by repetitive thoughts about the diagnosis and its implications. This usually lasts for a week or so.

Unfortunately, this is about the time when the patient must make critical decisions about treatment. For this reason, it is helpful to have a relative or close friend go along on doctor visits. This "buddy" serves as a second pair of eyes and ears to ensure that all the important information is digested, pertinent questions are asked, and the issues involved in making decisions are fully understood.

Once treatment begins, usually within a few weeks after diagnosis, most patients return to a more normal psychological state. Their emotional maturity, strength of personality, courage, and sense of humor will determine how well they adapt to the cancer in the long term. A person's responses to previous crises are the best predictors of how well she or he will cope with cancer. Another important factor is how the particular cancer affects the pa-

ALTERNATIVE CANCER TREATMENTS

Americans spend an estimated $4 billion annually on alternative can-
cer treatments. The spectrum of such therapies extends from benign
techniques designed to improve the patient's sense of well-being, to
dangerous, outright frauds. Treatments based on hypotheses about the
mind's role in illness are often mixed together with others based on
unproven nutritional or physiological theories.

Even the umbrella terms for these treatments—*alternative* or *un-
orthodox*—are confusing. Both imply a treatment used instead of conventional therapy, which isn't always the case. Many practitioners prefer the term *complementary therapies*, indicating that they should be
used in addition to—not in lieu of—standard medical treatment. (Although some alternative practitioners reject conventional medicine
entirely, others are M.D.s who combine some alternative therapies
with standard medical care.)

Patients intrigued by alternative therapies are often confronted
with a variety of approaches. Sociologist Barrie Cassileth and colleagues at the University of Pennsylvania identified six types of unor-
thodox therapies in common use today. None has been scientifically
proven to be an effective treatment for cancer. They are:

- Mental imagery treatments. These use guided imagery specifically to
  envision the immune system destroying tumor cells, based on the
  belief that such imagery can actually stimulate the immune system.
- Spiritual or faith-healing approaches.
- "Metabolic" therapies. These are based on the belief that the cancer
  is caused by a toxin or chemical imbalance that can be treated
  through a "detoxification" program.
- Diet therapies. These view cancer as symptomatic of an unhealthful
  diet; treatment entails overhauling your eating habits.
- Megavitamin therapies. These regard cancer as the result of a vitamin deficiency and treat the illness with multiple doses of various
  vitamin supplements.
- Immune therapies. A grab-bag term, which can encompass treatments ranging from meditation techniques to multivitamins and di-

etary instructions designed to strengthen or stimulate the body's immune system.

The researchers also encountered 40 or so other remedies, including a range of herbal and detoxification treatments. Sometimes, a variety of approaches are combined into a broader program.

The current cultural climate, which emphasizes taking personal responsibility for health, coupled with a growing mistrust of the medical establishment, has contributed to the number of patients who consider alternative treatments when first diagnosed with cancer. One attraction of these treatments to patients is that they are touted as naturalistic and "nontoxic," in contrast to standard cancer treatments, such as surgery, radiation, or chemotherapy, which do have well-known, adverse side effects. A recent study from the Office of Technology Assessment (OTA) found that sophisticated and affluent patients are more likely to pursue these alternatives than poor, less well educated ones.

While the OTA study found no evidence that alternative therapies are physiologically effective, some of these treatments may help enhance the quality of life for some patients. Any patient considering an alternative treatment should first discuss it with her or his physician. If the regimen is not harmful and would not interfere with conventional treatment, the physician may support its use.

tient's current stage of life and goals. For example, a tumor that leads to sterility will be far less distressing to a grandparent than to a newlywed.

Like patients facing other life-threatening illnesses, people who have cancer experience several common emotions, brought to popular attention by Dr. Elisabeth Kübler-Ross in her book *On Death and Dying*: denial (discussed above), anger ("Why me?"), bargaining ("Just let me live to see my children graduate"), depression, and acceptance of the prospect of death. It is important to know that there are no fixed, predictable stages of adjustment. For example, individuals who are cured of cancer or who live with it as a chronic disease for years will undergo a far different psychological adjustment. However, Kübler-Ross's concepts are useful for helping cancer patients and their loved ones become acquainted with feelings that often arise when life is in jeopardy.

Usually, close friends and loved ones experience the same emotions concerning the illness as the patient. In one study we did 15 years ago, even the *intensity* of their emotions was as strong as the patient's. In addition, the relative may feel the need to be the "strong one" who carries on family and work activities while also caring for the patient. If a family member or a close friend of yours has cancer, it is important to respect your own psychological reactions and needs as well as the patient's. Support for the relative is as critical as for the patient, and support groups and counseling are available to spouses and friends.

Some people have special difficulty coping with cancer because of prior experience with cancer. The following case shows how a childhood memory influenced—and endangered—early cancer treatment.

After Katherine, a 35-year-old teacher, discovered a lump in her breast, a biopsy showed that it was malignant. Her doctor recommended removal of the lump (lumpectomy) followed by radiation treatment. Because the tumor had been detected at an early stage, he considered her chances for cure to be excellent.

Nevertheless, Katherine became so depressed that she was unable to sleep or take care of her two small children. She was haunted by memories of her own mother's illness and death from breast cancer when Katherine was ten. Now she awoke each morning with a sense of certainty that breast cancer would kill her as well. Convinced that treatment would be useless, she canceled her initial appointment with her doctor. Katherine's husband was deeply concerned that her fear and depression were harming her chances for life-saving treatment. He persuaded her to see a psychotherapist.

During several therapy sessions, Katherine broke down and cried as she recalled her mother's death. With the therapist's assistance, she confronted her long-standing fear of dying from cancer at a young age as her mother had, leaving *her* children as she had been left. She soon realized her assumption that her breast cancer would be fatal was unrealistic. It had been caught at an early stage, and there had been significant advances in treatment since the time of her mother's illness. After several therapy sessions, Katherine called her doctor and arranged to have her operation and radiation treatments. Years later, her doctor considers her cured.

HOW COUNSELING HELPS

Beyond the anxiety engendered by the illness itself, cancer exposes patients to physical and emotional stress from painful and sometimes emotionally difficult treatments and their side effects. Various types of counseling can lighten the load. Among the most useful are the following.

PROFESSIONAL COUNSELING

A range of health professionals offer counseling for patients and their families, whatever the stage or type of cancer. Some people consider it a weakness to ask for help. On the contrary, reaching out requires a great deal of courage and offers enormous rewards. Counseling is especially important if the person with cancer—or a loved one—becomes very depressed, feels that the situation is hopeless, or is too anxious to carry out everyday tasks. Counseling is best provided as part of overall medical treatment, but if it is not offered at your hospital, it is worth seeking from an outside source.

For serious problems, several sessions of one-on-one psychotherapy with a mental health professional may be best. Ideally, the therapist should have experience working with cancer patients or others with serious illnesses. Most health insurance plans cover the consultation fee and a percentage of each therapy session. (For information that can help you find a qualified therapist, see Chapter 22 and Resources.)

SEXUAL COUNSELING

Many people are reluctant to confide in their doctors about sexual problems that occur after treatment. (Some doctors are also uncomfortable discussing sex with their patients.) Yet a couple can encounter problems if their sexual relationship is overwhelmed by physical discomfort, fear, anxiety, or feelings of unattractiveness in the aftermath of cancer. Treatments that affect sexual organs or function, such as removal of a testicle, can be most threatening. Often, the patient's partner also needs help coping. More counselors now specialize in treating patients with sexual problems resulting from physical illness. You can find a referral through your doctor, a cancer support agency, or the national association of sex therapy counselors (see Resources).

The case of Margaret, a 45-year-old executive, illustrates the benefits of sexual counseling after cancer treatment. Margaret was leading a full life, balancing her time between career, home, and family, when a routine Pap smear revealed she had cervical cancer. Margaret was treated with radiation therapy, which offered a high likelihood of cure. During her treatment, she and her husband were so concerned about the threat to her life that they didn't think about sex. However, after treatment, Margaret discovered that her sexual feelings returned. The first few times she and her husband attempted intercourse, Margaret found it painful. Out of anxiety, she began to avoid lovemaking, which her husband interpreted as rejection. He then stopped approaching her, which she believed meant that he was repulsed by her.

Eventually, the couple realized that the sexual issue was responsible for a growing distance in their relationship. They consulted a sex counselor, who quickly determined that the underlying problem was Margaret's physical pain during intercourse. The counselor offered exercises and advice for reducing the pain and Margaret's anxiety. In a couple of months, their marriage returned to normal, with a bonus: They had gained a heightened appreciation for each other by successfully surmounting a challenge together.

SUPPORT GROUPS

Groups in which cancer patients or survivors help each other, either with or without the guidance of a health professional, are another common form of counseling that can be extremely beneficial. People in support groups share information of all kinds, including information on alternative and experimental treatments. Some practice particular techniques, such as imagery, meditation, or yoga. Finally, these groups provide a safe environment in which patients can explore what it means to have cancer and learn from the perspectives of others.

Historically, the first cancer self-help groups tended to be for patients adjusting to extreme physical changes after surgery, such as a laryngectomy or colostomy. In the 1950s, the American Cancer Society began its Reach for Recovery program, in which volunteers who had had mastectomies visited fellow patients soon after their surgery. The program is now available worldwide. Today, there are support groups specific to particular cancers, treatments, and survivors of cancer of various types, as well as groups for spouses or parents of cancer patients.

People with chronic or life-threatening illness frequently say to others, "You can't possibly know how I feel." But support groups are filled with people who really do. These groups usually arise from grass-roots efforts of individuals who all had a particular type of cancer or experienced the same treatment and are making a similar adjustment. For example, after business-man Bob Fisher developed chronic lymphocytic leukemia in the 1970s, he began reaching out to others with the disease at Memorial Sloan-Kettering under the guidance of his doctor. Despite their ongoing anxiety, the patients tended to be reassured by talking to him. Because he'd "been there," too, he had a credibility the doctors and nurses didn't. After informally counseling other leukemia patients for a while, Fisher formed the first veteran patient counseling program at Memorial Sloan-Kettering. By reaching out, Fisher helped not only others, but himself as well.

Support groups are not for everybody. Some patients complain that the meetings serve as a painful reminder of their illness. But most find the close bonds that develop and the good feeling derived from helping others out-weigh the negatives. These groups can improve a patient's coping ability, strengthen family relations and communication with doctors, and instill a greater sense of self-confidence, competence, and control. (For a list of orga-nizations offering self-help and support groups for people with cancer and their families, see Resources.)

COPING WITH TREATMENT

Treatment for cancer can be extremely arduous, but various relaxation strate-gies can help patients tolerate it. Specifically, these tactics can reduce pain, as well as the anxiety, nausea, and vomiting that may develop from the mere *anticipation* of chemotherapy.

Depending on the chemotherapy regimen, between one-quarter and two-thirds of patients develop anticipatory anxiety and nausea, usually after un-dergoing three or four treatments, but often continuing well after the treat-ments are finished. Patients may become nauseated whenever they encounter something that reminds them of the treatment—smelling alcohol, seeing the hospital or a highway exit sign, even looking at the calendar can trigger a wave of nausea. Such reactions are the result of classic behavioral condition-ing: Anything strongly associated with the nausea-producing drugs begins to elicit nausea even if the person is not actually receiving any drug—a learned, or conditioned, response.

Anticipatory nausea sometimes worsens as treatment cycles continue. Pa-tients who have the greatest anxiety at the beginning of treatment seem to be the most likely to suffer anticipatory nausea. And not surprisingly, those who experience severe nausea and vomiting *after* a treatment as an actual chemical side effect are more likely to develop anxiety or anticipatory nausea before the next treatment. But in most cases, anticipatory symptoms can be significantly reduced or even eliminated through relaxation techniques.

Several studies have evaluated the benefits of relaxation used in conjunction with soothing guided imagery. (This imagery is used not to imagine battling the cancer, but simply to enhance relaxation.) In one experiment, researchers at Sloan-Kettering and two other cancer centers gave patients who became highly anxious or depressed from the side effects of radiation or chemotherapy a relaxation tape to use three times a day. Another group of equally distressed patients received a tranquilizer instead. After ten days, both the drug and relaxation exercises had substantially reduced anxiety and depression. Two-thirds of the patients in each group said they felt better, and both treatments were found effective, though the drug was slightly more so.

This study shows how a minimal intervention can help people "hang in" while undergoing treatment. It also shows that therapy can be tailored to the patient's needs: One may prefer a nondrug treatment, while another would rather take a pill.

A wide range of other relaxation methods can be used successfully by cancer patients. Progressive muscle relaxation (described in Chapter 14) has been shown in two studies to markedly reduce the frequency of anticipatory nausea and to reduce its duration and intensity when it does occur. Hypnosis, biofeedback, and meditative techniques, including the simple "relaxation response," can also be used effectively.

One behavioral technique that can be particularly useful for cancer patients, called *systematic desensitization*, uses relaxation methods to help the patient confront fears related to treatment. First, the patient and therapist together rank the various aspects of treatment from least frightening to the most fearsome and painful. Then the patient uses a relaxation technique to induce a tranquil state. Once thoroughly relaxed, he or she imagines various aspects of the treatment as vividly as possible, starting with the least frightening. When the patient is able to remain relaxed while imagining a particular scene, he or she progresses to the next most disturbing procedure, and so on, until it becomes possible to remain calm while clearly imagining the most frightening one. In one study, patients who used this method experienced shorter and much less severe bouts of anticipatory nausea.

ESPECIALLY FOR CHILDREN

Research has also led to special techniques for children, who are particularly fearful of treatments. Young leukemia patients, for example, must repeatedly face such painful procedures as bone marrow aspirations and lumbar punctures (spinal taps). Some children live in a state of such intense fear that nurses, parents, or doctors must physically restrain them to provide treatment. Several methods can help these children cope better. At Rainbow Babies and Children's Hospital in Cleveland, pediatrician Karen Olness has pioneered the use of self-hypnosis and guided imagery to reduce the distress of children going through painful procedures (see Chapter 16).

Another approach, developed by psychologist William Redd at Memorial Sloan-Kettering, is referred to as *cognitive/attentional distraction*. In this method, the patient's perception of anxiety and nausea is blocked by involving her or him in an engrossing, distracting activity. Redd and his colleagues have had great success using video games to divert children's attention before treatment and to prevent anticipatory nausea, in older children, playing the games also blocks anxiety. Distraction techniques can also be helpful in controlling or reducing pain.

Other distractions used during treatment include pop-up books and bubble blowing, developed by psychologist Leora Kuttner at the Vancouver Children's Hospital, and party blowers, used by Redd and psychologist Paul Jacobson at Memorial Sloan-Kettering. These methods can help children gain a sense of control in very difficult, even overpowering, circumstances. Positive incentives—using special treats or privileges—can also motivate children to cooperate with unpleasant or distressing treatments.

One innovative strategy is *emotive imagery*, in which the therapist or parent guides the child in creating a tale in which the character triumphs over the child's fears. The child identifies with the heroine or hero, and feels self-assertive, proud, and secure. The feared stimuli can even be brought directly into the story by the therapist.

Like hypnosis, emotive imagery works through the child's ability to make believe. One of Redd's patients, a seven-year-old boy with leukemia, had a terrible fear of needles. When David's turn came to go into the treatment room, he would kick, scream, and hide behind a chair, holding on with all his strength. To help the boy keep his mind off the needle and stay calm, a therapist helped him make up a story about Batman and Robin:

One time, Batman and Robin went on a trip and found an invisible magic glove that made the wearer very strong and able to withstand any pain. One day, Robin asked Batman if he could borrow the magic glove for a doctor's visit, because Robin didn't like getting shots. Batman lent Robin the glove, and when Robin got a shot, he didn't feel a thing.

The therapist then offered the invisible magic glove to David. From then on, David always put on the magic glove before his chemotherapy. To the relief of his parents and nurses, this greatly reduced his terror.

LEARNING TO CONTROL PAIN

Pain is the worst fear most cancer patients have. It may result from the tumor itself, from surgery, or from the side effects of chemotherapy and radiation. Pain also leads to emotional suffering when the patient believes it is a sign that the cancer is progressing—and emotional distress, in turn, can exacerbate pain (see Chapter 6).

Pain, like depression, is most common during advanced stages of cancer. Treatment must be geared first to control the pain that stems directly from the cancer itself, which requires drugs, including narcotic analgesics. Unfortunately, patients may limit the amount of pain medication they take because they are afraid of becoming addicted and erroneously equate being unable to tolerate pain with a weakness of character. Relaxation techniques are frequently used in cancer treatment as supplements to medication, but behavioral methods alone are not adequate to control severe cancer pain.

The emotional aspect of severe pain can be treated through psychological strategies that help patients cope with the meaning of the pain. For example, patients may learn a cognitive approach in which the pain is reframed—looked at from a different perspective. If the patient describes the pain as burning, the therapist might suggest imagining the pain as cold instead. If the pain feels jarring, the patient tries to think of it as spread out and dissipating. These coping strategies combined with relaxation—and, when indicated, anti-anxiety medication—can help reduce the fear that often heightens pain.

However, cancer pain often requires medication to control it, as well as these behavioral interventions. If medication is needed to control pain, the patient should accept it. Patients often have a greatly exaggerated fear of addiction, and children often go undertreated because their doctors share that fear. But the risk of addiction is far less than generally believed, and some of the new short-acting analgesics, in particular, are remarkably effective without being addictive.

COPING WITH ADVANCED DISEASE

After treatment is over, all patients feel anxious about the possibility of recurrence, although some feel it more intensely than others. These fears are normal and expected. The key is to prevent them from becoming disabling. Some patients say they put the "bad thoughts" out of their mind by thinking of something else (distraction) or using self-control methods, such as relaxation and suggestion (self-hypnosis). For some individuals, however, the fears may be so great that professional help is necessary.

If cancer does recur, the patient is thrown back into the sense of crisis and emotional turmoil experienced when the illness was first diagnosed. However, the depression and anxiety tend to be far more intense the second time around. Ordinarily, most patients can handle a recurrence better once they shift their hopes from curing the cancer to controlling it as long as possible.

At this phase of illness, mutual respect and trust between doctor and patient become even more important. Medical oncologists—internists trained in cancer care—are particularly skilled at attending to the medical and psychological issues that come with recurrent illness. The family physician who has known the patient over many years is often best suited to support her or him psychologically.

People face the possibility that their illness is terminal much the way they've faced other crises in life. Though they know that death is not the inevitable consequence of cancer, some are comforted by planning their funeral and the caretaking of their children. Others appear to deny the possibility that they could die. The important consideration for friends and family to remember is to respect the choices an individual makes concerning death. This is not the time to try to change his or her means of coping.

Today, more effort is being made to treat patients at home during terminal stages of illness rather than in the hospital. Since 1970, an increasingly popular approach in the United States has been the hospice program, which keeps the patient at home for as long as possible, followed by care in a comfortable, homelike environment. The focus is on comfort, pain control, and emotional support rather than treatment. Bereavement counseling is available for the patient's survivors.

There is a growing movement to offer hospice support while keeping the patient at home throughout. Some hospitals have home care units in which nurses provide 24-hour telephone consultation and home visits. Home care works well if patients and their families can reach assistance rapidly and know they will not have to deal with frightening situations alone. As more home care agencies develop and as insurance carriers recognize the value and economy of covering home care services, this model of hospice care may become more widespread.

THE CANCER SURVIVOR

Fear is almost universal among people who have survived cancer. They continue to worry, "Do I still have cancer? Will it return?" The anxiety that the tumor will come back never fully disappears. It does tend to decrease over time, but it often heightens before checkups. Survivors also face other problems as a result of the illness. Because they feel "damaged" in some way, they may feel less desirable, which can lead to difficulties finding or living with a spouse or loved one.

Their medical history can also interfere with their career advancement in two ways. First, survivors (and parents of a child who had cancer) may avoid changing jobs out of fear that they will not be eligible for health insurance under the new company's policy. If survivors do search for a new job, they may find they are discriminated against. Some companies erroneously believe that a previous cancer diagnosis makes someone a hiring risk, even if that person has been cancer-free for 20 years. Several studies have shown this to be mistaken, but the prejudice still exists. The National Coalition for Cancer Survivorship can help people who are grappling with these problems (see Resources).

THE BOTTOM LINE

Although a growing number of people believe that the mind and emotions play a significant role in causing cancer, research has not supported this popular conception. There is no conclusive evidence that specific emotions, personality types, or stressful events predispose a person toward the illness. Although expressing one's emotions and maintaining a fighting spirit are intrinsically helpful in the face of any crisis, their value in fighting cancer specifically is also an open question. However, there is early, encouraging evidence that social support may actually lengthen survival for cancer patients, probably because they cope with the illness more effectively and have a better attitude toward it.

Support groups and other psychological approaches can definitely help cancer patients improve their quality of life. Once the illness is diagnosed, patients and their loved ones often have difficulty coping; some patients may become so depressed or anxious that they are unable to pursue treatment. In such cases, individual or group therapy can make a tremendous difference.

Relaxation, guided imagery, hypnosis, biofeedback, meditation, distraction, and other behavioral techniques can all help people cope with the side effects of treatment for cancer, as well as with pain from the cancer itself. Special techniques can be especially helpful for children who have cancer.

We have only begun to explore cancer's emotional landscape, but we can already offer patients social and psychological treatments to help them cope with the illness. One day, we may be able to harness the mind to help them fight it.

CANCER DO'S AND DON'TS

Here are guidelines to keep in mind to prevent cancer or to better cope if you or a loved one has the disease.

1. DO what you can to prevent cancer by eating a low-fat, high-fiber, vegetable-rich diet. Avoid obesity. Drink only in moderation, and quit using tobacco in any form. Refrain from undue sun exposure.
2. DO follow the guidelines for early detection suggested by the American Cancer Society—especially, for women, monthly breast self-examinations, mammograms, and regular Pap smears.
3. DO see a doctor immediately if you notice a suspicious symptom.

Usually it will turn out not to be a sign of cancer, but if it is, this act alone may save or prolong your life.

4. DON'T believe the old saying that cancer equals death. Today, most cancers are curable if detected early. Even some that are detected at advanced stages are curable.

5. DO insist on a full partnership with your doctor in treating the disease. To make educated decisions on any treatments proposed, obtain all the information you need, including opinions of other experts. However, it is important that you finally choose one physician with whom you feel a mutual respect and trust so you can undertake treatment feeling fully committed and optimistic.

6. DON'T keep your worries about illness a secret from loved ones. They are your most important source of support, particularly when it comes to interpreting a doctor's advice or treatment plan. It's best to bring someone close to you to doctor appointments. Research suggests that people who feel supported can better tolerate illness, often cope better with treatment, and even have a better prognosis.

7. DO re-explore any spiritual values and beliefs that helped you through past crises. They may be especially beneficial during a time of illness.

8. DON'T panic about undergoing treatments that your doctor recommends. The most anxious period for cancer patients is often before treatment begins, when you may hear horror stories from others about surgery, chemotherapy, and radiation therapy.

9. DO ask about any potential side effects from treatment and discuss them with the doctor and nurse when they occur. Today, most side effects can be far better controlled than in the past. Remember that most of these reactions, even hair loss, are transient, but the treatment's potential benefits are not.

10. DON'T blame yourself for the cancer. There is no scientific evidence that emotional problems, personality characteristics, or trauma cause cancer.

11. DO use coping methods that have helped you in the past. Some common techniques: gathering information about the illness and

treatment, keeping your perspective, actively putting fears out of your mind, laughing at yourself and the issues of illness, exercising, listening to music, learning relaxation exercises, and concentrating on books or entertainment. It can be hard to muster the concentration and commitment necessary for some of these activities when you're feeling especially bad. If so, don't force yourself to continue, but don't reject the strategy completely. Simply put it aside and try again later when you're feeling better.

12. DON'T worry that you can't maintain a positive attitude 24 hours a day, seven days a week. Nobody can. Everyone has periods of fears and concerns, even depressive symptoms, when facing a serious illness. This is not a sign of weakness. No scientific data indicate that such down periods cause cancers to grow faster.

13. DO seek out a support group or self-help group that can provide you with an opportunity to talk with others in your situation.

14. DO consult with a mental health professional if you experience severe feelings of depression, anxiety, or guilt.

15. DO use any of the mind/body methods that you find help you cope, make you feel you are fighting for your health, and instill a greater sense of control over your emotions. Use only the parts that make you feel better. *Disregard* any that upset you. If you use an alternative therapy that includes diet or medications, be sure to ask your doctor if they might interfere with your cancer treatment. Good nutrition is particularly important during cancer treatment.

16. DON'T abandon standard medical treatment in favor of a holistic or alternative method. Anyone who encourages you to do so should be viewed with skepticism and alarm.

6

CHRONIC PAIN: NEW WAYS TO COPE

BY DENNIS C. TURK, PH.D., AND JUSTIN M. NASH, PH.D.

DESPITE THE IRRITATION, DISTRESS, OR OUT-AND-OUT AGONY THAT PAIN can cause, it is essential to our survival. Step barefoot onto hot pavement, and the jolt immediately sends you fleeing to cooler ground. A stabbing abdominal pain prompts you to get immediate medical care, which can be lifesaving if the pain signals appendicitis. While acute pain can be excruciating, it often serves a function and usually goes away: It's dissipated by time, by over-the-counter medication, by rest, or by appropriate medical treatment.

But when pain persists, it ceases to be the useful warning of an underlying physical problem and becomes a problem itself. Some 10 to 30 percent of Americans suffer to some degree from pain that serves no function and can become a tremendous burden. Such *chronic* pain can last for months or even years and have a devastating impact on an individual's quality of life. Pain may directly affect physical health as well; there is now some evidence that unrelenting pain can suppress the body's immune system.

Chronic pain also has a high social cost. More than 11.7 million Americans are significantly impaired and 2.6 million are permanently disabled by back pain alone. One national survey found that more than 550 million days are lost from work each year because of pain. According to a recent estimate, the cost in disability compensation and loss of productivity may be as high as $100 billion annually.

DENNIS C. TURK, PH.D., is director of the Pain Evaluation and Treatment Institute of the University of Pittsburgh School of Medicine. JUSTIN M. NASH, PH.D., is a psychologist at Miriam Hospital in Providence, Rhode Island, and at Brown University Medical School.

When their pain can't be cured, people often feel abandoned by the medical community and angered by the bills for treatments that were not effective. As their frustration mounts, their complaints can alienate their doctors, friends, and family members—making chronic-pain patients feel even more isolated, anxious, depressed, and preoccupied with their plight. Although pain begins as a physical problem, it soon takes on a psychological and interpersonal dimension. Consider three typical stories:

- Mary, a 24-year-old legal secretary, has temporomandibular joint (TMJ) pain. For the past three years, she has experienced pain in her jaw, difficulty in opening her jaw wide, and grating sounds when she does move it. She has consulted a dentist, a neurologist, an internist, and an otolaryngologist; none has been able to identify the precise cause of her pain, let alone treat it effectively. Mary has called in sick so often that she is in danger of losing her job. She may also lose her fiancé: He feels frustrated because he cannot help her and irritated when her pain forces her to back out of social activities he has planned. Mary's pain comes and goes, but it seems to worsen when she has conflicts with her fiancé, family, boss, and coworkers, which creates a vicious circle that leaves her ever more miserable. "People just don't understand what I'm going through," she says.
- Frank, a 52-year-old former construction worker, injured his back four years ago in a fall from the roof of his home. Diagnostic tests found a "bulge" in one of his disks—the soft-tissue cushions separating the vertebrae that form the spine—and mild arthritic changes in the vertebrae themselves. Most people with similar physical injuries do not experience disabling pain. But four years after his accident, Frank is still in great pain despite multiple treatments, including two spinal surgeries. He can no longer work, and, to make matters worse, Social Security has denied his application for disability payments. He spends most days dozing off in bed or on a recliner, a pattern that keeps him from sleeping well at night. Frank's former employer, his physicians, and some members of his family wonder whether he is exaggerating his pain or even making it up. As these people become more and more impatient with Frank, his frustration, depression, and anger deepen.
- Susan, a 32-year-old homemaker, has severe migraine attacks about once a week, although she takes medication every day to prevent them.

Several times in the last six months, her husband has had to take her to a hospital emergency room for injections of the potent narcotic meperidine (*Demerol*). During her agonizing attacks, Susan becomes extremely irritable and, she feels, virtually incapable of caring for her three-year-old son. When she is headache-free, she feels guilty and tries to compensate with frantic efforts to become a "supermom" that leave her exhausted. She also indulges her son—giving in to his tantrums or letting him eat junk food before dinner—but she knows these indulgences aren't good for him, and that compounds her guilt.

These patients' stories are like countless others we hear at the University of Pittsburgh's Pain Evaluation and Treatment Institute. Since 1985, we have studied the effects of pain on thousands of people in the hope of helping them and their families to cope. Studies performed at our institute and elsewhere have documented the important role that thoughts, feelings, and other people's responses can play in chronic pain. Perhaps the most vital message of this research is that psychological problems rarely cause pain; but the longer chronic pain exists, the more likely it is that emotional factors are prolonging it. Fortunately, there are also psychological interventions that can help make the pain much more manageable, if not totally eliminate it.

THE ROOTS OF PAIN

As the potholder slips, your finger grazes the inside of the oven. In the moment before you feel the burn, a complex biochemical and electrical process has taken place. It begins when nerves in your finger send messages through the spinal column to the brain and ends when the brain registers and interprets the sensation as pain. What happens between these two points, however, is still widely debated.

Currently, many researchers subscribe to the gate control theory, first proposed in 1965 by psychologist Ronald Melzack and anatomist Patrick Wall. They suggested that there is a "gating system" in the central nervous system that opens and closes to let pain messages through to the brain or to block them. It now appears that psychological factors such as attention to to pain, a person's emotional state, and the way a person interprets a situation can both open and close the gates (see "The Path to Pain"). For example, many athletes do not experience pain during the intense activity of the game,

THE PATH TO PAIN

According to the gate control theory of pain, your thoughts, beliefs, and emotions may affect how much pain you feel from a given physical sensation. The core of this theory is the idea that psychological as well as physical factors guide the brain's interpretation of painful sensations and the subsequent response. Here's how the gate control theory works (see the illustration on the facing page):

First, sensory messages travel from stimulated nerves to the spinal cord—the body's pain highway. There, they are reprocessed and sent through open gates to the thalamus, the brain's depot for tactile information. (Sharp pains, such as a sudden burn, stimulate different nerves than gnawing, dull pains.)

Once the nerve signal reaches the brain, the sensory information is processed in the context of the individual's current mood, state of attention, and prior experience. The integration of all this information influences the perception and experience of pain, and guides the individual's response. If the brain sends a message back down to close the gate, the pain signals to the brain are blocked. (That message may be carried by endorphins, natural painkillers in the body that are chemically similar to morphine.) If the brain orders the pain gates to open wider, the pain signal intensifies.

but only afterward, when they turn their attention to their injuries. Similarly, many pain patients find that their pain is worst when they feel depressed and hopeless—feelings that may open the pain gate—and that it's not so bothersome when they are focused on doing something that demands attention or is enjoyable. Although the physical cause of pain may be identical, the *perception* of pain is dramatically different.

Psychological differences between people may help account for their different perceptions of pain. It is impossible to gauge scientifically how much discomfort one individual is in, compared to another; there is no such thing as a "pain thermometer" to give an objective measurement of pain. A doctor can only infer how much pain people feel from their own reports or their

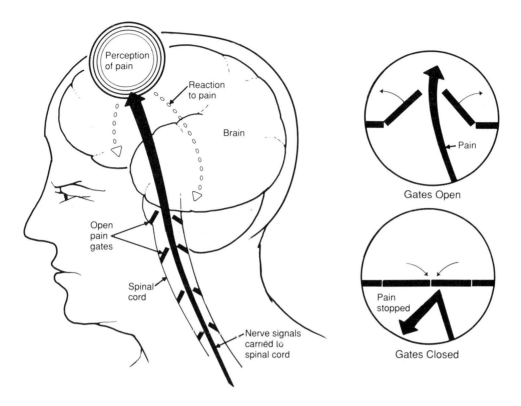

behavior. Even so, it's clear that two people with the same physical injury can experience the pain very differently. In Frank's case, for example, several of the spine's vertebrae had degenerated from arthritis, and he suffered from a bulging disk. Yet while Frank experienced incapacitating pain, many other people with the same physical problems experience no persistent pain at all.

The gate theory offers a partial explanation for such great variation in the experience of pain. But psychological factors can also affect pain in other ways, beyond opening or closing the "gates."

For one thing, thoughts and emotions can *directly* influence physiological responses—including muscle tension, blood flow, and levels of brain chemicals—that play important roles in the production of pain. Experiments conducted by one of us (Dennis Turk), with psychologists Herta Flor and Niels Birbaumer, suggest that stressful thoughts lead to pain only in those parts of the body that are already physically vulnerable. We placed muscle tension sensors on the lower backs, forearms, and foreheads of three groups of volunteers: patients with back pain, patients with other types of pain, and pain-free people. Their muscle tension was monitored while they recalled and described in great detail the last time they experienced extreme pain and their last episode of severe stress. When discussing these events, people with back pain had a higher tension level in their back muscles—and only in their back muscles—than they did when the experiment began. The other two groups showed no change in back tension. In a similar study of TMJ patients like Mary, recalling stress and pain elevated tension in the subjects' jaw muscles, but not in their lower backs.

Psychological factors can also *indirectly* influence pain by affecting the way you cope with it. Anticipating pain before it strikes, for example, can worsen the situation. Whenever a migraine begins, Susan feels helpless and fearful that she will be incapacitated for the rest of the day. Her stress then creates physical changes in blood flow and muscle tension that make the headache a severe and long-lasting ordeal.

This sense of helplessness can augment pain indirectly as well. Feeling a lack of control over your physical condition can sap you of the inner strength to fight back. It may lead you to catastrophize—overreact to relatively minor problems and view them as very serious—when you are faced with pain episodes and the stressful situations that trigger or worsen them. Hence, you may be tempted to turn to passive and harmful ways of coping, such as inactivity, and even damaging ones, such as excessive medication or alcohol, rather than using the more effective stress management strategies such as relaxation and distraction.

You can also increase your pain indirectly by refraining from certain activities or movements out of fear that they will hurt. For example, following the accident in which he hurt his back, Frank avoided all forms of exercise. The result: loss of muscle strength and tone, flexibility, and endurance. Frank also changed his posture and distorted his movements to evade pain. But these shifts actually caused further aches unrelated to his initial injury. Limping, for example, strained the muscles on the other side of his back, and they became painful as well.

Sometimes your interactions with other people can augment your discomfort by inadvertently rewarding it. Moans, groans, grimaces, and limps are part of the behavioral vocabulary of pain—they help communicate your distress to others. But friends or family members may respond to these signals in ways that harm you in the long run. For example, when Frank's pain rises, he lies on the floor and holds his back. In response, his wife gives him extra attention, offering to rub his back or bring him something to eat. She may even suggest that they cancel dinner plans with her brother—who has never been one of Frank's favorites. If Frank's pain often leads to such extra care and attention, he may unconsciously learn to express his pain to get what he wants from his wife. This pattern can develop even if neither he nor his wife is aware of it.

Although mental and emotional factors can greatly affect the experience of pain, it's important to realize that they are rarely if ever its root cause. When sophisticated diagnostic tests such as the CT (computed tomography) scan or MRI (magnetic resonance imaging) are unable to pinpoint the cause of chronic pain, some doctors and patients conclude that the discomfort is psychological. But most pain experts now believe that almost all unexplained chronic pain, at least initially, was rooted in a physical problem. The current cause of pain may be undetectable by available medical technology. Mistakenly attributing your pain to stress or other psychological troubles can just make you feel worse. (For a description of what's known about the physiology of common forms of chronic pain, see "Head, Jaw, and Back Pain: The Basis in the Body," at the end of this chapter.)

WHY TREATMENTS FOR PAIN OFTEN FAIL

Despite the growing awareness that psychological factors can contribute to chronic pain, conventional medical treatments rarely take them into account. The standard therapy combines potent analgesics with brief periods of rest to promote healing or to prevent further muscle damage. Resting too much can worsen your condition by diminishing your physical endurance and making you more prone to injury, and painkillers can also backfire.

Narcotic medication is very effective for acute pain and terminal-cancer pain, and a recent spate of research shows that very few patients become addicted to painkillers they receive while hospitalized. But giving hefty doses of painkillers for chronic pain can still be problematic. Even if addiction proves not to be a threat, you can develop a physical tolerance to a painkiller: You may need ever greater quantities to achieve the same degree of relief. If used excessively, some drugs—such as the analgesics and ergotamines used by headache sufferers—can cause "rebound" pain as the dose wears off. Unaware that withdrawal is triggering the pain, the pain sufferer may take increasing amounts of the drug, compounding the problem.

Even when narcotic medication does provide safe relief, it may not improve your ability to function, according to research on patients evaluated at specialized pain clinics. A drug may mute the pain, but it may also disrupt sleep patterns and alter concentration and thinking. In contrast to the "high" reported by recreational users of narcotics, some pain patients report that these drugs actually depress their mood.

Despite the drawbacks of medication for chronic pain, many people still believe that there must be a magic pill that will eradicate their problem. Many enter our clinic in search of a sorcerer rather than a doctor. The difficult truth for pain patients is that only their active participation in their treatment and their hard work are likely to help them improve and increase their functioning. One of their greatest weapons in the battle will be psychological interventions that rely on their inner strength.

SELF-MANAGEMENT STRATEGIES

Some psychological strategies for coping with pain, such as relaxation training and biofeedback, work by helping control physiological responses that contribute to pain production. Others help patients manage stress-inducing thoughts, emotions, and behaviors that can open the pain gates. All help increase the sense of control over pain and the factors that influence it. Patients who use these techniques often find that they can reduce their dosage of medication—under their physician's supervision, of course.

We have used all of the following strategies successfully at the University of Pittsburgh, often in varying combinations.

RELAXATION

Perhaps the most common and useful technique for controlling pain is muscle relaxation. It decreases or prevents muscle spasms, reduces and controls muscle tension, and helps control other physiological mechanisms (altered blood flow, changes in brain chemicals) involved in nervous system arousal and pain production. Muscle relaxation may also reduce anxiety and distress, improve sleep, and distract a person from the pain.

There are many relaxation methods, including progressive muscle relaxation, biofeedback, meditation, and the use of imagery. There is no one best approach; all can work for common forms of chronic pain. Research by psychologist Francis Keefe at Duke University has shown that relaxation can be effective for patients with low back pain. In addition, studies by psychologists Kenneth Holroyd at Ohio University and Edward Blanchard at the State University of New York (SUNY) at Albany have shown the efficacy of relaxation for people with chronic headaches.

The SUNY/Albany research also showed that pain patients can learn relaxation mostly on their own. In one study, headache patients attended ten clinic sessions over two months and were taught to reduce their muscle tension through progressive muscle relaxation. At the end of treatment, 96 percent had significant improvement in the frequency, intensity, and duration of their headaches. Another group of headache patients showed similar improvement when they learned relaxation primarily at home, with only three sessions in the clinic.

A recent review of several studies—conducted by Ohio University's Holroyd with psychologist Donald Penzien of the University of Mississippi Medical Center—found that relaxation training alone, on average, produced a 38 percent improvement for people with migraine headaches and a 45 percent improvement for those with tension headaches. (Improvement was measured on a scale that took the intensity, frequency, and duration of headaches into account.) Relaxation treatments for chronic headache may be still more effective when they are combined with cognitive restructuring (described below) or, in the case of migraine, with biofeedback training to alter blood circulation by warming the hands. Studies conducted by Holroyd and Blanchard, among others, have demonstrated that these combined treatments are effective to some degree in 50 to 75 percent of all chronic headache cases.

BIOFEEDBACK

Two types of biofeedback procedures are often used for pain. The more common type is electromyographic (EMG) biofeedback, which alerts you to electrical activity from muscle tension, thus helping you control it and diminish the pain it causes. The other method is thermal biofeedback, used mostly to treat migraine headache. Here you are "fed back" your skin temperature (usually from a finger); the process of learning to raise your skin temperature is associated with relaxation, which may lessen the pain of migraine.

Research by a number of investigators in the United States, Holland, and Sweden has shown that biofeedback helps between 40 percent and 60 percent of patients with headaches or TMJ pain. Fewer studies have been conducted with back pain patients using biofeedback alone. In one innovative experiment, Herta Flor and her colleagues treated patients suffering from chronic back pain with 12 one-hour sessions of biofeedback. They were compared to a second group, who received the same amount of treatment but were given false feedback—the information they received came not from their own muscles, but from other patients'. The patients given accurate biofeedback reported at least a 40 percent reduction in pain intensity, and half of them experienced a drop of 75 percent; the other group reported no change. Following the biofeedback, patients were encouraged to practice relaxation at home on a regular basis. After two-and-a-half years, the first group's improvements still held.

What remains unknown is exactly how biofeedback produces positive results in pain patients. Some scientists still believe it directly reduces physiological processes that contribute to pain. But several studies have found the technique beneficial even when it leads to no physical changes. One explanation is that biofeedback gives you a sense of control over your body and the pain. Therefore, whether it has a beneficial physiological effect or not, it can lead to a change in attitude that can help reduce discomfort.

COGNITIVE RESTRUCTURING

Few people realize how profoundly their thoughts alone can affect their mood and physical state—including their perception of physical pain. If you constantly tell yourself, "I don't see how this pain is ever going to get better," or "I can't take it anymore," as many pain patients do, you may exacerbate your pain in three ways. First, it becomes hard to develop the sense of power and control necessary to fight the pain. Second, these self-defeating, stressful thoughts can further tense your muscles. And finally, such thoughts may alert the nervous system to widen the pain gate and increase the discomfort.

Cognitive restructuring entails revising the way you think about your problem by rewriting your internal "script." It has been successful in treating a number of psychological problems, most notably depression. In the treatment of chronic pain, cognitive restructuring is usually used together with other approaches, such as relaxation.

In cognitive restructuring, pain sufferers use a diary to record when their pain was particularly severe; what the situation was at the time of the pain; what they thought about and felt before, during, and after the pain episode;

and what they tried to do to decrease the pain. By examining these diaries, perhaps with the help of a trained professional, the pain patient can identify negative thoughts and feelings and learn to change them. For example, they may learn to identify cues that trigger tension and anxiety and find out how to view stressful situations calmly and realistically rather than as catastrophes.

Evidence that cognitive restructuring can help improve chronic pain comes from psychologists Kenneth Holroyd of Ohio University and Frank Andrasik of the University of West Florida. In one study, patients with recurrent tension headaches were trained in cognitive restructuring and compared with a group of similar patients who were not. The trained patients reported at least a 43 percent improvement, and some as much as 100 percent improvement, in their headaches, while the untreated group showed no improvement.

Cognitive restructuring has not been formally tested on people with migraine headaches. However, we have used it in combination with relaxation training and biofeedback in our clinic and have found it to be valuable for many migraine sufferers, as well as people with other kinds of pain.

PROBLEM SOLVING

This approach is often used in conjunction with cognitive restructuring: As patients identify situations that trigger their pain, training in problem solving helps them deal with those situations.

For example, Mary, the legal secretary, has a supervisor who often loads work on her very close to deadline, which increases her stress and intensifies her TMJ pain. She copes by venting her frustrations to her fiancé after work, which helps her feel better temporarily, but doesn't resolve the issue and may alienate her fiancé over time. An alternative strategy—relaxing her muscles to keep tension from building up at deadline time—may be helpful for immediate pain reduction, but it does nothing to prevent future episodes.

A third option, a problem-solving approach, calls for Mary to identify the problem—time pressure, work overload—and then think of a reasonable solution and try it out. For example, she could let her supervisor know how overwhelmed she feels at deadline time and suggest spacing out the workload. Such open and assertive communication may itself prevent the episodes of pain.

No study has directly tested the effectiveness of problem-solving strategies separately from other stress management approaches to dealing with pain. In general, problem solving is used as part of a comprehensive approach to pain, which may include such strategies as cognitive restructuring, exercise, relaxation, and biofeedback. It can be a useful and important aid in dealing with any type of pain.

DISTRACTION

Many people with chronic pain become isolated and are left with nothing to focus on but their pain and misery. Learning to fill their minds with other thoughts may actually help lessen their distress. That's not an entirely new idea; by his own account, the philosopher Immanuel Kant would focus on the Roman philosopher Cicero whenever gout pain kept him awake at night, to distract his attention from the pain in his leg. Recently, researchers have systematically evaluated several different kinds of distraction strategies for dealing with pain.

In a review of these studies at Pittsburgh, we classified distraction approaches into five groups. All have now been shown to be effective for mild-to-moderate pain:

- *Pleasant images:* Conjuring up peaceful, pain-free visions.
- *Dramatized images:* Envisioning situations that use the pain as part of the script (for example, imagining that you are a wounded spy trying to escape your captors).
- *Neutral images:* Thinking of your weekend plans or recalling a movie you saw last week.
- *Focusing on the environment:* Instead of paying attention to your body, counting ceiling tiles or planning how to redecorate the room.
- *Rhythmic activity:* Counting or singing, for example.

Although none of these coping strategies was consistently more effective than any other, the imagery strategies collectively seemed to be more effective than other strategies that included no imagery. In our experience, the more individuals are able to become involved in the mental image, the more useful it is as a distractor. Vivid, detailed images, involving as many senses as possible, seem to work best. Although imagery is not a substitute for more active ways of coping with pain, it can be a valuable part of an overall plan. It can be particularly useful when one is tired or alone, such as after waking in the middle of the night and having difficulty falling back to sleep.

EXERCISE

Patients with muscular-skeletal pain, such as backaches and TMJ pain, often avoid exercising certain muscles because movement can hurt. But strengthening muscles despite discomfort can diminish pain by improving muscle tone, strength, flexibility, and endurance; it can also bolster your sense of control over your body. There is some evidence that workouts can also ease pain by facilitating the release of neurotransmitters called endorphins, morphinelike substances that serve as natural painkillers in the body.

Exercise regimens for people with chronic pain usually entail working each day toward a specific goal, one that is difficult but still attainable. (For someone with chronic back pain, for instance, a beginning goal might be to walk half a block a day and increase the distance gradually over time.) Physicians and physical therapists can help determine safe and effective ways for pain patients to recondition their bodies. When muscles have not been used for a long time, they may hurt when exercised. But for chronic pain patients, aggravation of pain during exercise does not necessarily mean that harm is being done; it may simply mean that the muscle being exercised has been weakened by disuse.

People with chronic pain need to learn to pace their activities and to rest only after attaining their goals, rather than stopping as soon as exercise begins to hurt. Using a chart to monitor exercise and keep track of progress can help pain patients increase their physical functioning in a careful, gradual way, enabling them to become more active without increasing their level of pain.

SHOULD YOU TRY A PAIN CLINIC?

Many people with persistent pain can successfully manage by using mind/body techniques on their own. But others will need professional help. In the past decade, a number of clinics devoted exclusively to treating pain have sprung up across the country. The best are interdisciplinary facilities that offer personalized treatment tailored to your specific physical and psychological needs.

Recently, we worked with a group of German researchers to review 65 studies including about 3,100 pain-clinic patients. On average, the clinic patients showed a 56 percent improvement in pain and disability compared with a 14 percent improvement for people in the control groups (only some of the studies were controlled). The clinic patients also showed significantly less psychological distress and higher levels of increased physical activity and were more likely to return to work.

The length of treatment can vary from several weeks to several months and may be conducted on an inpatient or outpatient basis. Here are some of the professionals you are likely to see at a clinic and the services they provide:

PHYSICIAN AND NURSE
Identify physical limitations, monitor medication, and help you improve aspects of healthy living (for example, diet, level of alcohol use, amount of sleep).

PHYSICAL THERAPIST
Provides treatment to increase muscle strength, tone, and flexibility and to improve body mechanics (how you move while performing such activities as lifting).

OCCUPATIONAL THERAPIST
Focuses largely on how you perform tasks of daily living—both at home and at work—and how you pace your daily activities.

PSYCHOLOGIST
Teaches many of the stress management, problem-solving, and coping skills discussed above. Works to help you improve your communication with family members, coworkers, and health-care providers.

Not all clinics offer the same range and quality of services. The unfortunate truth is that anyone can advertise as a pain expert. Here are criteria to help you assess a clinic:

ADEQUATE SIZE OF STAFF
Some doctors who call their practices pain clinics really offer only one method (say, anesthetic nerve block) that is supposed to work for everyone.

At a *minimum,* the clinic should have a physician, physical therapist, and psychologist and should offer a range of different treatments.

AFFILIATION WITH A TEACHING HOSPITAL
Many of the best clinics develop in an academic environment and benefit from the up-to-date knowledge generated there.

LICENSED PHYSICIANS, PSYCHOLOGISTS, AND PHYSICAL THERAPISTS
Check for this especially if the clinic is private. In clinics linked to teaching hospitals, a fully licensed staff is virtually guaranteed.

CERTIFICATION
The Commission for the Accreditation of Rehabilitative Facilities (CARF) sets general standards for pain clinics and certifies those clinics that meet its standards. CARF certification may be an especially useful guide in examining private, non-university-based pain clinics. The Joint Commission on the Accreditation of Health-Care Organizations (JCAHO) also certifies that clinics meet appropriate standards. The American Pain Society and the American Academy of Pain Medicine jointly publish a directory that describes the professional staff and the treatment available at each clinic and tells whether the facility is accredited (and by whom). For these organizations' addresses, see Resources.

THE BOTTOM LINE

Between 10 and 30 percent of Americans suffer from chronic pain. In many cases, the specific cause remains unknown and no medical remedy exists. Although psychological factors by themselves rarely cause persistent pain, they can trigger or worsen attacks of pain and contribute to distress and disability.

Although people who suffer from chronic pain are likely to feel helpless and hopeless, they can take an active role in managing their condition effectively. Research demonstrates that a number of self-management approaches—including biofeedback, exercise, imagery, and cognitive strategies—can help people develop a sense of mastery over the pain. If you have trouble battling pain on your own, an interdisciplinary pain clinic may be helpful for you.

HEAD, JAW, AND BACK PAIN: THE BASIS IN THE BODY

For the three most common forms of chronic pain—headache, temporomandibular joint (TMJ) disorder, and back pain—it's often difficult to find a precise cause. Here are the best current theories on the ways these types of pain develop.

RECURRENT HEADACHE

The two most common types of headache are *tension-type* and *migraine*. Tension-type headaches are mildly to moderately painful and are usually experienced as a pressing or tightening in the back of the neck or in the forehead. (Most people with chronic tension headaches have them three or more times a week.) Migraine headaches, which commonly occur two or three times a month or more, usually bring moderate to severe pain that is throbbing or pulsating; they usually affect only one side of the head, and the pain may be focused in or around the eye. Migraines are made worse by routine physical activities, light, and conversational noise levels, and they can be associated with nausea and vomiting.

Although these two types of headache seem to have distinct symptoms, our clinical experience is that many headache sufferers have some symptoms of each. Jes Oleson, a neurologist at the University of Copenhagen, has proposed a physiological model that would explain this overlap. He suggests that headaches result from nerve stimulation at three different sites around the head: the arteries in and around the brain, which change patterns of blood flow as they constrict or dilate; the muscles in and around the head, which may contract painfully; and the nerve cells within the brain itself, which can be stimulated by changes in brain chemistry. All of these sites can be affected by stress. Depending on which source produces the strongest pain message— the arteries, muscles, or brain—the individual will experience either a migraine headache, a tension-type headache, or some combination of the two. According to this theory, pain messages from the arteries are likely to produce the sharp, pulsating pain of a migraine, while signals

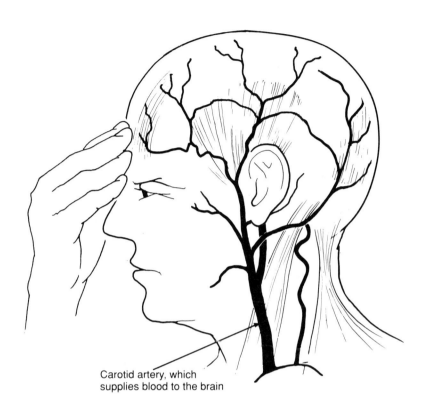

Carotid artery, which
supplies blood to the brain

from the muscles will produce the dull, aching pain of a tension-type headache.

TEMPOROMANDIBULAR JOINT DISORDER

In temporomandibular joint (TMJ) disorder, a person feels pain in the temporomandibular joint—the joint, located in front of the ear, that connects the upper and lower jaws—which can radiate to include the same side of the face, head, and neck. In addition, the ability to open the jaw may be limited, and opening the mouth may be painful and produce clicking, popping, or grating sounds.

TMJ disorder may be caused by arthritis or physical damage to the bone or soft tissue of the temporomandibular joint, which in turn can irritate the nerves in the jaw. But it may also be caused by stress or

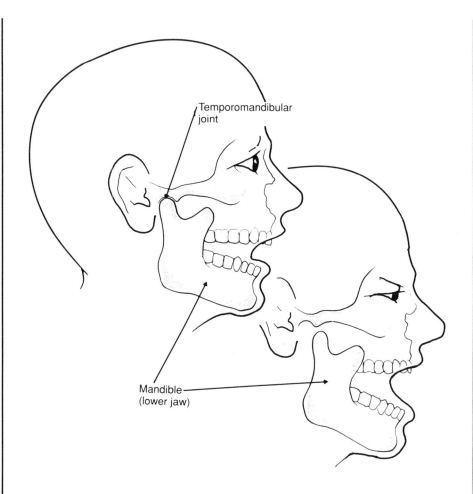

Temporomandibular joint

Mandible (lower jaw)

behavioral problems. When someone habitually grinds his or her teeth (usually during sleep), juts the lower jaw forward, or chews nervously on gum or pencils, the way in which the upper and lower teeth meet can be disrupted. The problem can sometimes be handled by a dentist; adjustment of your bite or a biteplate worn at night may help. However, in many cases dental treatment must be combined with psychological treatment, such as biofeedback or stress management.

CHRONIC LOW BACK PAIN
Chronic low back pain can develop from an acute injury, from gradual wear and tear, or from chronic muscle tension, although the pre-

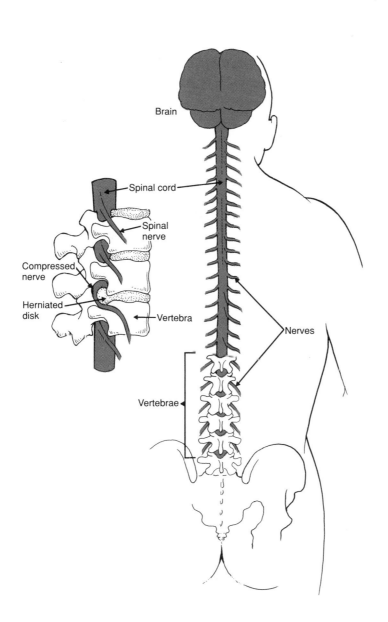

cise physical cause is usually impossible to determine. Whatever the initial cause, it can trigger a vicious circle, involving both mind and body, in which the pain becomes more and more difficult to control.

The problem may start when an individual begins to experience painful muscle tension or muscle spasms in the back. In response, she or he tries to decrease the pain by becoming less active and restricting movement. A short period of bed rest (about two to three days) may be beneficial after an acute back sprain. But prolonged inactivity makes the muscles become shorter, tighter, stiffer, and weaker, putting them at greater risk for muscle fatigue, muscle spasm, and pain. Soon other muscles (usually on the side of the body opposite the pain) will start to compensate for the restricted muscles and become overactive. This asymmetrical pattern can make the spine unstable; if there is pre-existing spinal degeneration, the imbalance can put pressure on the spinal nerves, leading to pain, numbness, loss of reflexes, and further muscle weakness. The spinal nerves can also be affected by pressure from other sources, including slippage in the vertebrae, slippage or bulging of the disks between vertebrae, or overgrowth of bone.

With the exception of cases where there is serious pathology, most chronic back pain (extending beyond three months) is most successfully treated at a pain clinic that emphasizes rehabilitation and improved function.

7

DIABETES: MIND OVER METABOLISM

BY RICHARD S. SURWIT, PH.D.

JANICE, A NORTH CAROLINA WOMAN IN HER EARLY THIRTIES, WAS THE first patient with diabetes I treated. I met her in the the fall of 1978 after her endocrinologist, Mark Feinglos, admitted her to Duke University Hospital because of severe complications from the disease. Despite intensive therapy, her blood-sugar level had skyrocketed, and she was suffering from bleeding in her eyes that threatened to leave her blind. At the hospital, Feinglos was able to bring her diabetes under control. But he was concerned that she would relapse once she returned home because she was under a great deal of stress, which could drive her blood sugar up again.

Feinglos knew I had worked with cardiovascular patients at Duke to help them learn to relax, and he asked me to create an emergency stress reduction plan for his patient. He hoped that teaching her to manage stress better would be the key to keeping her healthy.

The idea was intriguing, but it seemed like a long shot. Countless diabetic patients and their doctors had noticed that blood-sugar levels rose during stressful times of life, and some researchers had shown that experimental stress could raise blood sugar in diabetic patients. Physiological studies, too, showed that high levels of stress hormones could raise the level of sugar in the blood. But no one knew whether stress management techniques could actually bring blood sugar back under control.

Though there was no clear-cut evidence that stress reduction could help Janice, there was little to lose by trying. For one week, we trained her in two

RICHARD S. SURWIT, PH.D., is a professor of medical psychology at Duke University Medical Center and research director of the Duke Neurobehavioral Diabetes Program.

relaxation techniques that can decrease levels of stress hormones: progressive relaxation, in which you tense and then relax major muscle groups (see Chapter 14), and biofeedback, which uses electronic devices to help you assess and control your degree of relaxation (see Chapter 18). At the same time, Janice continued to receive traditional medical treatment. After she left the hospital, Feinglos was happy to discover that her condition did not deteriorate. We'll never know for sure the reason for her continued recovery, but the consensus of those involved in this medical crisis—including the patient herself—was that stress management was the key to her success.

The happy ending to Janice's story altered the course of my career. That same year, Feinglos and I began to collaborate on research in psychology and diabetes. Eventually, in 1989, our efforts led to the creation of the Duke Neurobehavioral Diabetes Program. Over the years, our team has conducted numerous experiments involving hundreds of patients nationwide. We have looked at the role that emotions and personality play in blood-sugar levels of everyone from the Pima Indians of Arizona to young Southern children playing video games. Our work is part of a nationwide research effort to explore whether and how attitudes, behaviors, and feelings can influence the development and course of diabetes. Although this research is relatively new, enough studies have been completed to offer encouraging information and advice to anyone with diabetes.

WHAT IS DIABETES?

Diabetes mellitus, the full medical term for this illness, means "excessive sweet urine." The sweetness comes from glucose, a sugar that is a major source of energy for the body's cells. Glucose in the urine is one of the signs of diabetes.

Normally, glucose enters the cells from the bloodstream with the help of the hormone insulin, secreted by the pancreas. In diabetes, this sugar delivery system breaks down, because either the pancreas produces too little insulin, or the body's cells have become resistant to the hormone, or both. (See "The Key to Diabetes.") Because glucose cannot readily enter the cells, it accumulates in the bloodstream; when it exceeds a certain level in the blood, it spills over into the urine. Although the evidence is not conclusive, doctors have long theorized that a high blood-sugar level is the culprit behind many of the disease's severe long-term complications, including nerve and eye damage and accelerated cardiovascular disease.

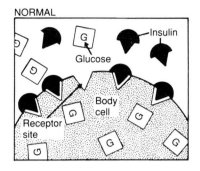

NORMAL

Insulin

Glucose

Body cell

Receptor site

THE KEY TO DIABETES

Diabetes develops when the body's cells are unable to process glucose, the form of sugar that is their major energy source. In normal cases, the hormone insulin, produced by the pancreas, acts like a key—it acts on specific receptors to "unlock" the cell walls so that glucose can be transported from the bloodstream into the cells.

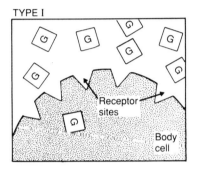

TYPE I

Receptor sites

Body cell

In Type I, or insulin-dependent, diabetes, the pancreas makes little or no insulin—not enough to allow much glucose to enter the cells. This type of diabetes must be treated with insulin injections to compensate for the body's lack of the hormone.

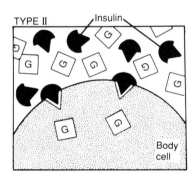

TYPE II

Insulin

Body cell

In Type II diabetes, the pancreas does produce insulin, but the cells are resistant to it; for some reason they do not respond normally to the hormone. Even with insulin present, glucose is not adequately transported into the cells. The result: Too much glucose remains in the blood. Type II diabetes is usually controlled through diet and exercise. Oral medication to stimulate insulin release and reduce insulin resistance may be necessary, and insulin injections are used in some cases.

There are two major types of diabetes. Type I, or insulin-dependent, diabetes affects approximately 1 million Americans. It has been called "juvenile diabetes" because it most commonly develops during childhood and adolescence. In this condition, the immune system mistakenly destroys the insulin-producing cells in the pancreas, resulting in a complete loss of the hormone.

In Type II diabetes, insulin is produced, but a defect in the body's cells makes them resistant to the effects of insulin. Even when they are exposed to the hormone, they don't take up glucose normally. The pancreas produces more and more insulin to compensate, but the hormone remains ineffective and blood sugar rises. Eventually, the pancreas may become exhausted and decrease its production of insulin. Because this problem becomes more common with age, the number of people with Type II diabetes is rapidly increasing as our average life expectancy is extended. More than 8 million Americans now have known diabetes, and 4 million more probably have it but are as yet undiagnosed. The great majority of diabetics have Type II.

Early signs of diabetes are frequent urination—the body's response to excess glucose in the urine—and constant thirst as a result of the water loss. Fatigue and weight loss may follow, as the body tries to compensate for the loss of glucose by breaking down protein, fat, and glycogen (the form of sugar stored in muscles). Those symptoms are more likely to be caused by Type I diabetes. Type II diabetes usually comes on more slowly and is often first spotted in the course of a routine physical exam.

It may be possible to minimize the complications of diabetes with medical treatment to carefully regulate the body's blood-sugar level. People with Type I diabetes need injections of insulin to make up for the body's lack of the hormone. Some Type II diabetics also require insulin injections, but most can be treated with a special diet, exercise to improve the body's ability to handle glucose, and oral medications that increase insulin production in the pancreas and reduce the body's resistance to the hormone. For both types of diabetes, however, stress control may also play a key role in keeping sugar levels in check.

THE CHEMICAL CONNECTION

Janice was hardly the first patient whose diabetes seemed to worsen in times of stress. Physicians have noted such a relationship for centuries. In his classic 1679 textbook, British physician Thomas Willis even attributed diabetes to "nervous juice."

Recently, I treated a minister whose blood-sugar level seemed to rise and fall in close step with his anxiety level. On Sundays, when he faced the stress of preaching to his congregation, his blood sugar was twice as high as it was the rest of the week.

Just how does stress cause such physical responses? In some cases, the route may be indirect. During times of tension, people with diabetes may overeat, abandon their exercise routines, and forget to take their medication, all of which may increase their blood sugar. But there is also evidence that stress directly creates physiological changes that exacerbate the illness.

Evidence of a biochemical link between diabetes and high stress levels was found just after World War I at Harvard Medical School by Walter B. Cannon, the pioneer of stress research who studied the stress hormones adrenaline and cortisol, produced by the adrenal gland (see Chapter 2). In one of his first experiments on diabetes, Cannon noted that cats who had been angered or frightened by the presence of a dog passed sugar in their urine, a sign of diabetes.

Why did stress produce this reaction? Cannon found that at times of heightened anxiety, large quantities of stress hormones are released into the blood by the adrenal glands. Their mission: to provide extra energy for battling the source of stress or fleeing the scene, the "fight-or-flight" response. One of its major components—along with an increase in heart rate, perspiration, respiration, and blood pressure—is an increase in the blood-sugar level.

In normal people, this sugar is readily used by the cells as extra fuel. But in people with diabetes, it simply accumulates in the blood, aggravating their condition.

CAN STRESS *CAUSE* DIABETES?

While most doctors now acknowledge that stress can aggravate diabetes, it is doubtful that psychological tension can actually lead to the illness. True, medical literature is filled with anecdotes of diabetes occurring soon after a tremendous stress. In 1879, Henry Maudsley, a physician and founder of modern psychiatry, described the case of a Prussian military officer, returning from the Franco-Prussian War, who developed diabetes within days of learning that his wife had been unfaithful during his absence. Recently, I was contacted by the attorney for a woman whose diabetes was discovered soon after she was seriously injured in an auto accident. The lawyer hoped to sue the driver for causing his client's diabetes.

While it is possible that stress could trigger the disease, in most cases of this sort, the apparent link between stress and the onset of diabetes is coincidental. It is a well-known psychological phenomenon that we tend to associate uncommon life events with each other. So if diabetes strikes around the same time as a car crash or a spouse's infidelity, we may erroneously attribute the disease to the stress.

Stress alone can't determine whether a person will get diabetes: Genetics plays a crucial role. Both major forms of diabetes tend to run in families, as studies of twins have dramatically shown. The chance of developing Type II

IS STRESS MANAGEMENT FOR YOU?

If you are diabetic, the following self-test can help you and your doctor decide whether relaxation techniques might help you control your disease. For this assessment to work, you must strictly adhere to your diet, exercise, and medication regimen. You must also know how to test your glucose level with a home blood-glucose monitor.

Throughout the day, every time you prepare to check your blood-glucose level, first rate your degree of stress on a 1-to-10 scale: 1 means you feel very calm and hassle-free, 10 means you are experiencing the most extreme stress you can imagine. Plot both your stress level and your blood-glucose level on graph paper; you may want to use different-colored pencils (see graphs opposite). Do this for two weeks. If your stress and blood-glucose levels rise and fall in parallel lines, chances are that stress may be affecting your diabetes control. If the two lines cross or each simply goes its own way, then stress is probably not a factor.

You can also use this technique to evaluate the effects of a stress management program in helping control your diabetes. A change in your stress level—preferably downward—should be accompanied by a similar change in your blood-sugar level. Be sure to show these graphs to your doctor and get an opinion of how you are doing.

diabetes if you have an identical twin with the illness is estimated to be as high as 90 percent. The rate is somewhat lower, but still high—50 percent—for Type I diabetes. If you do not have a genetic predisposition to diabetes, you are unlikely to get it, no matter how stressful your life is.

But in people who *are* vulnerable to diabetes, stress and tension may indeed be aggravating factors in the onset of the disease. Experiments with rats that carry the genetic predisposition for Type I diabetes show that stress can increase the number of animals that develop the disease and lower the age at which it strikes. And human studies have shown that people with Type I diabetes experienced more traumatic events in the three years before their

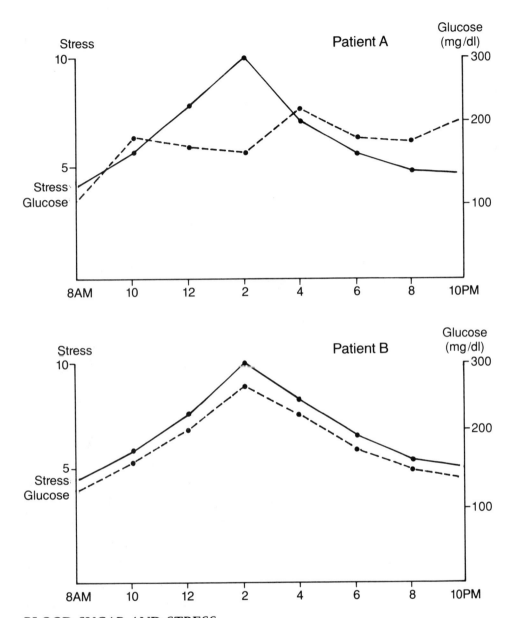

BLOOD SUGAR AND STRESS

In Patient A, blood-glucose levels do not surge in times of stress. Relaxation techniques, therefore, would probably not help her control her diabetes. In Patient B, higher blood-sugar levels are closely related to stress: During highly stressful periods her blood sugar shoots up. Stress reduction techniques may help this patient. (On these graphs, stress is measured on a self-rated 1-to-10 scale; glucose is measured in milligrams per deciliter, or mg/dl.)

diagnosis than did a random group of other, healthy people over a similar period.

Stress may also help trigger Type II diabetes when there is a genetic tendency to the disease. Some evidence for this comes from a Duke University study on a special strain of obese laboratory mice. These mice had been creating some consternation at various research labs around the country. Although some labs had reported that the mice had high blood-sugar levels characteristic of severe Type II diabetes, others were finding that the animals' blood-sugar levels were close to normal. Because these mice came from the same genetic stock and all had the genetic potential to become diabetic, we thought that different levels of stress in the different lab situations might explain why only some mice developed the disease.

To test the hypothesis, we drew blood from a group of the mice that had just spent a stressful hour confined in a very small restraining device. We compared their blood-sugar levels to those in a group that had been left in their home cages before blood was drawn. Sure enough, the restrained animals had blood-sugar levels twice as high as the others. However, when we subjected "nondiabetic" strains of mice to the same test, they did not show this stress effect.

With the help of the Pima Indians of Arizona, we have also tested our theory in human beings. The Pima tribe, which has been inbred for many generations, has the highest rate of diabetes of any self-contained population in the world. By age 40, a Pima Indian has a 60 percent chance of developing Type II diabetes. We wondered how stress would affect the blood sugar of young Pimas who had not yet shown signs of the disease, so we did an experiment to find out. We subjected 13 Pimas in their twenties to a computer-driven math test in which they had to solve problems of increasing difficulty at five-second intervals. To add to the tension, the computer tick-tocked maddeningly throughout the exam. We also gave the same test to eight non-Indians, also in their twenties, who did not have a genetic susceptibility to diabetes.

Both sets of volunteers took the test two hours after eating, when blood sugar should be falling back to normal levels. We found no significant difference in how well or how quickly these two groups performed the math problems. But there was a dramatic difference in their blood-sugar levels after the test: Blood sugar went up in approximately 75 percent of the Pimas, while the control group showed the drop that is normal two hours after a meal.

This experiment adds further credibility to the theory that stress can trigger high blood sugar in predisposed individuals and perhaps influence the time at which they develop overt diabetes. However, the role of stress shouldn't be overemphasized. Other variables—such as poor diet, obesity, lack of exercise, and other illnesses—probably play a more significant role. For stress alone to bring on diabetes, it would probably need to be both frequent and intense—far beyond the everyday hassles most of us experience.

IS THERE A DIABETIC PERSONALITY?

"Apathetic, hypochondriacal, clingy and passive, immature and masochistic." So ran a description of the "diabetic personality type" in a 1936 psychoanalytic journal. Today, doctors dismiss the notion that people with diabetes have specific character traits. We also know they do not have higher-than-average rates of most forms of mental illness. However, certain psychological disorders may pose special problems for people with the illness. And personality may be one factor that determines which patients are likely to develop high blood-sugar levels under stress.

The one emotional disorder that may afflict people with Type II diabetes more than it does the general population is depression. Since Type II diabetes becomes more common with age, diabetes and depression may be linked simply because both diseases are most common among the elderly; depression is not necessarily a cause of diabetes. Yet depression can heighten complications of the disease. Seriously depressed people experience hormonal changes similar to those brought on by stress. The result is that more glucose accumulates in their blood, which aggravates diabetes.

Fortunately, depression is now a very treatable illness. Early diagnosis can be difficult, however, because most people are unaware of the true symptoms of depression. Not all people who suffer from depression feel sad or hopeless. However, they may experience appetite changes, inability to concentrate, memory loss, and insomnia—particularly early-morning awakening. Anyone with these symptoms should not hesitate to discuss the possibility of depression with her or his doctor.

Psychologists and psychiatrists are also beginning to realize the great danger that bulimia (binging and purging) and anorexia (self-starvation) can create for people with diabetes. Although these eating disorders are always serious, they can be disastrous if you have diabetes because they interfere with the intricate metabolic balancing act required to control the disease. If your diabetes is stabilized by insulin injections and you don't eat well-balanced meals at regular intervals, too much insulin will accumulate in your blood, causing hypoglycemia (excessively *low* blood sugar) and, in severe cases, insulin shock, leading to brain damage and death. On the other hand, if you skip insulin injections as a way to lose pounds, your blood-sugar level can spin out of control and also lead to severe physiological damage, coma, and death.

Eating disorders are particularly common among teenagers, so it's especially important for parents of children with diabetes to be aware of them. If you notice any dramatic drop in your child's weight or a sudden change in eating habits, contact his or her pediatrician; you may also want to arrange for a consultation with a psychiatrist or psychologist.

No personality traits can cause diabetes, but some may exacerbate the illness. Our research suggests that shy, withdrawn people who don't have much curiosity about the world are less likely to adhere to the diabetes care regimen than are outgoing, fun-loving, curious people.

Our research also suggests that patients with Type A personality—characterized by aggressiveness, hostility, and a sense of time urgency—may experience more problems from diabetes during times of stress than do other people with the illness. We tested the blood sugar of children with Type I diabetes immediately after they played the video game Super Breakout. About half of the children had Type A personalities (according to ratings by their teachers and parents), while the others were Type B—more phlegmatic, calmer, and less easy to anger. In general, the Type A children showed an increase in blood sugar after the game, while the Type Bs showed a decrease.

Despite such intriguing findings, it will take more study before we'll fully understand why personality type seems to influence the effect of stress on diabetes or on the diligence with which patients follow their treatment plans.

MIND/BODY TREATMENTS

Before the discovery of insulin in 1921, the most common remedy for diabetes was rest. Some physicians even prescribed opiates to relax patients. Once insulin was discovered, these "psychological" treatments were dismissed as folk medicine. Were such therapies abandoned prematurely? Because stress hormones play a major role in the regulation of metabolic processes, including the release of insulin and the regulation of blood sugar, controlling excessive stress-hormone activity could theoretically be helpful in the treatment of diabetes. Now, preliminary studies at Duke and other medical centers suggest that stress management techniques can indeed help some people with the disease.

In our early experiments, we gave tranquilizers known to decrease stress-hormone levels to diabetic, obese mice. During times of stress, the drugs kept the animals' blood-sugar levels from rising as they normally would. But tranquilizers are not a useful stress management tool in human beings: They can be habit-forming and often lose their effectiveness when taken over a long period of time. To help people manage stress, we decided to try psychological rather than chemical methods.

Progressive relaxation and biofeedback, the techniques used with Janice, are common relaxation tools known to lower levels of stress hormones. Can they help control diabetes?

We first attempted to find the answer through a study of 12 patients with Type II diabetes who complained of high stress levels. For nine days, the patients remained at Duke University Hospital. Half received progressive relaxation training and EMG (electromyographic) biofeedback along with a standard diet and exercise regimen, while the other half received only the diet and exercise. At the end of the experiment, the patients who were taught relaxation techniques showed better metabolic control than the others. However, a similar study by another group of investigators did not find relaxation helpful.

In a more recent study, we followed 40 people with diabetes for up to one year; half were given relaxation training, and half were not. On the average, patients who were taught relaxation showed no greater diabetes control than patients who did not receive relaxation training. However, the metabolic response to relaxation was very variable; some patients showed a large response, others none at all. We discovered that people who reported significant anxiety in their lives were the ones who showed improved diabetes control from relaxation, while people who did not complain of anxiety showed little improvement from relaxation. The logical conclusion: While stress management may be helpful to people with Type II diabetes who are under stress, it is not for all people with diabetes.

The effect of relaxation techniques on people with Type I diabetes is not yet clear. One long-term study reported that patients who practice relaxation

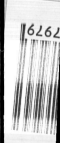

have fewer swings between high and low blood sugar and may even require less insulin to remain in control. But the study was very small and the results inconclusive. Other research has failed to find any benefit of relaxation in Type I diabetes.

In reality, the potential of psychology to help us understand and treat diabetes has hardly been realized. Most experiments have taken place in the last 10 to 15 years—a blink of an eye in the world of medical research. Recently, the American Diabetes Association formed a Council on Behavioral Medicine and Psychology to coordinate the activities of scientists working on this problem. In the years ahead, we should learn more about how stress affects diabetes control and how techniques to control stress can be useful in reducing the effects of the disease. When this occurs, stress management may find its way into most diabetes clinics.

THE BOTTOM LINE

If you have no family history of diabetes, your chances of developing the disease are small. But if you are genetically predisposed to the disease, numerous environmental factors—including infection (for Type I diabetes), weight gain (for Type II diabetes), and stress—may play a role in triggering it. High levels of stress have physiological effects that influence glucose metabolism and can increase your blood-sugar level, making diabetes more difficult to control once the disease has developed.

There is some evidence, though still preliminary, that relaxation techniques may help control the disease in some people with Type II diabetes who also experience significant stress. The methods tested to date include biofeedback (see Chapter 18) and progressive muscle relaxation (see Chapter 14). Other forms of relaxation, such as meditation and the basic "relaxation response," have not been tested for diabetes treatment. The self-test, "Is Stress Management for You?" (given earlier in this chapter), can help you determine whether relaxation techniques might be helpful.

CAN YOU "FEEL" YOUR BLOOD SUGAR?

One useful new advance for diabetics is the development of techniques to learn to recognize when blood sugar is high or low. Psychologist Daniel Cox and his colleagues at the University of Virginia have designed a method that allows you to relate your feelings, emotions, and sensations to blood-sugar levels. Many people with diabetes think that they can do this, but it usually requires experimentation and practice. What one person feels when his or her blood sugar is high may be the same as what others feel when their blood sugar is low.

To learn your own responses, use a portable blood-glucose analyzer to monitor your sugar levels throughout the day. Before each check, assess how you are feeling, using the checklist given below. While variations in blood sugar evoke different feelings in different people, the sensations listed below include the most common ones. Over time, you may be able to correlate your sensations with your blood-sugar level. However, you should only use your subjective experience as a possible warning sign, never as a substitute for actual measurement of blood-glucose levels.

The following list gives some common symptoms and moods associated with high and low blood sugar.

Hypoglycemia (low blood sugar)
Trembling
Sweating
Pounding heart
Mental confusion
Slurred speech
Anxiety/nervousness
Lightheadedness
Hunger

Hyperglycemia (high blood sugar)
 Dryness in mouth or throat
 Sweet or funny taste in mouth
 Need to urinate
 Pain, tingling in extremities
 Alert, energetic feeling
 Relaxed feeling

Either hypoglycemia or hyperglycemia
 Blurry vision
 Fatigue
 Weakness
 Numbness
 Heavy breathing
 Queasy stomach
 Headache
 Salivation
 Frustration
 Irritability/anger

8

THE SKIN: MATTERS OF THE FLESH

BY TED A. GROSSBART, PH.D.

ELSA, A 20-YEAR-OLD STUDENT FROM A CLOSE-KNIT FAMILY, WANTED TO become a concert violinist. Her sense of duty, however, demanded that she stay home to care for her elderly grandmother. Opting to follow her musical aspirations, Elsa left for conservatory anyway. But within a semester, she was back home, forced to give up her studies because of severe eczema on her hand that failed to respond to medicine. The irony of Elsa's predicament was not lost on the young woman. Recognizing the possibility that her skin condition might have an emotional component, she sought my help. As a psychotherapist specializing in skin disorders, I helped her explore her relationship with her family, while also teaching her visualization exercises aimed at soothing and protecting her hand. Within months, with a renewed sense of self-assuredness and an improved ability to negotiate family politics, the eczema cleared up, and she resumed her studies.

Another patient of mine, a 28-year-old artist, thought he wanted to become a father. But he had genital herpes, which flared up whenever his wife was ovulating. When the "coincidental" timing of his outbreaks became too blatant to ignore, he entered therapy. There he discovered his doubts about his willingness to become a parent. When he confronted these doubts directly, the virus went into remission.

To those of us who study the emotional as well as the physical components of health and disease, skin is a particularly fascinating organ. At once intimately private and blatantly public, skin is the ultimate interface between

TED A. GROSSBART, PH.D., is a clinical psychologist in private practice in Boston and an instructor in psychology at Harvard Medical School.

self and other—between our inner being and the outer world. And as the boundary between our inside and our outside, the skin sees as much action and intrigue as any border town. It is both the portal through which we feel the world and the movie screen upon which we project our personal feelings for the world to see.

Our skin is the one suit we never take off, but like everything else we wear, we change it to fit the mood or the occasion. Virtually every act of love or hate involves a dynamic interchange at the skin. So it shouldn't be surprising that the skin often provides the first manifestation of trouble when emotional problems spill over from the heart and mind.

As a clinical psychologist, I was struck early on by how frequently major medical conditions in my patients appeared and disappeared as their psychological state changed. I began to wonder how people could better be taught to protect their bodies from the emotional buffeting to which life subjects us. Specifically, could people be helped to feel hurt in their hearts instead of in their skin, and could treatment aimed at their emotional turmoil clear up their skin problems?

Answers began to emerge as I surveyed the clinical and research literatures and as I accumulated years of experience working with patients. Typically, the people who come to me with a skin problem have been through treatment after treatment; each approach may have helped a little, but none has helped enough. By the time they come to me, these people are ready to give up the fantasy that "the *next* cream may be the one that makes the problem vanish" and are prepared to try a more demanding psychological approach.

I only accept patients who have already had a good medical evaluation of their skin condition. Most skin problems have a clear biological or infectious component, and treating that component is essential. In many cases, dermatologists, allergists, or other health-care providers can treat skin problems effectively simply by using antibiotics or anti-inflammatory, antifungal, or antiviral drugs. In other cases, these simple, standard treatments are ineffective.

In every case, however, it's critical to get the best conventional treatment before exploring the psychological dimensions of a skin problem. Even if conventional therapy does not work on its own, it may become much more effective when combined with a psychological approach. Many studies now suggest that mind/body techniques can be helpful for a spectrum of skin problems, either as stand-alone therapies or as adjuncts to standard treatments. Although these studies have often involved relatively small numbers of patients, the overall number of positive studies is growing, and many dermatologists are finding them increasingly persuasive.

HOW THE SKIN WORKS

Despite its rather simple outer appearance, skin is remarkably complex. A section of skin about the size of a quarter contains, on average, an incredible 3 feet of blood vessels, 12 feet of nerves, 25 nerve endings, 100 sweat glands, and more than 3 million cells.

Skin is not merely a passive, protective integument, but a key player in the body's sophisticated armed forces. It lives a stressful and volatile life. As the largest of our organs (spread flat, it would cover about 20 square feet), the skin provides the first line of defense against a constant onslaught of microbes, physical traumas, and environmental irritants. It is well populated with roaming immune system cells that engulf invading microorganisms and are always on the lookout for weakened areas vulnerable to attack. What's more, recent research indicates that these cells use chemical messengers to remain in constant communication with the thymus—one of the immune system's major control centers in the body—as well as with the nervous system.

As might be expected of so complex an organ, disorders affecting the skin are quite diverse medically. Bacteria, viruses, hormones, chemical and environmental irritants, immune and autoimmune reactions, and hereditary influences all contribute to many diseases of the skin. The role of psychological factors in the cause and cure of skin conditions is equally varied.

In the absence of any clear behavioral link, such as compulsive scratching, how is emotional turmoil translated into physical symptoms? The mechanisms remain poorly understood. But with an increasing number of studies showing that emotions can have powerful effects on the immune system (see Chapter 3)—and with skin serving as one of the body's front-line immunological defenses against disease—it makes sense that the skin might be subject to a convergence of biological and emotional challenges.

SKIN AND SYMBOLISM

Although we all have stress in our lives, some people are more predisposed than others to develop stress-related skin conditions. While there is no simple

COULD MIND/BODY APPROACHES HELP YOUR SKIN?

Ask yourself the following questions. The more of these questions you answer positively, the more likely you will benefit from mind/body approaches.

☐ Do your symptoms get worse with emotional turmoil?

☐ Is your condition more stubborn, severe, or recurrent than your doctor expects?

☐ Are usually effective treatments not working for you?

☐ Do most treatments work, but not for long?

☐ Is each disappearing symptom quickly replaced with another?

☐ Do your symptoms get worse in a very erratic, seemingly nonsensical way?

☐ Do you see striking ups and downs in your symptoms with changes in your social environment: vacations, hospitalizations, business trips, or the moods of family members and bosses?

☐ Is your level of distress and concern about the problem unusually high?

☐ Do people find you puzzlingly stoical, unruffled, or computer-like in the face of stressful life events?

☐ Is your skin worse in the morning, suggesting that you rub or scratch unintentionally at night?

☐ Do you have trouble following your health-care provider's instructions?

☐ Do you do things you know will hurt your skin, like squeezing pimples or overexposing yourself to sunlight?

☐ Do you feel excessively dependent on your dermatologist or excessively angry with him or her? (Even if the faults are real, are you overreacting?)

☐ Does it seem that others notice improvements in your skin before you do? Is it hard for you to acknowledge when your skin has improved?

way to tell who is most susceptible, the checklist given here—"Could Mind/ Body Approaches Help Your Skin?"—can help you determine whether a psychological approach is likely to be productive for you. My experience as a clinical psychologist also suggests that some skin problems are most likely to be linked to emotional conflicts when the skin disorders themselves reflect the conflict symbolically. Often, skin problems provide their own clues about the possible emotional trigger.

Consider one woman I saw as a patient, a music teacher whose first baby had severe colic. For a year, he cried nearly nonstop night and day. As her son became more demanding, her husband became more withdrawn. Soon she developed a severe rash on the ring finger of her left hand, where she wore her wedding band. (Other fingers with gold rings were fine.) Eventually, the rash became so severe that she had to have her wedding ring cut off—as if to say with her skin what she felt she couldn't say in words.

Of course, many skin problems develop without such overt symbolism. Yet even in these instances, the symbolic meaning a disease develops *after* it appears can make it more difficult to treat.

Two good examples are herpes and warts, each of which can occur at virtually any skin location. Biologically, oral and genital herpes are similar. They are caused by nearly identical viruses; in fact, about one-fifth of genital herpes symptoms are caused by the virus that usually causes oral herpes. Psychologically, however, these are very different disorders: Oral herpes is generally dismissed as the nuisance of "cold sores," while genital herpes can become a source of devastating emotional turmoil.

Similarly, venereal warts have an impact very different from that of warts on a hand or foot, though caused by a nearly identical virus. Much of the extra suffering that comes with the genital versions arises from an interaction between the disease itself and feelings of anxiety, confusion, and guilt. Genital herpes or warts can trigger emotional stress that should then be alleviated in order to best treat the condition, because the stress itself can make the condition worse.

Appearance-altering skin problems like acne, eczema, psoriasis, and vitiligo can make people feel extremely embarrassed and want to isolate themselves. Like venereal warts and herpes, these conditions can trigger a vicious circle: The emotional distress they cause can make the condition more resistant to medical treatment, until the psychological factors at work are dealt with and the cycle is broken.

HOW TO BREAK THE CYCLE

Fortunately, psychological approaches can be very effective in helping people deal with the emotional side of skin problems and eventually find relief. The most effective approaches use a combination of the following six strategies:

RELAXATION

Relaxation techniques can be helpful in dealing with stress and the physical symptoms it causes. These techniques should be learned, however, with an awareness that the stress causing the problem does not necessarily stem from an obvious painful situation. It is just as likely to come from a struggle to *avoid* such a situation and the feelings it arouses.

DISTANCING YOURSELF FROM SYMPTOMS

Your skin condition and the suffering related to it are two separate things. Even if the condition itself remains unchanged, you can react to the condition in a different way. If you focus anxiously and incessantly on pain, itching, or irritation, those symptoms will tend to snowball. If you can distance yourself from the symptoms, they're likely to lessen. (For an example of how to do this, see "Itching: Unlinking the Chain" at the end of this chapter.)

VISUALIZING PHYSICAL CHANGES

The body often responds to an intensely imagined situation as if it were real, whether the situation is eating a lemon or having an erotic encounter (see Chapter 17). As you begin to identify situations or environments that can help your skin, you can fashion an "ideal imaginary environment." You may be able to improve your skin by repeatedly transporting yourself in your mind's eye to a sunny mountaintop or to a special resort where you are free to take a leisurely swim in a soothing vat of yogurt.

UNDERSTANDING THE MEANING OF THE SYMPTOM

The skin lives an emotional life that reflects much of what is happening in our hearts and minds. In a very real sense, it rages, cries, judges, remembers, and punishes for real or imagined sins. As we have seen, symptoms often seem to have very eloquent, personal symbolic meanings; understanding those meanings on an emotional level can help the healing process.

LEARNING TO LET GO OF THE CONDITION

The prospect of change, even the most ardently wished-for change, has some fear mixed in. A major skin disorder becomes interwoven into the fabric of daily life; it can affect where you work, what you wear, whom you see or avoid, and where you go on vacation. In some cases, it may reflect an unconscious attempt to resolve overwhelming dilemmas—a respectable way to avoid work or ask for love or a distraction from deeper emotional pain. As painful as the condition may be, losing the condition can threaten your equilibrium, and even patients with debilitating skin diseases sometimes sabotage treatment out of fear of change. Every dermatologist has a list of patients who stopped coming in just as their skin began to improve.

RECEIVING COACHING AND EMOTIONAL SUPPORT

Under the best of circumstances, your dermatologist would be not only a superb technician but a wise and supportive human being who is available at any time. Whatever your physician's skills in this regard, you may be able to get more of the emotional support you need from a psychologist or counselor or from a self-help group whose members have coped with the same disease you're suffering from. Whether in an individual or group format, these kinds of relationships can often help you heal.

Keep in mind that the best psychological treatment for one person's skin condition may differ substantially from that for another person's outbreak of the same disease. Hippocrates warned, "Who has the disease is more important than the disease he has." Different people channel psychological and emotional difficulties in different ways, and your hives could well have more in common with your neighbor's psoriasis than with your uncle's hives.

That said, it can still be helpful to review the research that has been done on mind/body approaches to skin diseases, to see what has worked for others and get some sense of what might be best for you. One caution, however: Success stories in which problem A was solved with biofeedback, problem B with psychotherapy, and problem C with hypnosis may tell us more about what was tried in each instance than they do about a special relationship between that disease and that technique.

STOPPING ITCHING AND SCRATCHING

Few skin symptoms have as devilish an ability to cause torment as a relentless itch-scratch cycle. Although much of the research in this area has focused on atopic eczema (dermatitis), there are many conditions and circumstances that can make the urge to scratch irresistible. Yet as doomed as itchers and scratchers typically feel, this is a skin syndrome that responds well to psychological approaches.

Several researchers have found that the key to breaking free of the itch-scratch cycle is to recognize that this syndrome is both a behavioral problem and an emotional problem and to treat both. In a sense, treatment for itching sits at the crossroads of two important avenues of psychotherapy—the psychodynamic and behavioral approaches—and both these approaches have proven quite useful.

In one study, Swedish clinical psychologists took 17 adults who had suffered from atopic dermatitis for at least three years and divided them into two groups. Both groups received a soothing medical cream, but the experimental group also used psychological techniques. At the end of a month, the experimental group was scratching less and had clearer skin than the cream-only control group.

How did they do it? Patients in both groups were given a golf counter to track the episodes of scratching. They were asked to identify those situations that produced the strongest urge to scratch, to determine the intensity of the urge, and to note where it was localized on the body.

But people in the psychological treatment group received additional training to help them become more aware of how, when, and where they began to move their hands when the urge to scratch took hold. They made a careful study of situations in which they scratched especially often or vigorously.

Having learned to recognize the subtle cues that led up to a scratch, these individuals then practiced a repertoire of behaviors incompatible with scratching. At first, they were taught to put their hands firmly and motionlessly on the itching area for one minute when they were tempted to scratch, then to move them to their thighs or to grip some object. When they felt confident with this approach, they skipped the step in which they would touch the area and just moved their hands to an object or gripped their thighs. Within weeks, these people had a new and powerful weapon with which they could counter previously irresistible urges to scratch.

The married team of Caroline and Peter Koblenzer—both are dermatologists, and she is also a psychiatrist—have developed a somewhat different approach. In one recent study, they treated eight children with chronic atopic eczema. All had been through multiple unsuccessful treatments, and both the children and their parents had become obsessed by the youngsters' incessant scratching. Yet the Koblenzers were able to help almost all of the children stop scratching.

Their program combined the best medicine available with weekly psychotherapy for each mother and child. The Koblenzers found that the mothers of these children (and some fathers) overcompensated for their angry feelings toward the children by becoming overly solicitous and unable to make appropriate demands. Therapy allowed the parents to express their negative feelings, helped them see that their compensatory reactions only made matters worse, and lowered their stress levels overall.

To get the kids to stop scratching, the Koblenzers strongly urged the parents to *permit* scratching, reasoning that the children had kept scratching partly to gain their parents' attention and concern. The children were also required to stay in their own beds at night, a time when both scratching and the resultant family turmoil were particularly intense. Because anxiety heightens both itching and scratching, the children also benefitted from the lower level of tension in the family overall.

When one person has a severe itching problem, the spouse, like the parent of a young child, can become both overprotective and judgmental. The Koblenzer approach has potential for breaking this kind of cycle in adults as well.

PSYCHOPSORIASIS: A NEW FOCUS

People with psoriasis are the fastest-growing part of my practice today, reflecting a new openness among dermatologists to psychological approaches to this disease.

In psoriasis, skin cells are rapidly overproduced, coming up to the surface before they've had time to mature fully. The red, raw cells then dry out, causing constant flaking. Until this century, the disease was poorly understood; it wasn't until 1908, for example, that psoriasis was distinguished from leprosy in the United States and Europe. In the Middle Ages, people with the disease were declared dead by the church or burned at the stake. Interestingly, the seeds of modern successes were discernible even then: We have at least one report, from medieval Persia, of psoriasis successfully treated with an approach resembling psychotherapy.

For psoriasis sufferers, the emotional impact is great. A study of 100 long-term patients by a Scottish dermatologist noted that the majority considered embarrassment the worst feature of their disease. Stares (real or imagined) and fears of contagion among the uninformed took a severe emotional toll. Patients surveyed by Dartmouth physicians Richard Baughman and Raymond Sobel also ranked embarrassment as the most severe consequence. (Interestingly, dermatologists surveyed in the Dartmouth study ranked embarrassment as the *least* important feature of the disease.)

Do emotions play a role in maintaining psoriasis? The English physician R. H. Seville found in a 1987 study that among 62 patients with psoriasis, the ones who did best medically were those who could identify the stressful events that triggered their outbreaks.

Good results in treating psoriasis have been obtained with a wide variety of mind/body techniques, including hypnosis, psychotherapy, relaxation, and biofeedback. Group psychotherapy, support groups, and mutual-help groups (listed in Resources) have proven helpful as well, particularly in cushioning the psychological impact of the disease.

Conventional ultraviolet-light treatments provide a good opportunity to add a psychological component to psoriasis therapy. Many of my patients take individualized audiotapes into the light box. Jeffrey Bernhard and his colleagues at the University of Massachusetts Medical Center, including Jon Kabat-Zinn (see Chapter 15), did a controlled study of a similar approach with patients receiving standard ultraviolet therapy. Their preliminary results indicate a quicker resolution of skin lesions in patients who, during their treatments, listened to audiotapes that included music and mental exercises that asked them to focus on their breathing, muscles, and body sensations. The tapes also guided the patients to visualize the mechanisms and cellular effects of the treatment.

In a major address to the 30th annual meeting of the North American Clinical Dermatologic Society in 1989, Eugene Farber, professor emeritus of dermatology at Stanford University, asserted the central role of stress (particularly anxiety, depression, and grief) as a trigger of psoriasis. He strongly endorsed a therapeutic role for clinical psychologists and for stress reduction, biofeedback, and discussion groups in treating the disease.

WARTS AND HERPES: A TALE OF TWO VIRUSES

In *Tom Sawyer*, Mark Twain described an elaborate American folk remedy for getting rid of warts, one that involved taking a dead cat into a cemetery at midnight. Other cultures have evolved equally bizarre treatments for this common affliction, and all probably work to some degree. Warts are notoriously amenable to psychological suggestion, a familiar phenomenon that is nevertheless far from fully understood. The eminent biologist Lewis Thomas was so impressed by it that he suggested that warts were worthy of the highest level of study—perhaps, he wrote, through establishing "a National Institute of Warts and All."

Warts, like herpes, are caused by a virus, and psychological factors help determine whether the virus is causing problems. There's a great difference between having the virus in your body and actually having a visible wart. We all swim in a sea of viruses, and there are many different viruses swimming within each of us. (If you have ever had chicken pox, for example, the virus that caused it is still in your body.) Usually, its presence has no impact. In fact, perhaps two-thirds of the people infected with the virus that causes genital herpes never experience another outbreak after their first few bouts of symptoms.

Similarly, the 50 or 60 variants of the human papilloma virus that can cause warts are often inactive in the body. Although the story is not as clear for warts as it is for herpes, the papilloma virus is a common inhabitant of our personal zoos; as many as 30 percent of American women may have the virus for venereal warts within their bodies, while many others carry the virus for the nonvenereal variety.

When the immune system is functioning well, it keeps all of these microscopic predators in their place. It quashes or prevents herpes recurrences and often produces spontaneous remission of warts. So to the extent that psychological factors can influence one's immune status, they can also affect viral recurrence rates or disappearance rates.

Evidence for a psychological role in warts and herpes goes back to the early part of this century. In 1928, two Viennese physicians used hypnosis to alleviate oral herpes symptoms and also demonstrated that hypnotic suggestions could experimentally trigger recurrences. Similar reports appeared sporadically over the next 50 years.

The first well-controlled experimental demonstration of hypnotic treatment of nonvenereal warts was directed in Boston by psychiatrist Owen Surman in 1973. After five weekly hypnotic sessions, 53 percent of patients who started with one or more warts were wart-free, while the untreated control group was unchanged. Since then, several researchers and clinicians have found that mind/body techniques can help speed the disappearance of warts. In fact, common warts, which often arise at times of challenge or transition, are probably the most responsive of all skin problems to a psychological approach.

Unfortunately, the treatment of warts and herpes is much more complicated when these diseases attack the genital region. From 26 to 31 million Americans have genital herpes, while 40 to 50 million Americans have venereal warts—all part of the fallout from a worldwide epidemic of sexually transmitted diseases. The fear, guilt, and anxiety that accompany these outbreaks can make their treatment especially difficult.

With non-sexually transmitted warts representing probably the best-researched and best-accepted application of mind/body techniques in all of dermatology, it is puzzling that almost nothing has been done to apply these techniques to people with venereal warts. The few clinical reports that have been published are very promising, however.

Herpes can carry a special stigma. I think of genital herpes as two diseases: *medical herpes*, an infection caused by a virus; and *psychological herpes*, the emotional impact of the disease, caused in part by the media, which have portrayed people with herpes as players in a modern morality play.

A positive change in attitude could have real clinical benefits. Margaret Kemeny, a psychologist at the University of California, Los Angeles, found that depressed people with herpes had lower levels of certain immune system cells and more recurrences of the disease than did other people with herpes who weren't depressed. And Paul Silver, then a clinical psychology graduate student at the Virginia Commonwealth University, studied people with ten or more herpes recurrences a year and found that those who believed they had little control over their outbreaks or who simply "wished" the disease would go away had more frequent and more serious recurrences than did those who practiced positive coping skills. Although large-scale controlled studies remain to be done, several clinicians have now published reports showing that psychological techniques can help reverse outbreaks of oral and genital herpes.

STRESS AND ALOPECIA

Loss of hair is neither life-threatening nor physically painful, but the good news about alopecia areata stops abruptly there. This cause of hair loss is markedly different from male pattern baldness, which is both more common and more predictable. For most people with alopecia areata, the loss is limited to one or two areas of the head, but this can be very traumatic. In some related conditions, the areas of hair loss expand until all of the scalp hair has disappeared (*alopecia totalis*), or until no hair is left anywhere on the body (*alopecia universalis*). At any level of severity, hair may regrow, often after a year or two, and that regrowth may be permanent or temporary. Such unpredictability only serves to heighten the already potent emotional impact of this mysterious disorder.

The cause of alopecia is unknown, although some studies suggest it may be an autoimmune disorder in which the immune system mistakenly reacts to the hair follicle as if it were an intruder. Whatever the physiological underpinnings, emotional stress—especially traumatic loss—frequently triggers alopecia. But unfortunately, despite this psychological connection, there have still been few attempts to apply mind/body techniques to alopecia.

One promising though preliminary study was done by psychologist Susan Eppley at the University of Cincinnati. Eppley worked with three men and seven women, all with alopecia, and taught them relaxation and mental imagery exercises. Despite several limitations in the study, the researchers were able to document a measurable acceleration in hair growth and a significant reduction in anxiety.

"SIMPLE" ALLERGIES AREN'T

Allergy itself is not a disease, but rather a *mechanism* that causes problems such as asthma, hay fever, or hives. An allergy represents an overreaction of the immune system; you may get an allergic skin eruption from exposure to certain plants or animals or after eating a food to which you are sensitive. But while allergies reflect a biological oversensitivity, psychological factors are major players as well.

Some allergic reactions may even be triggered by a harmless substance to which a person believes he or she is sensitive. Japanese physicians Yujiro

Ikemi and Shunji Nakagawa hypnotized allergic volunteers and told them that a leaf applied to their skin was toxic, like poison ivy. The leaf was actually harmless, but the subjects' skin became red and irritated anyway. In addition, when the researchers told the hypnotized subjects that a real toxic leaf was harmless and then applied that leaf to the skin, they showed a dramatically *reduced* allergic response. The power of belief was greater than the power of the toxin.

Hives—itchy, red, swollen spots that afflict about 20 percent of people at some time in their lives—can result from a true allergic reaction or can be triggered directly by the emotions with no apparent physical allergen. Some evidence of the potential role of emotions in hives comes from Ziro Kaneko and Noboru Takaishi of Osaka, who treated hives successfully with hypnosis. Fourteen of their 27 patients made complete or near-complete recoveries; only five found no benefit. The doctors were also able to recreate the skin symptoms experimentally, either by giving the patients direct suggestions of skin irritation or by bringing to mind situations that aroused anger.

To be sure, allergies are complex and have different bases in different people. But by recognizing the role of the mind in the allergic response, we can at least open the door to the possibility of taking some control over these debilitating immune system responses.

THE BOTTOM LINE

Skin problems are caused by a wide range of factors that often work together, including genetics, hormones, and infectious agents. But the skin is also highly responsive to emotional changes.

A variety of mind/body techniques, including simple relaxation training, hypnosis, imagery, psychotherapy, and biofeedback, can help relieve skin conditions. Itching and scratching, even severe cases, can be relieved with a combination of psychotherapy and behavioral techniques. Warts are clearly treatable by hypnosis, and herpes may be as well. There is also growing interest in psychological approaches to psoriasis and a number of other skin problems, because clinical experience—and some formal research studies—show that mind/body techniques can be a major resource for people with these problems.

ITCHING: UNLINKING THE CHAIN

Often, an effective part of the psychological approach to a skin condition involves combining relaxation with imagery specific to the problem. As an example, here's how imagery can work in the case of itching, one of the most common skin problems.

Many people with chronic itching suffer from a "chain reaction": They begin by scratching an ankle, say, and then feel the itch move up the calf, to the knee, through the thigh, and onto the upper body. With imagery, you can allow yourself to itch and scratch just a little, without having it become an out-of-control problem. (This technique is often used as part of a comprehensive program and should not generally be used in isolation; it is presented here only as an example of imagery instruction applied to skin problems.)

First, get yourself into a state of deep relaxation, using one of the techniques in Chapters 14, 16, or 17, or similar techniques. Then think of the image of a chain, imagining that each link is *totally separate* from the others. Unlike a real chain, if you shake one link—no matter how hard—the others will be completely unaffected. When you have this image firmly in your mind, use it in the following ways:

- Unlink the itch in one part of your body from the rest of your body. If the back of your wrist itches, separate that itch from feelings in the front of your wrist, the back of your hand, your fingers, your forearm, or your palm. Then, even if you do scratch the back of your wrist, and that spot alone, it doesn't matter.
- Unlink *today's* itch from all other itches, past and future.
- Unlink the *urge* to scratch from the action: See if you can let it remain only an urge.
- Unlink the rest of yourself from the itchy piece of skin, and even imagine that piece of skin floating across the room. That itch has nothing to do with you.

You can also visualize your hand as a healing instrument and use that image to help counteract itching. Again, you start by achieving a relaxed state. Imagine yourself in the environment most likely to make your skin comfortable and healthy—a cool lake, a warm bath, or whatever feels best—and then unlink the chain, as described above.

Next, imagine your hand as a deep reservoir of whatever sensations are most healing and soothing to your skin. Focus on the idea that your hand will *automatically* be transformed from an agent of scratching to an agent of healing. When your hand feels full almost to bursting, move it to each area of your skin that sometimes itches. Rest the soothing hand lightly on your skin; don't rub or press. Feel the soothing power flowing out of your fingers, spreading throughout the sensitive area, so there's no room left for the sensations of itching. Spend as much time on each area as you need to. If the sensations diminish, take your hand away long enough for the reservoir to refill.

9

GUT FEELINGS: STRESS AND THE GI TRACT

BY WILLIAM E. WHITEHEAD, PH.D.

LIFE WAS GOOD FOR TED, A 50-YEAR-OLD CLERK AT THE SOCIAL SECURITY Administration, until he was promoted to a managerial post in which he supervised a dozen people. A somewhat anxious, unassertive person, he found his new job stressful, especially because he had to discipline employees when they performed poorly or broke the rules. Soon after his promotion, Ted began to experience severe abdominal pain and frequent, loose bowel movements. On many days, his condition forced him to stay home from work. His symptoms disappeared during a two-week vacation, but they quickly returned afterward. At that point, he came to our clinic at the Johns Hopkins University School of Medicine.

We found that Ted had no detectable physical problem other than abdominal tenderness and excessive contractions in his lower colon. The diagnosis was irritable bowel syndrome (IBS)—a chronic or recurrent disorder than can cause irregular bowel movements (either constipation or diarrhea) and abdominal pain. The physiological basis for IBS is not well established, but emotional factors often play a major role.

Because his tension level at work was high and his symptoms cleared during his vacation, we thought Ted's problem might well be influenced by stress. To confirm this, we asked him to keep a diary of his symptoms for four weeks. Each week, his pain was highest on Monday through Thursday, de-

WILLIAM E. WHITEHEAD, PH.D., is a professor of medical psychology in the Departments of Psychiatry and Medicine at the Johns Hopkins University School of Medicine.

clined on Friday, and reached its lowest level on Sunday morning. But by Sunday night, he was often so sick that he knew he wouldn't be able to work on Monday.

Ted's case is a classic example of the part stress can play in what are called *functional* gastrointestinal disorders—conditions of the gastrointestinal (GI) tract for which there are no detectable organic or physical causes. Clearly, work-related tension and anticipation of work stress were intensifying his illness.

His experience is hardly unique. An estimated 30 million Americans suffer from IBS, and the great majority of them find that stress makes the condition worse. In a survey at the University of North Carolina, Chapel Hill, gastroenterologist Robert Sandler and his colleagues found that stress caused abdominal pain or a change in bowel patterns for about 85 percent of patients with IBS.

But Ted's story also typifies a more recent discovery about functional GI disorders: The symptoms can worsen when people find that the illness brings them benefits, enabling them to sidestep unpleasant situations (such as stressful work), bringing them financial compensation, or increasing the attention they get from others. People don't consciously use these illnesses to get what they want. But inadvertent, unconscious learning may trigger them—evidence of just how subtle mind/body interactions in gut problems can be.

At Johns Hopkins, my colleagues and I have focused on problems of the lower GI tract: the small intestine, colon, and rectum. Although we see patients with many illnesses, IBS offers a model for describing the psychological component of these types of conditions. It is the most common reason people consult gastroenterologists and has been studied more extensively than any other functional gastrointestinal disorder.

NOT "ALL IN THE MIND"

One important research question, and a complex one, is whether IBS stems from true psychological problems rather than simply being linked to stress. At Johns Hopkins, we found that 47 percent of the patients referred to our medical clinic with IBS could be diagnosed as having a psychiatric disorder. Other research groups have reported that as many as 100 percent of their IBS patients have psychiatric problems, including depression, generalized anxiety disorder, panic attacks, and phobias. Psychiatric problems are also common in patients seeking treatment for other functional GI disorders, particularly Crohn's disease—a chronic inflammatory condition that affects primarily the lower small intestine and sometimes the colon.

Although it may seem that psychiatric problems *cause* gastrointestinal disturbances, the most recent research shows this is probably not true. Rather, patients who suffer from both IBS *and* an emotional problem are simply more likely to seek medical treatment than other people with IBS.

In a recent study, our team at Johns Hopkins surveyed 149 women in the Baltimore suburbs who had the same social and educational background as the average female patient who came to our clinic with IBS. Of these community women, 26 percent had the same symptoms of IBS as our clinic patients, yet 80 percent of the suburban women with IBS had *not* consulted a physician. When we studied that 80 percent, we found to our surprise that they were as psychologically healthy as people with no bowel symptoms. In contrast, the IBS patients who came to our clinic did have a higher-than-average rate of psychological problems. When gastroenterologist Douglas Drossman conducted a similar study at the University of North Carolina, he found comparable results.

While IBS itself is not a symptom of psychological conflict, psychological problems may influence the course of the illness by increasing a person's vulnerability to stress. Anxious or depressed people tend to feel far more stress than other people do during difficult interpersonal encounters. As a result, they may often be in a state of physiological arousal, which can worsen gut troubles.

The type of stress that worsens IBS tends to be simple, everyday unpleasantness that most of us experience—such as work deadlines and marital spats—which may have a particularly strong impact on people with emotional problems. Some patients with chronic IBS may have a biological susceptibility to the condition, which is exacerbated by their emotional state. In general, IBS patients have bowels that seem to overreact to many triggers, including certain gut hormones and a high-fat diet. For some people, however, the impact of stress alone may be great enough to trigger IBS.

Finally, research has shown that childhood traumas may predispose people to develop certain gastrointestinal conditions. For example, the early loss of one or both parents, either through death or divorce, is more common in patients with IBS and peptic ulcer disease than in the general population. Women with IBS are also more likely than other women to recall a history of sexual or physical abuse. We do not yet fully understand how these childhood experiences contribute to the development of functional GI disorders. Our belief is that these events increase a person's general sense of vulnerability, making her or him more susceptible to everyday stressors throughout life.

LEARNING TO BE ILL

Among patients who seek treatment for IBS, the condition is often part of an overall pattern that psychologists call *illness behavior* or *somatization* (see Chapter 13). People who fit this pattern have a multitude of physical concerns and visit doctors and clinics excessively. In IBS patients, other physical problems tend to include dysmenorrhea (painful menstrual periods), urgent and frequent urination, fibromyalgia (tender, painful areas in the muscles), and asthma. For somatizers, the pattern of symptoms appears to be perpetuated unconsciously by the rewards of being sick, such as increased attention or time off from one's job. IBS patients who are somatizers have a higher-than-average rate of illness-related absenteeism from work. They are also unusually likely to have surgery they may not need, especially hysterectomies and appendectomies.

Because somatizers may get operations and other treatments that are not medically necessary, researchers are especially eager to understand the origins of what might be called *learned illnesses* or the *illness habit*. Unnecessary medical treatment increases the likelihood that a person may develop an iatrogenic disorder—an illness that actually results from the treatment itself. In the case of IBS patients, hysterectomies, appendectomies, and colonic resections can all leave scar tissue in the abdomen, which in turn can create obstructions in the colon or small intestine. Moreover, with the current crisis in health-care costs, we can little afford to give people medical treatment when their needs are really psychological.

Although some people develop learned illnesses during adulthood (as Ted, the clerk, did), most research has focused on the ways parents may inadvertently encourage this behavior in their children. We now understand the common patterns well enough to offer some basic advice that may help parents avoid this pattern (see "Are You Teaching Your Child To Be Sick?").

ARE YOU TEACHING YOUR CHILD TO BE SICK?

At Johns Hopkins, we have carried out a number of studies to see how the illness habit may be learned in childhood. In our first study, reported in 1982, we asked a random sample of 832 adults to recall how their parents had responded to them during childhood when they had symptoms of a cold—an almost universal and frequent illness. People with IBS were more likely than others to say that their parents indulged them with toys, gifts, or treats when they were sick.

Over the last decade, working with more elaborate questionnaires, we have found that adults tend to experience the symptoms their parents paid attention to when they were children—or symptoms they witnessed in their parents themselves. Thus, in one study, women whose mothers allowed them to stay home from school and rest when they had bowel symptoms, but not when they had colds, were especially likely to have IBS (but not colds) as adults. Similarly, women whose menstrual symptoms had brought them maternal sympathy and attention in adolescence were more likely than other women to suffer from dysmenorrhea. This research implies that illness behavior can be learned when it is rewarded. It may also mean that parents can prevent later problems in their children by responding appropriately to their illnesses. Among the steps parents can take:

- Don't give the impression through your remarks or actions that you see illness as a way to avoid unpleasant tasks in your own life. Children imitate their parents.
- Deal matter-of-factly with sickness. It certainly makes sense to provide rest, comfort, and sympathy to an ill child. But if you offer the child gifts and treats as well, you may give the impression—both to the sick child and to his or her siblings—that an unhealthy child is loved more than a well one.
- Use good judgment. Frequent stomachaches that seem to crop up on school exam days, then miraculously disappear when the television is turned on, are probably better ignored than indulged. However, abnormal physiological responses—such as fever, abdominal distension, or rectal bleeding—do require attention. When in doubt, check with your child's doctor.

PHYSICAL PATHWAYS

While some researchers are exploring the role of learning in functional GI disorders, others are focusing on the physical mechanisms through which stress may influence the GI tract in susceptible people. Laboratory experiments confirm the fact that psychological stress and emotional arousal have physical effects on the digestive system. They can increase acid secretion in the stomach, associated with ulcers and inflammation of the esophagus; can influence the contractions of the small intestine and colon; and can affect the time required for food to move through different regions of the GI tract.

While several parts of the brain help regulate GI activity, the most important is probably the hypothalamus, which controls many bodily functions through the autonomic nervous system's two branches, the sympathetic and parasympathetic (see Chapter 2). Unlike most of the physical responses we associate with stress—racing heart, elevated blood pressure, sweating, and so on—gastrointestinal reactions are not stimulated by the "fight-or-flight" hormones and the sympathetic nervous system. Rather, colon contractions and excess gastric acid are triggered by the parasympathetic part of the nervous system, which we usually associate with relaxation.

These reactions, which can lead to GI disturbances, may once have had an evolutionary advantage. Increased colon contractions and gastric acid secretion could have survival benefits in the event of poisoning: Extra gastric acid can help destroy bacteria in food, while colon contractions will rid the body of toxins more rapidly. Perhaps our bodies are unable to distinguish between actual poisoning and the external, often symbolic threats that we normally think of as stressors.

To complicate matters, research shows that the effects of stress on the GI tract vary from person to person. In research at the University of Sheffield in England, gastroenterologists Paul Cann and Nicholas Read studied patients with IBS. In those who suffered mostly from constipation, food moved through the small intestine more slowly when the patients were under stress; in diarrhea-predominant IBS patients under stress, food moved more rapidly. Other researchers have found the same kind of variability.

EVERYDAY TROUBLES AND RARE CONDITIONS

You don't need to have a chronic disorder to experience gastrointestinal discomfort under stress. In Sandler's survey at the University of North Carolina,

SELF-HELP FOR IRRITABLE BOWEL SYNDROME

Most people with irritable bowel syndrome manage well; about 60 to 80 percent never even consult a physician. Here are some tips that can help you take control of the problem:

- Understand the natural history of your illness. Irritable bowel syndrome is a chronic disorder that will periodically get worse and then get better. Occasional bouts of symptoms are unavoidable, but they do not mean you were misdiagnosed or need a different treatment. The good news: IBS does not steadily worsen over time and will not predispose you to any other disease.
- Some people with bowel symptoms become afraid that they have colon cancer or inflammatory bowel disease such as Crohn's disease. Don't let this fear keep you from seeing the doctor. You're unlikely to have these disorders, but if you do, early treatment can make all the difference. If your doctor rules out these illnesses, accept her or his assurances and dismiss your worries.
- Recognize that diet can influence your bowel symptoms. If you have constipation, follow a high-fiber diet. If you have lactose intolerance, which makes it difficult to digest dairy products, minimize dairy products in your diet. (About 20 percent of all adult Americans and up to 70 percent of black Americans have this problem.) Other foods—such as carbonated beverages (in large amounts), spices, caffeine, alcohol, and high-fat foods—may aggravate bowel symptoms in some people.
- If you tend to have constipation, regular moderate exercise may help prevent or alleviate it.

66 percent of healthy people said that stress caused an altered bowel pattern—usually diarrhea—and 49 percent said that stress caused them abdominal pain. Although there is little concrete evidence, there are plenty of anecdotal reports that everyday stressors can lead to GI problems.

HEARTBURN

This common problem results when acid from the stomach leaks up into the esophagus, a process called *acid reflux*. You are more likely to have this problem if you overeat—which many people do under stress—because the excess food puts extra pressure on the esophageal sphincter, the valve that separates the two organs. Alcohol and nicotine also relax this sphincter, so more acid gets through if you deal with stress by smoking or drinking.

INDIGESTION (DYSPEPSIA)

Overeating may also lead to this problem, characterized by pain, a bloated feeling, and nausea. If stress causes you to gulp down your meals—swallowing air along with your food—you increase the amount of gas in the GI tract, which can lead to belching, bloating, flatus, and abdominal discomfort. About one-quarter of all adults say they suffer frequently from bloating and repeated belching.

STOMACH PAIN

Pain that occurs on an empty stomach, and is not caused by an ulcer, may be worsened when stress increases the flow of stomach acid. Again, smoking and drinking make the problem worse: Nicotine increases acid flow, and alcohol can cause inflammation of stomach tissues.

FUNCTIONAL DISORDERS OF THE ESOPHAGUS

A strong feeling of a "lump in the throat"—technically called the *globus symptom*—is a reaction of the esophagus that is almost always precipitated by strong emotion and that is more common in anxious people. Chest pain that begins in the esophagus also seems to be more common in people who are anxious or depressed.

FUNCTIONAL DYSPEPSIA

Troubling about 20 to 30 percent of adults, this is characterized by recurrent upper abdominal pain or discomfort—often associated with bloating, nausea, or vomiting—in people who do not have peptic ulcer disease or cancer. Abnormal movement of food through the stomach or small intestine seems to cause the symptoms in some, but not all, patients. Some studies suggest that

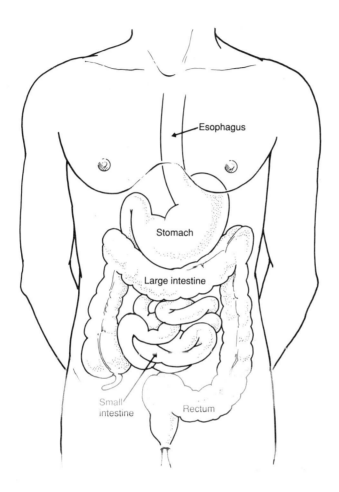

GASTROINTESTINAL TROUBLE SPOTS

The esophagus, the tube that carries food toward the stomach, is the site of heart-burn, caused when acid from the stomach backs up into it. Ulcers are most common in a spot just beyond the stomach proper: the duodenum, the first part of the small intestine. When food reaches the small intestine from the stomach, it is bathed in digestive juices and broken down into simple nutrients for absorption into the blood. Waste then passes into the large intestine, or colon, which stores and eventually eliminates undigested food. Dysfunction in the colon's muscles may lead to irritable bowel syndrome and other problems.

patients with functional dyspepsia experience more stress and have more anxiety and depression than the general population, although not every study has found this.

FUNCTIONAL ANORECTAL PAIN

About 9 percent of adults experience fleeting sharp pains in the anal canal or rectum, usually only a few times a year. More seriously, about 7 percent experience a dull and aching rectal pain, associated with muscle tenderness, which lasts for several minutes to days. Both conditions are believed to be linked to chronic muscle tension or spasm as well as to stress and anxiety, although not enough research has been done to be certain of this.

THE TRUTH ABOUT ULCERS

Peptic ulcers occur in the stomach or in the duodenum, the upper part of the small intestine. If left untreated, ulcers can perforate the wall of the stomach or intestine or cause other serious complications. Common ulcer symptoms are persistent gnawing hunger or upper abdominal pain. Black, tarry stools are a sign that the ulcer is bleeding.

Ulcers have long been thought of as a classic example of stress-induced illness. However, research shows that they are more biological than psychological in origin. One new theory holds that a contributing cause of ulcers may be a bacterial infection that irritates the stomach lining. While that theory is controversial, it is clear that excess gastric acid secretion and a decrease in the mucus that normally protects the stomach lining can both contribute to the development of ulcers.

Although stress alone does not seem to be a cause of ulcers, it may contribute to their development. People in stressful occupations—such as air traffic controllers, police officers, and truck drivers—do have a higher-than-average rate of ulcers. A new 13-year study of more than 4,000 people, done by researchers at the Centers for Disease Control and elsewhere, has also shown that people who experience their lives as stressful are almost twice as likely as others to develop ulcers over time. This difference held after the results were adjusted to account for age, gender, education, smoking habits, and regular use of aspirin, all of which can affect the risk of developing an ulcer.

One hypothesis holds that ulcers result when a biological vulnerability, such as a predisposition to produce excess gastric acid, is exacerbated by stress. However, the influence of stress on gastric acid secretion varies enormously from person to person. In two separate experiments, I measured changes in gastric acid in healthy volunteers who had to press a button at least once every 20 seconds to avoid electric shock—certainly a stressful situation. In the first study, I found that the task significantly increased gastric acid secretion. But when I repeated the experiment a year later with a different group of healthy people, I found significant *decreases*.

Although the role of stress in chronic ulcers is still being debated, the debate may be moot. Psychological remedies are rarely considered these days because ulcers can be treated with drugs that block gastric acid secretion, such as cimetidine (*Tagamet*) and ranitidine (*Zantac*). Most peptic ulcers heal rapidly with the use of these drugs, although recurrences are common, particularly in people who smoke, drink, or frequently use painkillers such as aspirin and ibuprofen. There is now some evidence that recurrences can be prevented with antibiotic treatment of the bacteria that help cause peptic ulcers.

PREVENTION AND TREATMENT STRATEGIES

For most functional GI disorders, there is not yet enough research to tell whether or not mind/body approaches can be helpful. However, several have been tested in the treatment of irritable bowel syndrome, with promising results.

PSYCHOTHERAPY

Two studies have shown that combining medical therapy with brief psychotherapy is superior to medical treatment alone for IBS. In both studies, psychotherapy was focused on identifying stressors that worsened the patient's symptoms and teaching the patient more effective ways of coping. The symptoms that improved most were pain and diarrhea; constipation was relatively unresponsive to psychotherapy. In each study, 12 months after therapy, most patients who received the combined treatments still had fewer symptoms than before. This suggests that the initial improvement was not due to the placebo effect or a desire to please the therapist.

RELAXATION TRAINING

Progressive muscle relaxation training, in which IBS patients are taught a set of exercises to induce whole-body relaxation, was evaluated by British psychologist Paul Bennett and physician Stephen Wilkinson. These investigators found that relaxation exercises and medical therapy were equally effective at relieving bowel symptoms, but that relaxation training did more to improve psychological symptoms. Other research has shown that a combination of relaxation training and medical therapy leads to greater reductions in abdominal pain and in medical consultations for bowel symptoms than does medical therapy alone. These studies have tested simple methods of stress management, using tape cassettes and minimal professional supervision.

A more complex stress management technique for IBS has been studied by psychologist Edward Blanchard and his students at the State University of New York at Albany. This approach combines progressive muscle relaxation and biofeedback with cognitive therapy to help people identify self-defeating thoughts and replace them with more positive ones. Blanchard's team found that patients who underwent this training fared better than a control group of patients who were waiting to receive therapy.

HYPNOSIS

Research by British gastroenterologist Peter J. Whorwell found IBS patients improved with the help of 30-minute hypnotherapy sessions in which suggestions for whole-body relaxation were combined with imagery that focused on relaxing the smooth muscle that lines the bowel. Participants went through seven or more therapy sessions, then practiced self-hypnosis at home using the same suggestions. By about the fourth week of training, people using hypnosis had greater improvements in pain and bowel symptoms than a control group given a placebo treatment. The results were well maintained after 18 months. Whorwell's findings have been replicated by other scientists, who have also shown that group hypnosis works as well as individual sessions.

BIOFEEDBACK

Experiments with biofeedback have shown that people can learn to control their rate of gastric acid secretion and stomach contractions (see "Training the Stomach"). Although these studies offer impressive proof of the brain's influence over GI functions, they have not led to practical treatments, perhaps

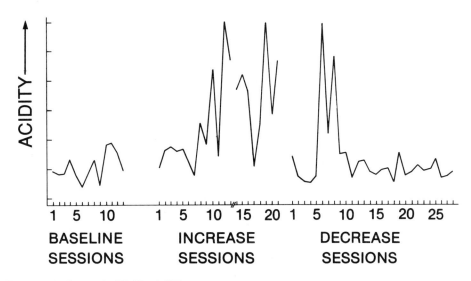

TRAINING THE STOMACH

In the past, doctors believed that various functions of the gastrointestinal tract could not be controlled voluntarily, and thus could not be treated through mind/ body methods. However, this chart shows how biofeedback did help one female volunteer to control the amount of gastric acid her stomach secreted. (An excess of gastric acid can lead to peptic ulcer disease.) In the experiment, the woman watched a meter that measured the acidity of her stomach's contents. In the "increase" sessions, she received a token reward for every measurable increase in stomach acid. It took the patient only about 10 sessions to master the skill. In the "decrease" sessions, she was equally rewarded for lowering stomach acid. Again, she learned to control this visceral response in about 10 sessions.

because more traditional stress management techniques seem to be more effective. In an experiment several years ago, I found that people with IBS could learn to inhibit colon contractions through biofeedback, but that this skill alone did nothing to decrease their pain. In contrast, people who received standard relaxation training did find that their abdominal pain improved, even though they were not able to control their colon contractions.

I believe that standard relaxation and stress management techniques are generally more helpful than biofeedback for people with GI disorders, for two reasons: First, learning to control involuntary processes is a difficult and lengthy undertaking. And second, stress management, unlike biofeedback, helps you to *prevent* stress from leading to a bowel symptom rather than just trying to control the symptom once it appears.

ARE YOU AT RISK FOR GI TROUBLES?

Studies suggest that the following characteristics may raise your risk of developing a functional gastrointestinal disorder:

☐ Childhood sexual or physical abuse.
☐ Loss of one or both parents during childhood.
☐ Parents who encouraged illness behavior.
☐ Parents who themselves had gastrointestinal symptoms of unknown cause.
☐ High levels of stress or tension.
☐ Low levels of social support from family and friends.
☐ Depression.
☐ A sensitive gastrointestinal system, shown by frequent gastrointestinal symptoms in the past.

Recent studies suggest that biofeedback may be helpful, however, in treating constipation that results from chronic constriction of the anal sphincter and muscles in the floor of the abdomen. This newly recognized syndrome may account for up to half of all patients who complain of chronic constipation. Although stress is not considered a culprit in this illness, biofeedback can help treat it by teaching patients to relax the sphincter and other voluntary muscles on the abdominal floor.

THE BOTTOM LINE

Stress and other emotional factors can play a role in functional gastrointestinal (GI) disorders—illnesses for which there is no known physical cause. The most common of these by far is irritable bowel syndrome (IBS), marked by abdominal pain and irregular bowel movements. IBS is not caused solely by emotional factors, but people who are psychologically vulnerable may be more likely to develop the condition or to see it worsen. There is growing evidence that learning "illness behavior," particularly in childhood, can also contribute to the problem. One mystery is why stress influences the GI tract differently in different patients with IBS: It may lead to diarrhea in one, and in another, constipation.

Tension may also play a role in some less common GI disorders and in the everyday gastrointestinal upsets often experienced by otherwise healthy people. And stress can contribute to ulcers, although it is not their primary cause.

Numerous mind/body treatments—particularly psychotherapy, relaxation training, and hypnosis—can effectively help prevent and treat GI disorders that have a psychological dimension. Biofeedback has been useful in documenting the mind's influence on the GI tract, but it is generally not a very effective treatment for stress-related symptoms (although it is the treatment of choice for fecal incontinence). As we learn more about the causes of IBS and other gastrointestinal illnesses, our understanding of the best treatments, including mind/body techniques, will certainly grow.

10

ARTHRITIS AND RHEUMATIC DISEASES: WHAT DOCTORS CAN LEARN FROM THEIR PATIENTS

BY THEODORE PINCUS, M.D.

THE ADVANCES OF 20TH-CENTURY MEDICINE OWE MUCH TO A CONCEPT known as the *medical model*. The underlying assumption of this model is that each disease has a single cause that can be identified by "objective" testing—including high-technology blood tests, X-rays, and scans—and that this information determines the best treatment. The model suggests that the solution to any health problem depends almost entirely on the actions of physicians and on the health-care system, and very little on the actions of the patient.

This medical model, which virtually ignores the patient's thoughts and emotions, is effective for acute diseases like pneumonia or bleeding ulcer, in which the outcome—recovery, decline, or even death—occurs over a period of days. But the model can have substantial limitations when applied to a chronic illness like arthritis, in which the effects of disease may be progressive over a period of years.

Arthritis, in fact, provides a prime example of some of the ways in which mind/body concepts can expand the medical model. Learning how arthritis patients *feel* about their condition—their pain, their difficulties in functioning, their fatigue—gives a more accurate picture of their health than high-technology tests. Furthermore, patients themselves often provide the most valuable information needed for diagnosis, treatment, and monitoring the course of their disease.

THEODORE PINCUS, M.D., is a professor of medicine at Vanderbilt University School of Medicine.

THE JOINTS IN HEALTH AND ILLNESS

Most rheumatic diseases occur at or near the joint between two or more bones (see the illustration on the next page). The joint is lined with a tissue called *synovium*, which produces fluid to keep the joint lubricated, and is covered with *cartilage*, which provides a smooth surface so that bone does not rub against bone. A number of sacs known as *bursae* also help to lubricate the joint. Muscles are connected to bone by structures known as *tendons*, and bones are connected to one another by *ligaments*.

Rheumatoid arthritis is an autoimmune disorder. For reasons that are not yet understood, the body's self-defense system acts as if there were an infection within the joint, producing enzymes that attack and gradually eat away at the cartilage that provides a surface for easy motion. Because the cartilage may be progressively destroyed over time, many specialists believe it is important to treat rheumatoid arthritis early and aggressively, before the inflammation has caused serious damage.

In osteoarthritis, damage is not done by inflammation, but by unknown mechanisms or trauma that wear down cartilage in an irregular, asymmetrical pattern.

The medical model emphasizes drug therapy as the primary treatment for arthritis, and that approach is also somewhat limited. To be sure, effective drugs are valuable in treating the various forms of arthritis, and often two or more drugs are needed to manage a condition effectively. But optimal treatment requires more than drugs to help a person function and cope with arthritis; it requires physical and occupational therapies, an exercise program, and attention to psychological issues.

Extensive research now indicates that the outcome for patients with arthritis depends at least as much on their own actions as on the actions of doctors and other health professionals. People who feel confident that they can manage their arthritis actually use the medical system and other resources

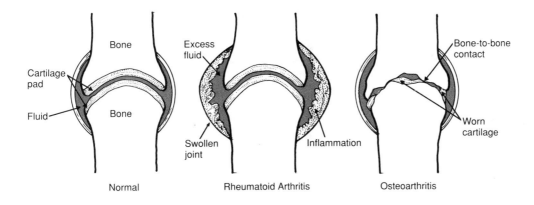

more effectively than people who lack confidence that they can fight their disease.

A VERY COMMON PROBLEM

Arthritis—the term literally means *inflammation of joints*—is the most common chronic health problem in the United States. Approximately one-fifth of all Americans under age 65, and half of those over 65, have some kind of painful condition of the muscles, bones, or joints that requires medical attention. These disorders are also called rheumatic diseases—derived from the Greek *rheuma*, meaning *flow*, which refers to a concept that flow of fluid in the joints is impaired.

Everyone has experienced some musculoskeletal pain from time to time; it's usually minor and gets better quickly by itself. But serious rheumatic diseases can make it difficult to do simple daily activities, such as bathing, getting in and out of a car, or even walking. Persistent, progressive arthritis can make it impossible to function effectively at home or to work outside the home. More than 2 million Americans under age 65 are permanently disabled because of arthritis, and the wages lost to the disease are estimated to be in excess of $50 billion. Furthermore, the most serious forms of arthritis may lead to a significantly shorter life expectancy.

The great variety of rheumatic diseases and their potential severity (although only a minority of cases are severe) often lead physicians to do extensive testing in an effort to pinpoint an exact label for what is causing trouble.

But that's where the medical model begins to break down. In many cases, elaborate diagnostic tests may provide little new information of value to treatment beyond what could be learned from the patient's history and a physical examination by an experienced doctor. The primary problems of people with musculoskeletal disease generally involve pain, fatigue, and difficulties in performing such activities of daily living as walking and dressing. These problems cannot be measured directly by any blood test or imaging procedure, and the most effective treatment may be designed in many cases without extensive testing.

Not only do extensive tests often fail to contribute to an accurate diagnosis, but they sometimes may lead to misdiagnosis and inappropriate treatment. X-rays and scans may show apparent abnormalities, including mild osteoarthritis or mildly ruptured discs, that do not explain symptoms in many patients. (In fact, these abnormalities are seen frequently in people who have no pain or symptoms.)

The interpretation of blood tests is also complex and may lead to inaccurate diagnosis. For example, gout, systemic lupus erythematosus (lupus), and Lyme disease, all important rheumatic diseases, each occur in less than 1 percent of the population. But abnormal blood tests associated with these diseases are found in about 5 percent of the general population. Many individuals with common problems such as tendinitis, bursitis, and fibromyalgia have blood tests and X-rays ordered in an attempt to identify gout, lupus, or Lyme disease. However, *most* of the people in whom these tests are positive do *not* have one of these diseases; they only have a positive blood test. By contrast, people with rheumatoid arthritis often have *normal* blood tests and X-rays early in their disease, when aggressive treatment might be most effective. A physician who relies only on these tests can miss an opportunity to treat the disease early on.

Blood tests, X-rays, and scans can be valuable when selectively applied to a problem, after a careful discussion and examination by a physician or other health professional. However, a battery of such procedures is rarely effective. In the hands of a knowledgeable physician, such as a rheumatologist, the patient almost always provides the most important information needed for a diagnosis.

RHEUMATOID ARTHRITIS AND LIFE EXPECTANCY

Our work, like most research on rheumatic disease, has focused primarily on rheumatoid arthritis, a chronic illness that affects about 1 percent of the population. This disease may lead to a decline in function, which can progress from a simple loss of the capacity to jog or play sports, to difficulties with activities of daily living, to total disability in some patients. Recent studies indicate that more than 60 percent of people who have had rheumatoid arthritis for more than 10 years are unable to work, and that rheumatoid arthritis may also shorten life expectancy by an average of 10 to 15 years.

This shortened life expectancy is comparable to the effect of untreated hypertension, an important risk factor in the development of cardiovascular disease, the major cause of death in the United States (and the Western world)—although hypertension is seen about 20 times as frequently as rheumatoid arthritis. The attributed causes of death in people with rheumatoid arthritis are similar to those seen in the general population, with cardiovascular disease the most common. However, death rates from infections and lung, kidney, or ulcer disease are higher in people with rheumatoid arthritis than in the population as a whole.

Because rheumatoid arthritis can shorten life expectancy, physicians are eager for any information that could help identify which individual patients are at greatest risk for an early death. As might be expected—and as researchers have documented only over the last decade—the risk of early death rises with how severe the arthritis is. Studies are now in progress to determine whether effective treatment of rheumatoid arthritis can improve life expectancy for people with the disease.

By using a simple questionnaire, my colleagues and I, including James Fries at Stanford University and Robert Meenan at Boston University, have found that patients' self-rating of their ability to function actually predicts mortality rates as effectively as medical measures of the severity of the disease, such as X-rays or blood tests. Apparently the *quality* of life is quite relevant to the *quantity* of life with this disease—and possibly other diseases as well.

LEARNING FROM PATIENTS THEMSELVES

Our work is part of a recent trend in arthritis research. Seeking to overcome some of the limitations of the standard medical approach, several researchers have searched for better ways to assess the severity of rheumatic disease and predict the likely course of the illness. One straightforward approach has been to get information directly from patients through standard structured questionnaires, often self-administered by the patients. This approach has proved

THE TYPES OF RHEUMATIC DISEASE

More than 100 types of rheumatic disease have been identified, including conditions caused by mechanical soft-tissue problems, trauma, inflammation, and degenerative processes.

Mechanical problems include inflamed tendons and bursae—*tendinitis* and *bursitis*—which usually get better by themselves, although they may become chronic and progressive. Trauma—injury—may damage ligaments or cartilage, sometimes requiring surgical repair.

The most common rheumatic disease involving inflammation is *rheumatoid arthritis*, in which the lining of the joint becomes inflamed. Other types of inflammatory arthritis include *ankylosing spondylitis* and related conditions, characterized by inflammation of the place where tendon enters bone. Inflammatory arthritis may also result from crystals deposited in the joint, such as uric acid crystals in *gout*, or infection by a bacterium or virus.

Connective tissue diseases—including *systemic lupus erythematosus, scleroderma, polymyositis*, and various forms of *vasculitis*—are related to rheumatoid arthritis, and are autoimmune in nature. These serious conditions can involve inflammation of the internal organs, which can be life-threatening.

Osteoarthritis, also called *degenerative joint disease*, has traditionally been blamed on the "wear and tear" of aging. But although it is more common in older people, it is not inevitable, and modern researchers believe some type of mild, slow-moving inflammation or metabolic disorder may be involved.

One of the most puzzling rheumatic diseases is *fibromyalgia*. This condition, which affects an estimated 2 to 5 percent of all women (and very few men), causes widespread musculoskeletal pain—most prominently in the neck and shoulders—and tenderness in muscles at many sites in the body. In fibromyalgia, X-rays, blood tests, and physical examination of the joints show no abnormality. The diagnosis can be made from the patient's reports of pain, fatigue, and trouble sleeping, and from physical examination (certain sites on the body will be tender to the touch).

Many health professionals misunderstand this condition; they question whether the patient has a "real" disease and give patients with fibromyalgia a battery of blood tests, X-rays, and other tests to rule out a wide range of rheumatic disorders. But false-positive results may lead patients with fibromyalgia to be mislabeled as having lupus, Lyme disease, or gout; and the high-tech approach to diagnosis can, in itself, make patients afraid that their disease is serious. Alternatively, a physician experienced in musculoskeletal disease, such as a rheumatologist, can usually make an accurate diagnosis on the basis of an interview and examination.

An aerobic exercise program, perhaps supervised by a physical therapist, can be the most helpful therapy for fibromyalgia, although drug therapy can also be useful in some cases. Antidepressant drugs may improve sleep and help people become more resistant to pain, while aspirin and other anti-inflammatory drugs may offer effective pain relief.

to be quite valuable in recognizing and monitoring the severity of disease. Over the last decade, more and more rheumatologists have begun to use their patients' own reports, which include assessment of pain, functional impairment, and fatigue, in planning and monitoring their care.

We have used a questionnaire, derived from one developed by James Fries, Halsted Holman, and colleagues at Stanford University, to gather a wide variety of information about our patients. We ask them how much pain, morning stiffness, fatigue, and other physical problems they experience. We ask how difficult it is for them to perform ordinary daily activities, such as dressing, getting in and out of bed, and turning faucets on and off. And we ask them about psychological issues—for example, how satisfied they are with their physical capacity, how they feel about their health in general, and how much they feel in control of their lives.

Our patients' answers tell us more about the ups and downs of their disease in most cases than laboratory reports and X-rays do. The information from self-administered questionnaires is correlated significantly with these medical measures. But the questionnaire results are more predictive of the course of the illness, the likelihood that people will become so disabled that they cannot work outside the home, and even how likely they are to die earlier than expected.

What can this mean? First, it suggests that a person's sense of his or her own health can be accurate and predictive. In addition to reflecting overall health status, the self-report questionnaires also measure psychological factors that usually are not assessed in the traditional medical evaluation.

In rating the difficulty of daily activities, for example, patients not only report their ability to function, but also reflect their thoughts and feelings about it. And there is now good evidence that a person's self-rating of health may be associated with a good or poor course of arthritis—which, in turn, could affect the risk of earlier death.

It's also possible that feeling pessimistic or out of control of one's life could shorten survival, either by making patients less motivated to follow effective medical treatment or perhaps through a direct negative effect on the immune system. To some extent, psychological state reflects the severity of disease: The sicker someone is, the more pessimistic she or he is likely to feel. However, when individuals with similar degrees of illness are compared, patients with poor psychological status have poorer outcomes over long periods, among both those with mild arthritis and those with severe disease.

CAN EMOTIONAL PROBLEMS CAUSE ARTHRITIS?

Over the last ten years or so, our understanding of a link between psychological factors and arthritis has become more sophisticated and productive than in earlier years. But the notion of such a connection is hardly new.

Half a century ago, when physicians were unable to isolate an infectious agent or other direct cause for rheumatoid arthritis, some doctors became intrigued by the possibility that psychological factors might trigger it. The psychoanalyst Franz Alexander and his colleagues theorized that individuals who repress anger and are unable to express emotion were particularly likely to develop the disease. However, little evidence was found to support the existence of this or any other type of "rheumatoid personality."

Further research was directed to identify particular psychological problems in patients with arthritis. One series of studies used the Minnesota

Multiphasic Personality Inventory (MMPI), a questionnaire of 566 statements to which the subject is asked to respond "true" or "false." These studies indicated that patients with rheumatoid arthritis were more likely than the general population to answer questions in patterns suggesting hypochondriasis, depression, and hysteria.

A few years ago, however, a reanalysis of those studies questioned that conclusion. People with rheumatoid arthritis, it seemed, had been identified as having emotional problems on the MMPI because they answered "false" to statements like these: "I am about as able to work as I ever was," "I am in just as good physical health as most of my friends," "During the past few years, I have been well most of the time," "I do not tire quickly," and "I have few or no pains." For a person in good physical health to answer "false" to these questions may, in fact, suggest a psychological problem. But for a person with arthritis to do so is appropriate; it's an honest report of the effects of the illness.

The same phenomenon may explain why people with rheumatoid arthritis may have significantly higher than normal scores on other questionnaires used to identify depression. In the widely used Beck Depression Inventory, for example, patients are asked whether they agree or disagree with statements like "I can work about as well as before," "I don't get more tired than usual," and "I am no more worried about my health than usual." Their wholly appropriate responses to such statements may have led to an exaggerated estimate of depression in patients with rheumatoid arthritis, although some patients may be depressed as a direct result of the disease.

While these notions about the psychological roots of arthritis have provided only limited advances, other approaches may provide important new insights into the link between psychological status and the severity of rheumatoid arthritis. Recent research suggests that three psychological traits may have a significant impact on the course of disease: self-efficacy, learned helplessness, and sense of coherence. Although these traits may sound abstract, all have practical significance for the way a person deals with illness. Each may relate directly to the individual's ability to cope with life's challenges, including the challenge of a potentially serious disease like arthritis.

COPING STYLES AND THE COURSE OF ILLNESS

How does a healthy coping style improve the course of arthritis? Although the associations are clearly documented, the mechanisms are only beginning to be understood. One possibility, of course, is that poor coping ability may be a sign that the disease is severe and has overwhelmed the individual's resources. Nonetheless, as noted above, when two people appear to have the same degree of physical impairment, the one with the more effective coping style generally will experience less pain and less difficulty getting around. Furthermore, strong coping abilities appear to lead to lower levels of functional and work disability and even longer life expectancy.

SELF-EFFICACY

Self-efficacy, first described by psychologist Albert Bandura at Stanford University, refers to the belief that one can perform a specific action or complete a task. Self-efficacy is like confidence—but the confidence to do something specific, rather than a general sense of self-confidence that you can do all sorts of things. For example, your feelings of self-efficacy may be high in regard to your driving—you know you have the skills to get where you're going despite rain and snow—but poor when you're faced with organizing your desk.

This kind of confidence appears to have real importance in the course of arthritis. In 1978, researchers at Stanford University developed a self-help course for people with arthritis that is now available throughout the country (see "The Arthritis Self-Help Course"). This course has been shown to reduce pain and depression, improve the ability to function day-to-day, and cut down on doctor visits.

The course is designed to help people make positive changes in a number of areas, including nutrition, exercise, and pain control. But when the Stanford researchers analyzed their results after a decade of work, they found that patients did not benefit primarily because they had learned more about their disease or changed their behavior. Instead, the main factor in their improvement was an increased sense of self-efficacy. The course had led them to feel more confident that they could cope with arthritis, and that in itself enabled them to deal with the disease much more effectively.

LEARNED HELPLESSNESS

A very different psychological concept from self-efficacy is learned helplessness, a phenomenon first described by Martin Seligman and his colleagues at the University of Pennsylvania. In a series of experiments (described in detail in Chapter 21), animals were exposed to painful electric shocks that they

THE ARTHRITIS SELF-HELP COURSE

The Arthritis Self-Help Course shows how much confident, educated people with arthritis can do for themselves.

The course was developed in 1978 at Stanford University by Kate Lorig (a nurse and health educator), Halsted Holman and James Fries (professors of medicine), and their colleagues. As of 1991, 120,000 people had completed it. It is given to groups of up to 15 individuals with all kinds of chronic arthritis, usually by nonprofessional people who have arthritis themselves.

In six two-hour weekly sessions, participants are taught about the different kinds of arthritis. They learn how to design their own exercise program; how to manage pain with techniques like relaxation; how to improve their nutrition; and how to fight depression and fatigue. They learn ways to solve the problems posed by their disease and to communicate more effectively with their physicians.

The course works. On average, participants report their pain is reduced by 15 to 20 percent. Those who were depressed when they started the program are less so when they finish. They see the doctor less often—even four years after taking the course, medical visits in one group were down by 43 percent. Although they may still have physical difficulty with daily activities, graduates of the course lead more active lives, going out and spending time with friends more often.

Follow-up studies have identified some reasons behind the course's success. The studies have shown that participants do make some of the healthy behavior changes taught in the course; they exercise more, for example. But the factor most closely linked to improvements in pain, depression, and activity level is a positive adjustment in attitude. Graduates of the course have higher levels of *self-efficacy*—the confidence that they are able to deal with their disease. In one group of patients, self-efficacy, as measured by psychological tests, was still 17 percent higher four years after they took the course.

The Arthritis Self-Help Course is available throughout the United States and in Canada, Australia, and South Africa. In this country, the course is given through the Arthritis Foundation—at 792 locations in 1991—at an average cost of about $20. See Resources.)

were unable to escape. The animals learned to be passive; in later situations, when given shocks that they *could* easily avoid, they lay down and didn't even try to escape.

Some people with chronic illnesses seem to fall into a similar state of learned helplessness. Feeling helpless in the face of their disease, they often fail to do things that they could easily manage and that they know would be likely to benefit their health.

Researchers have applied this concept to arthritis with a 15-item questionnaire, the Arthritis Helplessness Index, which includes statements like "My condition is controlling my life" and, conversely, "I am coping effectively with my condition." Among people with rheumatoid arthritis, those who score high in learned helplessness have lower self-esteem, greater anxiety and depression, and greater day-to-day difficulties with their disease. One study showed that when the sense of helplessness went up from one year to the next, so did patients' difficulty in performing activities of daily living. It is not clear whether functional impairment led to greater learned helplessness or vice versa; causation probably occurs in both directions. But evidence suggests that helplessness can contribute to pain and functional disability in individual patients.

Further studies have indicated significant links between learned helplessness and physical and functional measures of the severity of arthritis, such as the number of damaged joints, measurements of grip strength, the speed at which a person can walk, and a "button test"—how quickly a patient can fasten and unfasten five buttons. Current research is being directed to determine whether learning self-efficacy, as in the self-help course described above, may be an antidote to learned helplessness.

SENSE OF COHERENCE

A person's attitude toward life, too, may have a significant impact on his or her ability to deal with arthritis. One way to gauge that attitude is by measuring the sense of coherence, a concept developed after World War II by Aaron Antonovsky, a medical sociologist. He was studying individuals who had survived the Holocaust, in an effort to understand why some people do much better than others in the face of severe adversity. People who score high on sense-of-coherence tests feel that their circumstances make sense and, what's more, that *life* makes sense: It has enough meaning to justify the effort and investment of energy that its problems demand.

An analysis of nearly 900 people with rheumatoid arthritis found that those with a high sense of coherence had less trouble with activities of daily living than those with lower scores, and were in better overall health. To such people, life's demands seem manageable—they think they have what it takes to cope with their problems. People with a strong sense of coherence can choose the most appropriate strategy to deal with the stress of a particular situation. For example, a secretary with rheumatoid arthritis who finds it difficult to sit for hours at a computer terminal might simply switch her chair for one with arms and place a wrist bar under her keyboard to cope with the demands of her disease and her work environment.

EDUCATIONAL LEVEL AND RHEUMATIC DISEASES

In recent years, our own research has turned up another intriguing association: Formal educational level is correlated with the course of rheumatic diseases in individual patients.

We first observed this link in a group of 75 patients with rheumatoid arthritis. When we analyzed their records, we found that disease progressed significantly more quickly, and the mortality rate was higher, in patients with less than 12 years of formal education. Further analyses of 385 patients with rheumatoid arthritis showed that clinical status—measured by laboratory tests, physical examination of their joints, and self-reports—was significantly worse in patients who had not finished high school than in those who had.

We then found the same thing in patients with four other rheumatic diseases: osteoarthritis, fibromyalgia, systemic lupus erythematosus, and scleroderma. In each case, as with rheumatoid arthritis, less education went along with greater feelings of learned helplessness and greater difficulty with day-to-day activities. In all five diseases, the level of formal education was a better identifier of pain, disability, and helplessness than either the patient's age or the length of time she or he had the disease.

Our findings were similar to other research, both in the United States and elsewhere, showing that people with relatively little formal education have higher rates of most chronic diseases and poorer health in general. In part, this reflects the effects on health of employment and income, which are correlated with education. Nevertheless, associations between education and health hold even when other key factors are taken into account.

Several studies, summarized by epidemiologist Leonard Sagan in *The Health of Nations*, have shown that well-educated people are healthier even when income differences are accounted for. A recent report from the National Center for Health Statistics, drawing on a survey of more than 100,000 people, underscores the point: At every income level, education shows a major independent relationship to health. A low level of education is associated with higher levels of many chronic conditions—including arthritis, heart disease, and lung disease—in many countries, including Great Britain, Sweden, Norway, Italy, and Switzerland.

Does education itself somehow help people cope with arthritis and even live longer? If so, sending patients back to school to get a diploma should be part of the standard prescription. But as valuable as education is, we think more schooling itself could provide only a small part of the answer.

There probably is no single reason why lower education is associated with poorer health, any more than why higher age is associated with poorer health. Multiple factors contribute to the associations. Researchers have found that well-educated people have better health habits—regarding nutrition, exercise, and smoking, for example—and also use medical services more effectively.

In our efforts to use our findings toward improving health, we have observed that a person's formal educational level reflects those psychological strengths or weaknesses that have been found to influence health in general and arthritis in particular. The ability to complete one's education in youth partly reflects a general capacity to cope with challenging situations.

Research has shown that people with little formal education on average are at risk for a higher-than-average level of anxiety, depression, learned helplessness, and life stress, and a lower sense of coherence, self-efficacy, and social support. These difficulties in coping may determine how one responds later in life to a disease like rheumatoid arthritis. The most effective efforts to improve the results of medical care might be directed toward improving coping skills in individual patients.

THE BEST APPROACH TO ARTHRITIS

Anyone with a serious arthritic disease needs excellent medical care, which includes health professionals, drugs, an exercise program, joint preservation, and general health measures. Drugs, which are often prescribed in combination with each other, should be viewed as an important component of a treatment program for rheumatoid arthritis and other inflammatory conditions.

Nonetheless, simply being a "good patient" and hoping drugs alone can cure you is not the most effective approach.

If you have arthritis, several kinds of health-care professionals can help you deal more effectively with day-to-day challenges. First, it's important to have a knowledgeable and sympathetic physician, often a rheumatologist who specializes in the care of people with arthritis. A physical therapist can design, and guide you through, tailor-made programs for exercises and preservation of joints. An occupational therapist can help you in performing day-to-day activities, including such practical chores as bathing and cooking, and can provide a wide range of special devices to help you dress, undress, turn faucets on and off, and eat on your own. And a social worker can help resolve the family problems that may develop when a member has a disabling disease, as well as help with vocational counseling if your ability to work is limited by arthritis.

Besides the very practical help these professionals offer, working with them can be a real boost to your feelings of self-efficacy. Even Olympic athletes need a coach to guide their training. Everyone—including people with arthritis—can feel stronger by working with an expert in a "coaching" relationship.

Again, medication is valuable in treating many people with rheumatic diseases. Just as an emphasis on drugs alone will lead to less than optimal results, a reluctance to use pain medication, out of stoicism or fear, may make things worse. There's no advantage to feeling pain. In fact, research at the University of California, San Francisco, suggests that chemicals released when you're in pain, including one called *substance P*, can actually worsen inflammation in rheumatoid arthritis.

The Arthritis Self-Help Course is an excellent way to learn more about your disease and about strategies for coping with it. This course is conducted through local chapters of the Arthritis Foundation, found in your local telephone directory. Arthritis puts your body under a special kind of stress, so health-enhancing practices, from good nutrition to relaxation techniques, can be especially important.

THE BOTTOM LINE

Any understanding of arthritis, and of individual patients with arthritis, has to go beyond blood tests, X-rays, and other standard medical procedures. An arthritis patient's difficulty with day-to-day activities and state of mind can help determine the course of the disease. Conversely, changing one's attitude toward the disease can make a difference in the results of drug therapy for treating it.

A key to dealing with arthritis is self-efficacy—the feeling of confidence that one *can* cope with the disease is therapeutic in and of itself. One self-help group approach, available nationally to people with arthritis, seems to work by enhancing self-efficacy. People who go through these groups experience less pain and have fewer doctor visits.

The ideal approach to arthritis treatment, for most people, involves a combination of a supportive physician and other health-care professionals, appropriate drugs to relieve pain and inflammation, and learning and practicing new coping strategies. Any one of these approaches by itself is likely to be incomplete and less than optimally effective. Together, however, they can do a great deal to fight rheumatic disease.

11

Asthma: Stress, Allergies, and the Genes

by David A. Mrazek, M.D.

When in mental anguish, fear, mourning or distress . . . his agitation affects his respiratory organs and he cannot exercise them at will. The weight of the accumulated gas residue within him keeps him from inhaling a sufficient volume of air. . . . The cure of such conditions . . . lies not in food recipes, neither in drugs alone, nor in regular medical advice . . . psychological methods are a greater help.

These words from the *Book of Asthma*—the first major treatise on the disease, written in 1190 by the physician Maimonides—speak to an ancient fascination with the link between asthma and the mind. In our own century, several theories have been developed to describe the link, with varying degrees of success.

In the 1930s, the emphasis was on the psychoanalytic idea that asthma was linked to specific psychological patterns. The prevailing hypothesis was that intense anxiety associated with separation from an important person or people—beginning with separation from the mother—was the central conflict behind asthmatic episodes. The theory implied that "asthmatogenic parents" were responsible for the symptoms of their offspring. But while intense, unexpected separations may well precipitate some attacks, this is not a universal or highly specific trigger for asthmatic episodes. Studies of patients have never

DAVID A. MRAZEK, M.D., is chairman of psychiatry and chief of psychiatry and behavioral sciences at Children's National Medical Center in Washington, D.C.

found evidence of an "asthmatic personality" or a consistent pattern of psychological conflict.

In the 1960s, working from an entirely different perspective, behavioral psychologists proposed that asthmatic children are conditioned. One aspect of this view was that the special attention associated with the attacks reinforced them. Some researchers demonstrated that the frequency of asthma attacks could be reduced by using behavior modification techniques, without addressing underlying emotional issues. Many of these behavioral studies were simplistic, however, and difficult to replicate.

The current view is that psychological factors have a far more complex role in asthma. Anxiety about separation may be a trigger for some people, but so may any number of other psychological conflicts and stresses. "Rewarding" children for being sick may have a limited effect on the frequency of illness, but it isn't a basic cause of the problem.

Perhaps most important, psychological stressors must be understood as just one factor in asthma, along with physiological vulnerability and exposure to allergens. No amount of psychological conflict, conditioning, or stressful upbringing will cause asthma in a person who is not genetically predisposed to it. But although stress and psychological factors are not the whole story, they are an important piece of the puzzle, both in the development of asthma and in the triggering of attacks.

THE NATURE OF ASTHMA

Asthma, also described as reactive airway disease, is a common disorder whose basic symptoms are episodic attacks of chest tightness and wheezing. Physiologically, it is caused by dramatic, repetitive, intermittent inflammation and constriction of the airways. Asthma frequently begins early in childhood, although many patients report their first symptoms as adults. In the United States, approximately 7 percent of children have been diagnosed with asthma, but the total number of children who have had episodic wheezing spells is roughly twice that.

Many children have sustained periods of remission, during which they are essentially asymptomatic. (In fact, many people who seem to develop asthma as adults may actually have had very early asthmatic symptoms in the first two years of life that were either undiagnosed or ignored.) As many as 80 to 90 percent of people with asthma require no ongoing medical treatment to manage their illness. They learn that their mild episodes of chest tightness and wheezing tend to go away by themselves or respond quickly when a bronchodilator is used. Many very mild asthmatics are simply able to ignore their symptoms without any treatment at all.

Asthmatic attacks can be triggered by many different factors, and it is actually quite unusual for asthma to be precipitated by only one kind of trigger. In the great majority of cases, a single, simple cause cannot fully explain the illness, its chronic symptoms, or its course.

Asthma has a strong genetic component. Children with one asthmatic parent have approximately a 20 percent chance of developing the disease, while those with two asthmatic parents have nearly a 50 percent risk. Studies comparing identical twins (who share all the same genes) with fraternal twins (who do not) reveal that heredity plays a sizable role in both the symptoms of asthma and the bronchial reactivity that underlies it. But genetic studies of families with a high incidence of asthma have failed to find any single responsible gene.

Recently, researchers have hypothesized that several separate genes, working through different physiological mechanisms, might interact to cause asthma. One gene might control the tendency of the airways to narrow and make breathing difficult; another could determine susceptibility to allergic reactions, often a trigger of asthma attacks; and a third gene could control the sensitivity of the autonomic nervous system, which is activated under stress.

Perhaps due in part to the complex genetics involved, asthma follows different patterns in different people. In some, the mechanism is primarily allergic. Symptoms are triggered by allergens like pollen or dust mites. Other asthmatic patients are completely free of allergic reactions, but find that their wheezing is primarily linked to infection. A cold or flu can lead to a prolonged illness that requires bronchodilator therapy. In other people, symptoms are triggered only by certain physiological changes, most commonly those that accompany strenuous exercise. And still other people with asthma are extremely sensitive to environmental irritants, such as cigarette smoke, that act directly on the airways. Finally, there are people whose symptoms are primarily triggered by intense emotional stress.

HOW STRESS CAN TRIGGER ASTHMA

Although the experience of stress is universal, different people react to it in different and quite specific ways. Identical stressors can cause a racing heart in one person, intense stomach pains in another, and a stutter in a third. The

ANATOMY OF AN ASTHMA ATTACK

Air enters the lungs through the *trachea*, which branches into the left and right main *bronchi*. (See the illustration on the next page.) Those passages, in turn, are subdivided into smaller and smaller bronchial tubes and bronchioles, which finally end in air sacs called *alveoli*. In the alveoli, inhaled oxygen enters the bloodstream and carbon dioxide is removed to be exhaled.

During an asthma attack (left side of the illustration), the muscles that line the airways tighten, constricting the route through which air goes in and out. The lining of the bronchial tubes swells and becomes inflamed, blocking the passage of air still further. The mucus that ordinarily lubricates the airways becomes thick and sticky and may actually plug them up. It becomes harder and harder to breathe out; air depleted of oxygen is trapped in the lungs, leaving no room for fresh air.

Any number of things can trigger an asthma attack: direct irritation of the lungs by cigarette smoke or smog; an allergic response to pollen or other substances; or nerve impulses generated by the stress response of the autonomic nervous system. However, you will only suffer from asthma if the cells that line your airways are hypersensitive to the trigger, and this problem seems to be hereditary.

"organ specificity" of the individual patient—the way he or she responds to stress—is most likely due to an inborn vulnerability, not to personality characteristics.

In a person genetically programmed to have a hyperreactive autonomic nervous system, stress and arousal can send a barrage of nerve impulses to the cells that line the airways. If that person also has the gene for hyperreactive airways, those impulses could trigger the bronchial constriction that leads to a sense of chest tightness and shortness of breath—an asthmatic attack. This may be the way in which negative emotions like anger and anxiety trigger attacks in susceptible people.

Less dramatically, a time of protracted emotional turmoil or depression may be associated with a worsening of the disease. A child whose parents are

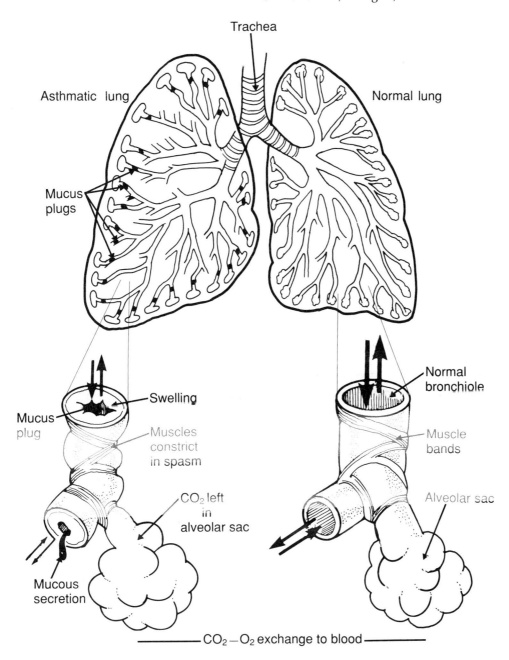

Trachea

Asthmatic lung

Normal lung

Mucus plugs

Swelling

Mucus plug

Muscles constrict in spasm

Normal bronchiole

Muscle bands

CO_2 left in alveolar sac

Alveolar sac

Mucous secretion

————— $CO_2 - O_2$ exchange to blood —————

in the middle of a bitter divorce may suffer more frequent and severe attacks. Late in life, an adult asthmatic who may have been in remission for ten years can develop symptoms again when her or his marriage falls apart. Extended emotional stress can destabilize respiratory functions that were previously un-der reasonably good control.

While it is possible to divide asthmatics into groups—those whose symptoms are primarily triggered by allergy on the one hand, and by emotion on the other—most people fall between these extremes. What's more, allergic and emotional factors can interact in asthma. In times of stress, a less severe allergic reaction may be enough to trigger an attack.

To complicate things still further, the airway constriction in asthma is subject to the process of conditioning: Asthmatics actually "learn" to react to substances to which they are sensitive. Asthmatics who are allergic to cats, for example, may feel their chest tighten as soon as they see a cat, even if the animal is too far away for any antigen to reach them. In a famous experiment a century ago, a researcher triggered attacks in asthmatics who were allergic to roses by presenting them with a paper rose! In such situations, it is easy to see the mind's effect on the body.

ASTHMA AND PSYCHOLOGICAL PREVENTION

Although the association between severe emotional stress and asthma attacks is now well established, my colleagues and I have been studying another component of asthma: the role of early stressors in the initial onset of the disease. The connection is proving to be a strong one—and one that could suggest effective strategies for preventing the disease.

Intense, early family stress is now one of five basic risk factors for the development of asthma that have been identified. The others are:

- Elevated blood levels of immunoglobulin E, the antibodies associated with allergy.
- Viral infections, particularly in the first or second year of life, that result in a wheezing illness.
- Exposure to highly allergenic substances, such as dust mites or animal dander.
- Genetic risk, reflected by the number of first- and second-degree relatives with the disease. If there is no genetic risk for asthma, the other four risk factors will have little effect.

In our own research, we have studied a group of 150 children who have a parent with asthma and therefore are at genetic risk for the disease. Using several complementary measures, we have consistently found that situations that disrupt the family and disturb children's earliest efforts to accommodate to disruptions in routine do increase the probability that asthma will develop.

First, we looked at the stresses that the families experienced—for example, the death of a close relative, an unexpected job loss or move, or trouble with the law. When such stressors occurred at a greater than average rate in the year before a child was born, the child was significantly more likely to develop wheezing at two years of age. Those families that experienced high stress before a child's birth tended to have roughly the same level of stress during the first months of the child's life. And a turbulent home life during this time may well have affected some of the children's early ability to regulate emotions.

We also analyzed in a more thorough way how parents responded to these stressors. When the children were three weeks old, researchers visited the home to observe the mother and child together. The mothers were interviewed to learn about their difficulties in caring for their babies, their general ability to cope with the stresses of their lives (such as juggling work and family demands), and the strength and turmoil of their marriages.

Here, too, there was a significant association. When the children were two years old, 21 of the entire group—14 percent—had developed asthma (This information was based primarily on the mother's report, but with some corroboration from the child's medical record.) The 52 children whose mothers had parenting problems had triple the risk of asthma: 25 percent, compared to only 8 percent for the others. Among the 67 children whose mothers were finding it hard to cope with life in general, 13 (19 percent) developed asthma, compared with 8 (10 percent) of those whose mothers were coping well. In the group whose mothers had no difficulty in either coping or parenting—nearly half the sample—only 3 children (4 percent) developed asthma, despite their genetic predisposition.

What's the explanation? The first few years of life may be a window of vulnerability, a critical time in determining whether asthma develops. If children who are genetically predisposed to asthma are exposed to viral respiratory diseases at this time, this may sensitize their airways; similarly, exposure to a high level of allergens like animal dander or certain foods may turn the predisposition to asthma into reality. Exposure to early emotional stressors may work in the same way.

A family history of asthma may stem partly from a genetic tendency toward a hyperreactive autonomic nervous system. If the family situation is stressful—and if, for example, the baby is allowed to experience prolonged periods of acute distress—this chronic arousal could lead to a pattern of physiological overreaction, which could stimulate asthmatic symptoms.

In contrast, attentive parenting can help a baby learn to regulate even a highly reactive autonomic nervous system. Parents who are sensitive and responsive to their babies' needs—who feed their children promptly when they are hungry and make sure they can rest when they are tired—will keep periods of intense distress to a minimum and diminish the arousal that could lead to airway hyperreactivity. In time, the babies learn to regulate themselves.

Can preventive measures protect babies at risk for asthma from developing the disease? On theoretical grounds, some advice makes obvious sense. Parents of children at risk should minimize their chances of catching flu, colds, and other viral infections by avoiding exposure to sick children—if possible, choosing a day-care arrangement that makes this easier. They shouldn't expose their children to environmental irritants like cigarette smoke. And they should avoid early exposure to common allergens, such as cat dander, and foods like dairy products and eggs that are especially likely to trigger food allergies. (Breast feeding provides one method to minimize exposure to food allergens early in life.)

In addition, parents can help prevent asthma by being sensitive to their infants' needs for emotional stability. The goal should be to help a baby to avoid experiencing intense, prolonged emotional distress. Parents can also try to minimize unexpected separations and the consequent emotional stress to babies, especially during the first two years of life.

A research project is now under way to test whether specific family interventions are effective in preventing asthma. We have taken families with newborn babies in which a parent has a history of asthma and randomly assigned them to four equal groups. Families in one group are regularly visited by a layperson trained to help the mother solve early parenting problems, resolve family conflicts, and cope with stressors such as returning to her job and finding adequate child care. Another group of families is given dietary advice for feeding their new baby, designed to minimize exposure to highly allergenic foods such as milk, eggs, and peanuts. A third group gets both the diet and home visits, while the fourth—a comparison group—gets only an educational session about risk factors for the development of asthma. In time, this research should provide evidence on which of these interventions—all of which should be effective in theory—actually work in practice.

AFTER ASTHMA DEVELOPS: SORTING OUT THE MIND'S ROLE

Although the effect of stress on asthma is real, it can be difficult to sort out in practice. Many people are convinced that they, or their asthmatic children, experience attacks when they're under stress. They often can point to a number of incidents that they believe prove the point. But sorting out the role that stress plays in any one person's asthma can be very difficult.

A classic example of that difficulty comes from the case of a 19th-century British physician who had been afflicted with the illness for most of his life and had made it the focus of his studies. Although his symptoms had always been relatively mild, he suffered a severe attack on a day when he was reviewing the financial accounts of his estate in his stables with his steward. As he read over the ledgers, he became convinced that his steward had been systematically defrauding him. He erupted in a fit of anger, which led to the worst asthmatic episode he had ever experienced.

From the physician's account of the episode, he was convinced that the steward's betrayal had triggered his attack. But the vignette is open to another interpretation. The physician's violent reaction probably stirred up a considerable amount of dust and hay—highly allergenic substances that could well have contributed to his severe attack.

In many ways, asthma is similar to headache—another physical problem with multiple causes. With the exception of severe migraines, headaches caused by tumors, and a few other conditions, headaches are usually self-limited and benign. As people with mild headaches learn to adapt to their headaches, they are likely to develop a personal, unscientific explanation for the origin of the headaches. One person may believe that her headaches are the result of stress and try to control them through relaxation, while another may decide that his headaches stem from a special sensitivity and will avoid a particular food substance or additive. If the headaches subside when the suspected trigger is avoided, that will be taken as proof of a connection—even though it may be only a coincidence—and soon the belief becomes fixed.

The situation with asthma is very similar. If a family notices that a child develops wheezing when they visit the grandmother, for example, the way they explain their child's symptoms is likely to depend on their view of the world. If they focus on the fact that the grandmother has a cat, they may interpret the child's wheezing as a "cat allergy" and begin to keep the child away from cats. When the symptoms then disappear—as they generally will on their own or after use of a bronchodilator—they will take this to be evidence that their diagnosis is confirmed. But the identical series of events can be interpreted in a totally different way by parents who believe in a psychological explanation: They may conclude that family conflict at the time of the visit was responsible for the attacks. In fact, it may well be that both family stresses *and* the presence of a cat triggered the child's symptoms.

DO ASTHMATICS HAVE MORE EMOTIONAL PROBLEMS?

People with chronic asthma have been reported to have more emotional problems than physically healthy individuals. However, the studies that support such a relationship have generally been flawed. For one thing, physical symptoms of asthma are easily confused with manifestations of psychological problems—anxiety, for example, can be caused by the sensation of shortness of breath. Careful studies have shown that adult asthmatics with mild or self-limited symptoms have neither more nor fewer emotional problems than the general population.

Among children with very severe asthma, however, psychological disturbance tends to be more common. For these children, the evidence suggests that the psychological problems are more likely to occur as a result of the illness, rather than having been involved in the onset of the asthma. The psychological risk is greatest when asthma begins early, is severe and persistent, restricts activity in school and sports, and requires regular steroid treatment and repeated hospitalizations. In one study of 75 severely asthmatic preschool children—all of whom had been hospitalized repeatedly—59 percent were experiencing emotional and behavioral problems, which was three times as many as in a comparison sample of children matched for age and sex who had no chronic physical illness.

Perhaps the most balanced view is that the link between asthma and psychological problems is a two-way street. Having any chronic illness is stressful—whether it is asthma, arthritis, or diabetes—and symptoms associated with the disease can increase the risk of emotional problems like depression. Conversely, being depressed can make the symptoms of asthma worse.

The process of conditioning can contribute to the problem. Once an emotional stressor, such as fighting with your spouse, becomes linked in your mind to the onset of symptoms, you may begin to wheeze more readily whenever that kind of conflict arises.

PSYCHOLOGICAL TREATMENT FOR ASTHMA

Given the link between emotions and asthma, it's not surprising that a number of psychological and psychiatric approaches can lessen the severity of asthma attacks, as well as improve the emotional symptoms that go with them.

A variety of relaxation techniques have been used as part of comprehensive treatment programs for asthma. Relaxation can help many asthmatics, both by helping to moderate the emotional response to stressful events that can trigger asthma attacks and by counteracting stress-related physiological changes that can constrict the airways.

Hypnotherapy has also been used with some success to reduce the frequency and severity of attacks. One strategy uses posthypnotic suggestion to reduce the body's response to asthmatic triggers. For patients who tend to have attacks at night, the suggestion might be made that they will have deep, restful sleep, with the capacity to move air easily in and out of their lungs, and will awaken rested and happy. Even an acute attack can be reversed in a person who can readily go under hypnosis.

Psychotherapy is often a productive approach for asthmatics. As people begin to deal with their emotional problems, their asthmatic symptoms often improve. For example, asthmatics who have been chronically depressed can come to feel better about themselves through therapy and may then find that they do not need as much asthma medication, even if the therapy has never dealt with their disease directly.

Although the improvement in symptoms may not be rapid, the lasting impact of long-term psychotherapy has now been well illustrated by the studies of Peter Knapp, at Boston University, and his colleagues. Psychodynamic, behavioral, and cognitive therapy (see Chapters 21 and 22) have all been reported to be helpful.

Psychiatric drugs can have beneficial effects on the disease as well. Tricyclic antidepressants, in particular, can not only relieve symptoms of depression but also improve respiratory function, perhaps an unintended side effect.

Group therapy is often quite helpful for asthmatics. It seems to work particularly well with children who have a relatively severe form of the disease. Not only are illness-related issues addressed, but children with the same illness can be particularly effective in providing vital support and encouragement. A child who feels sorry for her- or himself and constantly laments "I can't do it because I'm asthmatic" can develop a new set of expectations by sitting in a group with other asthmatics who are more active and optimistic.

There is also a long tradition of using family therapy for young asthmatics, based on the rationale that the family can be a major source of stress or a powerful force for emotional regulation. Even though there is no good evidence that an "asthmatogenic family" can single-handedly create asthma in its offspring, family factors often play a role and various family therapy approaches have been shown to be helpful.

Research on fatal asthmatic episodes has shown particularly dramatically how crucial the psychological aspects of asthma can be. Between 1 and 2 percent of severely asthmatic patients ultimately die of their disease. A study of severely asthmatic children has shown that chronic family conflict and overt symptoms of depression, particularly when triggered by recent separation and loss, are associated with an increased risk of a fatal episode in these vulnerable children. Young adolescent patients appear to be particularly vulnerable, perhaps because their respiratory control may already be destabilized by the hormonal changes of puberty. In these cases, psychological intervention can literally be lifesaving.

THE BOTTOM LINE

Asthma has a strong genetic component: Psychological factors alone are not sufficient to cause the disease. But in some people who have inherited a tendency for hyperreactive airways, stress and emotional factors may precipitate asthma attacks or make them more severe. Attacks may worsen in general during times of emotional turmoil or depression. Episodes of intense emotion, like a fit of anger, can trigger an attack. And in some people with a conditioned response, simply thinking that they have been exposed to something they are allergic to—for example, a cat—can bring on a bout of wheezing.

Family stressors also play a role. Recent research has shown that intense family stress in the first two years of life increases a young child's chance of developing the disease, if she or he has a genetic predisposition to it. Family conflicts have also been linked to the risk of fatal asthma attacks in adolescents and can trigger nonfatal attacks in many children and adults with the disease.

Hypnotherapy can help lessen asthma attacks through posthypnotic suggestion, and basic relaxation techniques may be effective for some people with asthma. Psychotherapy is often helpful as well, both in defusing the emotional factors that can trigger asthma attacks and in helping people deal with the emotional consequences of the disease.

12

INFERTILITY, PREGNANCY, AND THE EMOTIONS

BY MACHELLE M. SEIBEL, M.D., AND
JAMES A. MCCARTHY, M.D.

CONCEPTION, PREGNANCY, AND CHILDBIRTH ARE AMONG THE MOST deeply meaningful parts of our lives and arouse the strongest of feelings. So it is not surprising that these areas, so highly charged with emotion, are themselves sensitive to the effects of stress.

The link between emotions and fertility has been appreciated since biblical times. Consider the story of Hannah, from the first chapter of the first book of Samuel.

A man named Elkanah had two wives. Peninah, who had many children, and Hannah, who was ridiculed by Peninah for her inability to conceive. Eventually, Hannah became so distressed she would not eat. She prayed and wept bitterly; her lips moved, but she was unable to utter a sound.

A priest saw her in this state and accused her of drunkenness. But when Hannah explained the reason for her sorrow, the priest said to her, "Go in peace. May the God of Israel grant your petition." Comforted and calmed, Hannah returned home, began to eat, and shortly thereafter conceived a son, Samuel.

Unfortunately, infertility is rarely so simple, either in its cause or in its cure. Stress alone cannot cause infertility. But it can contribute to the problem and may also affect the course of pregnancy, the health of the fetus, and the process of childbirth itself.

MACHELLE M. SEIBEL, M.D., is director of the Faulkner Centre for Reproductive Medicine in Boston, where JAMES A. MCCARTHY, M.D., is a reproductive endocrinologist on staff.

HOW CAN EMOTIONS AFFECT FERTILITY?

Infertility affects some 10 million American couples of childbearing age. What is lost is something that has never been, and therefore the deep impact of infertility often goes unnoticed by other people. Alone in their grief, infertile couples have been described as a neglected, silent minority.

Ironically, some early attempts to study the link between emotions and infertility may only have made life worse for infertile people, particularly women. One theory held that infertility in women often reflected a hidden psychological conflict. Many infertile women lacked femininity, the theory said; deep down, they didn't want to be mothers, and their bodies were acting out their wishes. But this pessimistic theory was never based on good evidence, and experts in infertility have now abandoned it.

Moreover, we have come to understand that infertility is not a "woman's problem" to begin with, but a personal and family crisis shared by a couple, both of whom may require treatment and need emotional support. Rather than holding a simplistic view of an "infertile personality," we increasingly appreciate how the psychological and physiological interact.

Scientists have only recently pieced together the links between stress and fertility problems. The normal reproductive cycle depends on a carefully timed sequence of events, orchestrated by hormones released by the brain and pituitary gland. Stress can disrupt the sequence. In addition, nerve fibers connect the brain and reproductive organs directly, providing another avenue by which emotional stress may disrupt normal function in both women and men (see "How Stress Can Affect Conception").

Although stress can clearly affect reproductive physiology, there is little evidence that stress alone can cause lasting infertility. In fact, women have conceived under the most stressful conditions imaginable—during wartime and even in concentration camps.

Statistics have also disproved a persistent myth about stress and infertility: the belief that women who have tried in vain to conceive are more likely to become pregnant after they have adopted children, presumably because they are no longer so tense about being childless. Over the past 20 years, repeated studies have found this is simply not so. The frequency of conception among adoptive parents is exactly the same as it is among parents who do not adopt.

While stress is probably not a primary cause of infertility, it is a factor that can *reduce* fertility. In the presence of other problems—such as a dysfunction in the fallopian tubes—the additional burden of stress may be enough to shift the balance to infertility.

WHEN INFERTILITY BECOMES A CRISIS

Because infertility itself often causes enormous stress, a vicious circle can easily occur: The stress of dealing with infertility may worsen the physiological problem.

Infertile couples lament that they have lost a sense of control over their bodies and their destinies, that their sense of order in the world has been disturbed. Many women describe infertility and the sustained effort to overcome it as the worst experience of their lives. Their attempts to have children interfere with all other long-term goals. For example, ongoing doctor's appointments and medical procedures can mean significant time away from work, making it difficult to focus on a career.

Some women feel less than feminine if they are unable to bear children. Others worry that they are disappointing their partners or their families. Many feel a profound sadness. They may avoid seeing pregnant friends and family members and may even fight back tears when they see a pregnant woman in the supermarket.

Less is known about the effect of infertility on men. But many men, like women, may feel guilty or responsible for denying their partners the opportunity to have a child. Men are expected to be stable and calm and to provide support for their partners, but they often find it hard to accept support themselves. When a man is being treated for infertility, he must often cope alone with painful, stressful, and disruptive treatments, as well as with his partner's feelings.

For the couple, infertility can create a major crisis, particularly when the pain is not evenly distributed on both sides. A man who has three children by a previous marriage may be less eager than his wife to have children. If the wife has already had children and her husband is the last living bearer of his family name, he alone may view infertility with anxiety. Other factors can compound the turmoil: A woman who had an abortion years earlier or a man who impregnated another woman before he met his wife may see infertility as a punishment.

Under the stress of infertility, a relationship can crumble. The couple no

HOW STRESS CAN AFFECT CONCEPTION

Two organs that play a major role in the release of stress hormones—the pituitary gland and the hypothalamus, the tiny "control center" at the base of the brain—orchestrate the reproductive hormones as well.

The hypothalamus (see the illustration on the next page) releases periodic chemical signals that stimulate the pituitary to produce and release *luteinizing hormone* (LH) and *follicle-stimulating hormone* (FSH). FSH stimulates the ovum and the sac of fluid surrounding it—the follicle—to grow to maturity. When the follicle is large and mature enough, the level of the hormone LH rises rapidly, triggering ovulation: the release of the ovum into the fallopian tube.

But when hormones are produced in response to stress, the sequence goes awry. A variety of stress hormones can disrupt the orderly release of signals from the hypothalamus. The pituitary's secretion of LH and FSH is impaired. And as a result, menses may become irregular or ovulation may be suppressed altogether.

Nerve fibers traveling through the spinal cord also link the brain directly to the ovaries, uterus, and fallopian tubes. Through these connections, too, emotional stress may interfere with conception—for example, by disrupting ovulation or the activity of the fallopian tubes—or may have an adverse effect on pregnancy. Because of similar links between the brain and reproductive organs, in some men stress can reduce sex drive and cause impotence. Less commonly, it can lead to retrograde and sham ejaculation—the sperm is ejaculated backward into the bladder or is not discharged at all—perhaps by changing muscle tone along the male reproductive tract. There is also good evidence from animal studies that severe psychological stress can cause abnormal sperm development, which may impair fertility.

longer views intercourse as an expression of affection: Instead of making love, they work at making babies. The widespread use of home ovulation detection kits has, if anything, made things worse. Couples purchase these kits to gain control over their cycles, but then they feel required to respond sexually when an indicator changes color. It is not surprising that many infertile cou-

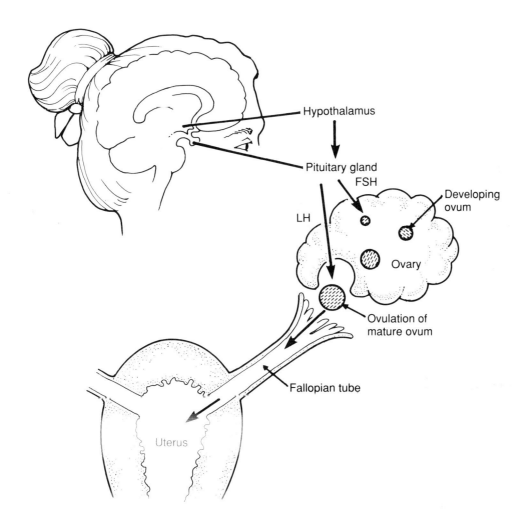

ples suffer some kind of sexual dysfunction. One major way in which stress interferes with fertility, in fact, may be by lowering the frequency of intercourse.

Although many patients who are treated for infertility do become pregnant, a substantial number must eventually recognize that they will never be biological parents. But this process has been greatly complicated by modern medicine. Virtually every year, there is a new treatment that makes it more and more difficult for couples to give up their struggle for parenthood. En route to accepting the inevitable, they must come to terms with a very real sense of loss, passing through the stages of surprise, denial, anger, isolation, guilt, and grief.

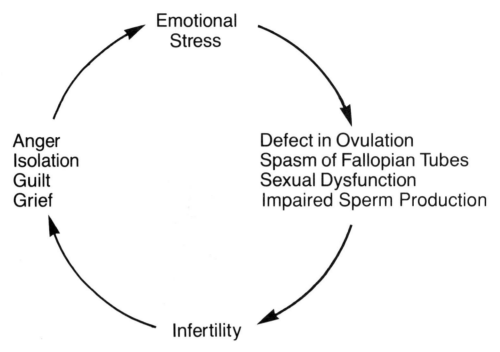

STRESS AND INFERTILITY: A VICIOUS CIRCLE
*Emotional stress can contribute to physiological problems that cause infertility—
and that, in turn, worsens the stress.*

CAN STRESS REDUCTION HELP?

If infertile couples experience such turmoil, will stress reduction help them to
conceive? Research on that question is still in its early stages. In one study,
we and our colleagues enrolled 54 women in a behavioral treatment program.
In ten weekly meetings, they were taught to elicit the relaxation response—a
technique known to reduce stress and tension (see Chapter 14)—and asked
to practice at home for at least 20 minutes, twice a day. By the end of the
program, they were significantly less anxious, depressed, and fatigued than
before.

In addition, 34 percent of these women became pregnant within six
months of completing the program. Women who had been infertile for a relatively short time (2.5 years on average) had a significantly higher rate of
conception than those who were infertile for longer (an average of 3.5 years).
This pattern is often seen with other infertility treatments as well.

Encouraging as these results sound, we can't say with assurance that the technique itself actually increased pregnancy rates because the study lacked a control group—a comparison group of similar women who were not taught relaxation. What's more, we found no correlation between psychological test results and conception: Whether women were especially anxious before the program or much less anxious afterward seemed to have no effect on how likely they were to conceive.

What we can say is this: The conception rate within the group—34 percent in six months—was higher than is typical among women under treatment for infertility, and the stress reduction technique may have been partially responsible. In any case, relaxation training clearly contributed something quite valuable in its own right: a significant improvement in emotional well-being and thus in quality of life. Considering the distress that accompanies infertility and its treatment, such a benefit is not to be taken lightly.

If our relaxation response program helped couples to conceive, it may have been by breaking the vicious circle of stress and infertility, each intensifying the other, that can make conception ever more difficult. If so, other stress reduction methods might work equally well: yoga, meditation, counseling, psychotherapy, perhaps even prayer (as in the story of Hannah).

A good working relationship with a physician can itself reduce stress. Ideally, the physician will offer empathy and compassion along with state-of-the-art medical treatment. Presenting treatment options fairly and evenly, a good infertility specialist will encourage both partners to share the responsibility of decision making. The physician should define infertility as a couple's problem, not just one partner's, and avoid weighted terms, such as *hostile mucus* or *habitual aborter*, that tend to evoke feelings of blame and guilt. He or she should also give the couple a realistic time frame in which treatments are likely to work, to help restore a sense of control.

If you are being treated for infertility, don't be surprised if your physician recommends that you see a mental health professional. All patients treated at our center are encouraged to have counseling, where they learn at least the basics of stress control. And counseling is required for all our patients receiving in vitro fertilization or other assisted reproduction techniques.

Often it seems that the people who least want to see a psychiatrist, psychologist, or social worker are those who have the most to gain. Having lost control of a bodily function so important to them—reproduction—they are afraid of an intrusion on their minds as well. But stress control and counseling can help individuals and couples gain control of their minds, their bodies, and their lives.

In particular, we encourage patients to join support groups of others who have similar problems or groups of people who are all going through the same procedure, such as in vitro fertilization. Sharing information and venting fears in a friendly, supportive atmosphere can reduce the stress of facing the un-known. In addition, sharing practical information on different treatments and physicians can help group members find the approaches that will be most effective for them.

Whatever the reason, a support group may increase a couple's chances of conceiving, according to a recent study at the University of Massachusetts. Of infertile couples who participated in support groups, 30 of 42, or 71 percent, achieved pregnancy, compared to 12 of 48 couples (25 percent) who did not participate. As with stress reduction techniques, there is a strong suggestion that support groups are beneficial.

STRESS DURING PREGNANCY

Once a woman becomes pregnant, her life and her body are intricately inter-woven with the life of her developing baby. It's not surprising, then, that a number of investigators have found a relationship between the psychological stress an expectant mother experiences and the health of her fetus.

Many studies have examined the link between stress during pregnancy and prematurity and low birth weight, which can cause serious problems in the newborn. Pregnant women under significant psychological stress gain less weight than would be expected for the number of calories they consume, perhaps because stress is affecting their metabolism. Studies have also shown that severe stress during pregnancy leads to lower birth weight in the infant.

Scandinavian studies have suggested that stress during pregnancy may have long-term effects. Using the Finnish population register between 1925 and 1957, researchers located people whose fathers had died before they were born—presumably a terribly stressful situation for their mothers. These peo-ple were significantly more likely to develop alcoholism, personality disor-ders, and schizophrenia—and more likely to commit crimes—than people whose fathers had died shortly *after* they were born. These unfortunate out-comes were particularly likely when the father's death occurred during months three to five, or months nine or ten, of the pregnancy.

A Swedish study followed infants born to women who were denied legal abortions in 1960 and compared them with other children born in the same wards. The women who had been forced to continue pregnancies they did not want bore significantly more infants with birth defects (1.8 percent, compared to 1.1 percent in the control group). Among women 25 years of age and older, the difference was striking: 3 percent, compared to 0.6 percent for the control group. However, it is unclear whether the increased birth defects were due to the stress of the unwanted pregnancy itself or to behavior linked to the stress, such as a poor diet, smoking, or drug or alcohol abuse.

While it is difficult to separate the effects of stress itself from related factors like these, experimental evidence suggests that the chemical changes caused by stress could have an impact on the fetus during pregnancy. In one study, the offspring of rats exposed to mild stress throughout pregnancy had abnormal levels of a chemical that regulates brain activity and showed persistent behavioral abnormalities after birth. In another study, stress reduced levels of the sex hormone testosterone in pregnant rats, a change that could affect the development of male offspring and alter their future ability to reproduce. And a study of pregnant women in especially stressful medical jobs showed that they had higher levels of stress hormones than women in less taxing positions—although the study was too small to show whether they also had a higher rate of complications.

Although these studies give reason for caution, they don't mean that pregnant women should cloister themselves for nine months and try to avoid any difficulties or challenges. In an area of great concern to modern women—the stress of working during pregnancy—the data are mixed. Although some groups of working women may be at increased risk, a demanding job in and of itself does not necessarily pose a threat to either mother or infant.

Some studies have found a clear link between job stress and difficulties of pregnancy. In one, a group of pregnant enlisted women on active duty in the military was compared with a control group, the nonworking wives of active-duty personnel. The enlisted women were more likely than the control group to develop high blood pressure during pregnancy and to deliver low-birthweight babies.

In contrast, however, a major national study reported in the *New England Journal of Medicine* found relatively little risk of work stress during pregnancy among nearly 1,000 highly stressed female physicians, compared to women with less demanding jobs. The physicians did have twice the rate of premature labor, which may require bed rest or hospitalization. But they had no more preterm deliveries, miscarriages, or stillbirths than the less-stressed women.

Not just what a woman does, but how she feels about it, seems to be critical. One study found that pregnant women who did not want to continue working reported more job-related stress than those who wanted to work, and had a significantly greater risk of preterm and low-birth-weight deliveries. (Interestingly, the same study found no increased risk in women subject to such stresses as poverty, traumatic life events, and psychiatric problems.) It appears that a feeling of helplessness—being trapped in a stressful situation—can have a more adverse effect than the stress of the situation itself. A woman who's working hard but likes what she's doing should have relatively little reason to worry about the effect on her pregnancy.

Despite the uncertainties, the research thus far provides a convincing argument for pregnant women to protect themselves against stress, with counseling, relaxation techniques, support groups, or the like. Studies have shown that such support reduces both the stress to the mother and the chance of having a low-birth-weight baby.

Psychological and social support can be especially important for women who are hospitalized for a week or more during their pregnancy (for premature labor, for example); they often suffer from heightened anxiety and find it difficult to follow medical instructions. The helplessness of being stuck in a hospital seems to add to the stress of dealing with obstetrical complications. Women who are poor, unemployed, young, poorly educated, unmarried, or have children at home have the most difficulty.

LABOR AND DELIVERY

Labor and delivery represent a short period of time compared to the rest of pregnancy, but it is a particularly important time, during which the baby must make its transition from life within the mother to an independent life outside. Uterine contractions during labor and delivery reduce blood flow to the fetus, and anything that reduces it further at this time is particularly worrisome.

Laboratory experiments have consistently shown that psychological stress can lead to increased uterine muscle activity, the potentially hazardous pattern that occurs during preterm labor. Lamaze training, on the other hand, appears to have a beneficial effect. One group of investigators found that women trained in Lamaze had significantly lower blood levels of beta-endorphin, a hormone released during stress, and progressed through labor more rapidly. The researchers suggested that this was due to a reduction of the fear, tension, and emotional stress associated with labor. Other studies have found that the presence of a companion shortens and eases labor (see "The Benefits of a *Doula*" at the end of this chapter).

Fetal monitoring has become an important technological support for modern obstetricians. But the use of an internal fetal monitor during or near the time of labor has been linked to a 50 percent increase in growth hormone, insulin, cortisol, adrenaline, and noradrenaline. Although this outpouring of stress-released chemicals has not been shown to affect the outcome of pregnancy adversely, it clearly indicates how stressful the procedure can be.

These physiological changes suggest that the possible adverse effects of fetal monitoring on labor and delivery should not be ignored. When monitoring is clearly indicated to make sure the baby is not in danger—during prolonged labor, for example—its benefits outweigh the risk posed by the stress of the procedure. But perhaps the routine use of fetal monitoring should be reconsidered, and the stress factor should be taken into account in deciding whether it is worthwhile.

THE POSTPARTUM PERIOD

With the birth of her baby, when pregnancy ends and parenting begins, a new mother typically experiences great shifts in mood. Some researchers feel that the common experience of postpartum blues may reflect a sudden fall in the brain opioids, the enkephalins and endorphins—mood-elevating chemicals maintained at high levels during pregnancy, labor, and delivery. But despite enormous hormonal changes, the overwhelming majority of women cope well during this transition period.

Others don't, and some suffer depressions that may be quite severe. Postpartum problems seem to be more common among women who have had emotional difficulties in the past, including severe premenstrual tension or emotional turmoil early in the pregnancy itself. A woman who is unusually anxious, preoccupied, or cautious in her first trimester may need additional emotional support all through the pregnancy. The obstetrician can help by scheduling more frequent prenatal visits for reassurance and by giving the woman the opportunity to ventilate her feelings; friends and family can help by being encouraging and sympathetic.

Such social support during pregnancy apparently pays off in the postpartum period. Emotional support in the months before the baby comes has been shown to help adolescent parents bond with the new infant. It has also proven to be of great value in helping men of all ages make the transition to fatherhood. In extremely stressful situations—if the newborn is critically ill or a previous child was stillborn, for example—an organized support program can help the family maintain stability during the first months of parenthood.

Postpartum stress can also arise from conflicting expectations of parenting. Anxiety escalates, for example, if the new mother expects the new father to take a more active role than he has in mind. If counseling *before* delivery can identify and address such potential conflicts, it may help reduce emotional distress during this period of adjustment and transition.

THE BOTTOM LINE

The desire to have children has profound emotional meaning and may involve deep emotional conflicts. In particular, the inability to conceive can create enormous stress, which may in turn worsen the problem of infertility. Stress reduction, including support groups, can help to break the cycle.

During pregnancy, prolonged emotional stress on the mother can affect her fetus—though the simple stress of working at a demanding job is not necessarily hazardous. In the critical period of labor and delivery, supportive measures that reduce stress, including the presence of a labor coach or companion, may ease the process and minimize the risk of complications.

The evidence that stress can have a negative effect on fertility, pregnancy, and childbirth is still not definitive. But in our opinion, emotional support and stress reduction should be incorporated into obstetric care from the time of conception through the first months of parenthood. In addition to the potential health benefits for mother and baby, such support can clearly enhance the new family's quality of life.

THE BENEFITS OF A *DOULA*

In most traditional cultures, women have been guided through labor and delivery by a *doula*—a female companion who has given birth herself. (The word comes from the Greek.) Now the benefits of this age-old approach have been confirmed in recent research by pediatricians John Kennell of Case Western Reserve University and Marshall Klaus of Children's Hospital in Oakland, California. Two studies in Guatemala and one in the United States found that women assisted by a doula—who offered encouragement, soothing physical contact, and emotional nurturance—needed significantly fewer cesarean sections and generally had an easier labor than women in a control group.

In a study of women at a Houston hospital, for example, 8 percent of those supported by the doula had cesarean sections, compared to 13 percent of women who were merely monitored by an uninvolved observer and 18 percent of the control group, who had no support during labor at all. Fewer of the women supported by doulas required epidural anesthesia (8 percent, compared to 23 percent in the observed group and 55 percent of controls). They had shorter labors and fewer forceps deliveries, and their newborns had fewer medical problems.

It seems likely that these benefits reflect a reduction of psychological stress during labor and delivery. If so, the doula is essentially another means to promote relaxation. Her supportive presence gives the woman in labor a focus for her attention, diverting her thoughts from contractions and pain, and helping her keep her breathing slow and steady. The research makes it clear that a supportive partner can make a great difference during labor. Lamaze classes may offer the same benefit, with the "labor coach"—often the woman's husband—representing a broader version of the doula concept.

13

SOMATIZATION: WHEN PHYSICAL SYMPTOMS HAVE NO MEDICAL CAUSE

BY NICHOLAS A. CUMMINGS, PH.D.

EVER SINCE HER ESTRANGED HUSBAND'S SUICIDE, LENORE, A 54-YEAR-OLD registered nurse, had experienced such intractable headaches that she was forced to go on disability. The pain was so excruciating that Lenore could fall asleep only when she was completely exhausted. Even then, the pain would usually awaken her after only 15 minutes. In a desperate search for relief, Lenore sought medical help every day—sometimes twice a day. Her medical bills, paid by her former employer's health plan, came to more than $75,000 a year.

Because a chronic headache could indicate any of a wide range of diseases, each of the doctors Lenore visited was compelled to subject her to a long list of laboratory tests and medical procedures. When nothing showed up and the physician became exasperated with her, Lenore would find another one and begin the long exploration again. Three different pain clinics tried to treat Lenore, giving her various medications to no avail.

Lenore could find no relief no matter how many doctors she visited because the cause of her illness was not physical. Patients like Lenore are known to mental health professionals as *somatizers*, people whose medical problems are actually a physical manifestation of emotional conflicts that remain unconscious. Like energy in physics, the stress caused by these conflicts

NICHOLAS A. CUMMINGS, PH.D., is president of the Foundation for Behavioral Health and of the National Academies of Practice, a former president of the American Psychological Association, and chairman and C.E.O. emeritus of American Biodyne.

cannot be destroyed, but it can be transformed; and somatizers translate it into physical symptoms that are easier for them to acknowledge than the psychological issues. Many people have physical illnesses that may be worsened by stress and emotional conflict, as described in other chapters of this book. But somatizers have a less common problem: Their physical symptoms are almost completely psychological in origin.

There are several theories as to why somatization occurs. One holds that somatizers lack the ability to express their feelings of distress in words, but instead express them as somatic perceptions—"gut feelings." One possibility is that the neuropeptides, chemicals that are active both in the brain's emotional centers and in organs throughout the body, orchestrate the connections between emotional distress and its expression in physical symptoms.

Another theory holds that the failure of parents to attune and respond to an infant's needs makes a child unable to distinguish between internal states (for example, telling anger from sadness). Later in life, this inability interferes with social connections, and physical symptoms become a means for reaching out for care and contact. In other cases, parents may inadvertently reward a child for having symptoms—for example, paying attention to recurrent stomachaches and letting the child stay home from school. Either way, physical symptoms may come to express a deep emotional need to be cared for.

At present, though, these are simply hypotheses; no one can yet say with certainty what the underlying mechanisms might be that translate emotional distress into bodily symptoms. Whatever the cause, rather than dealing directly with the emotional stress, somatizers may spend years going from doctor to doctor in search of physical relief. But those who do consult a psychotherapist may finally find help. Psychotherapy is a treatment that works for somatizers, because it breaks through their denial of the real problem.

After three years, Lenore found help through therapy that enabled her to face the psychological problems that had led to her physical complaints. Brought up in a traditional Japanese-American community in California, she had married an alcoholic who physically abused her for 30 years. When she finally left him, he threatened to commit suicide if she did not take him back. Lenore resisted his pleas, even though her neighbors strongly disapproved; in her community, wives were expected to remain dutiful to their husbands, even if they were unfaithful. After pleading in vain with Lenore for three months, her husband shot himself in the head.

Lenore's intractable headaches had begun shortly after her husband's death. In therapy, she came to realize that they were a physical manifestation of her guilt (and, perhaps, her rage), for she believed that she had killed him. Her psychotherapist proposed that had her husband shot himself in the heart, Lenore would probably have somatized a heart condition.

Although the therapist attempted to reassure Lenore that she was not responsible for her husband's death, Lenore's headaches only got worse. Finally, the therapist tried a paradoxical approach. He told her that she had, indeed, killed her husband, and then gave her the assignment of deciding how many years she should be punished with headaches. Considering that question brought home to Lenore the reality of why she had left him: the years of beatings and infidelity. As therapy continued, Lenore's headaches diminished in intensity and eventually disappeared altogether. She returned to work and began to enjoy her freedom as a single woman.

CHOOSING AN ILLNESS

When patients somatize, many factors may influence their "choice" of illness. These people are not intentionally faking a disease; their motivation is unconscious. In some cases, a patient chooses a particular malady because it best symbolizes his or her emotional plight. For example, romantic disillusionment may be expressed through an imagined heart ailment.

Often, though, a somatizer selects a symptom that has received wide media coverage as being treated with cutting-edge methods on the frontiers of medicine. The less medical science knows about a physical condition, the better candidate it is for a somatizer to mimic. Hence, there are fads in diseases that change with the growth in medical knowledge. Twenty years ago, many patients came to emergency rooms and physicians' offices with symptoms that resembled heart attacks but were not. As cardiologists advanced in knowledge and diagnostic sophistication, somatized heart symptoms gave way to a virtual epidemic of low-back pain. Then, with the development of more precise methods for diagnosing many back disorders, low-back pain began yielding successively to hypoglycemia, chronic fatigue syndrome, and strange and rare allergies that continue to baffle medicine.

In many cases, people with such complaints are suffering from actual physical illnesses. The difficulty is in separating those people from the somatizers. Physicians cannot risk missing a diagnosis, and when a patient complains of discomfort, they may order endless examinations and laboratory tests in search of a physical cause. But this medical attention just encourages the patient to keep channeling his or her conflicts into a physical condition rather than addressing them directly. The consequence is continued pain and suffering.

Somatizers often seem to choose particular symptoms because they are natural extensions of a physical problem they really do have, perhaps a stress-related problem. For example, some people tend to hyperventilate under emotional duress. This produces symptoms—such as shortness of breath, dizziness, and irregular heartbeat—that can resemble a heart attack, paving the way for a somatized heart condition. Somatizers with baffling allergies usually suffered previously from known allergies, but to a much lesser extent. As their stress escalated, mysterious allergies became an available route for expressing it.

THE SCOPE OF THE PROBLEM

I began to study somatization syndrome in the 1950s as a psychologist at the Kaiser-Permanente Health Plan in northern California—a forerunner of the modern health maintenance organization (HMO). In looking over their patient records, Kaiser-Permanente physicians discovered that 60 percent of visits were by patients who had no discernible physical disease.

At first, we thought there was something about the HMO approach that encouraged this type of patient to enroll. But when other researchers did follow-up studies by investigating somatization in traditional fee-for-service plans, they found similar results. In 1976, the American Medical Association testified before the U.S. Senate Health Committee that "in the United States on any given day, 60 to 70 percent of the patients who are waiting to see the physician either have no physical disease but are somatizing stress, or stress is impeding the treatment and healing of a physical condition."

Although many people have complaints that doctors cannot readily diagnose, only a fraction of them are true somatizers. According to recent estimates by Charles Ford, a psychiatrist at the University of Alabama School of Medicine, in Birmingham, roughly half the patients in doctors' offices have at least *one* symptom with no evident medical explanation, but only about 10 percent of patients have no evidence of any medical disease whatever.

Despite their relatively small number, however, somatizers account for a disproportionate share of the nation's medical bills. They repeatedly go to doctors in a fruitless search for diagnosis and treatment and have yearly medical costs 10 to 14 times higher than the national average, according to Michael Kashner, a medical economist at the University of Arkansas College of Medicine. Charles Ford, who has analyzed the problem for the American Academy of Family Physicians, estimates that somewhere between $20 and $30 billion a year is spent on unnecessary care for somatizers.

The prevalence of such patients may have first become apparent at Kaiser-Permanente because of the way this HMO-type plan reimbursed doctors at the time of our study. Then as now, Kaiser-Permanente physicians were paid a set fee in advance for each patient no matter how many visits that patient made. Hence, there was no financial incentive for a doctor to keep treating a patient with no physical disease, as there would be under a traditional health insurance plan. Also, in standard medical plans, physicians often record the diagnosis they are exploring—even if the diagnosis is still uncertain—because the patient cannot collect insurance if no diagnosis is written on the insurance form. In the HMO setting, however, there is no pressure to provide a diagnosis prematurely, and so records give a truer picture of the number of patients seeking treatment who have no medical problem.

THE NEED FOR THERAPY

Often, patients at Kaiser-Permanente who appeared to be somatizers were directed to psychotherapists who could finally help them. In traditional medical practice, this is less likely to happen. But without therapy, both the patients' distress and their medical costs can mount.

Ron's case is typical: A 48-year-old married man, he became convinced that he was having a heart attack—several times a month. In fact, Ron was suffering from stress-induced hyperventilation.

The fundamental problem was not his heart but his home life. Ron had been impotent for several years, and his wife was having an extramarital affair, which Ron consciously ignored and denied. Every time he saw some small evidence of her affair, he would begin to hyperventilate and rush to his doctor's office, thereby obliterating any thoughts of his wife's unfaithfulness.

Invariably, his physician would patiently examine him and then order an electrocardiogram (EKG) to reassure him. The EKG and other tests would be negative, and Ron would indeed be reassured—until the next time he had an unconscious need to deny his wife's infidelity. In 14 months, Ron underwent more than 90 EKGs, all with negative results.

Ron's physician was a sensitive, caring man who believed he was doing the right thing by reassuring Ron. But any qualified psychologist or psychiatrist would have concluded that the repeated cardiac testing merely reinforced Ron's conviction that he had heart trouble. Although the results were negative, the very process of having his heart tested reinforced Ron's notion that he was sick.

Ron's circumstances changed when his employer switched from traditional fee-for-service health insurance to an HMO plan. When Ron asked his new HMO physician for an EKG, the doctor refused because he had read the previous doctor's findings and concluded that Ron's problem was not physical. Instead, he referred Ron to a psychotherapist. At first, Ron refused to go and sought out another HMO physician instead. Finally, after three HMO doctors each referred him to psychotherapy, Ron reluctantly accepted their recommendation.

At the beginning of his first session, Ron was wary of the therapist because he expected her to challenge his belief that he had heart trouble. When she did not, Ron relaxed and began talking about his impotence. Then he gingerly mentioned the possibility that his wife was having an affair. It soon became clear to Ron that his marital troubles were the source of his "heart problem." After his second session, Ron experienced his last hyperventilation attack. After many more sessions, he was able to overcome his impotence, a symptom of his low self-esteem as a man.

THE EVIDENCE FOR EFFECTIVENESS

As Ron's story illustrates, traditional medical practice can inadvertently encourage patients to continue somatizing. The physician simply does what she or he has been trained to do: persistently hunt for a physical cause that would explain the patient's symptoms.

When that process proves futile, however, then psychology—not medical care—can often break the cycle. In 1979, the Federal Alcohol, Drug Abuse, and Mental Health Administration (ADAMHA) published a summary of 28 studies that had investigated the issue of psychotherapy and somatization. This research, which we had initiated 20 years before with our work at

Kaiser-Permanente, consistently showed that psychotherapy reduced the use of medical services for somatizers and that the decrease in medical care was usually enough—often more than enough—to pay for the cost of the therapy.

The following year, ADAMHA convened a conference attended by major researchers in this field. They concluded that the health-care system is burdened by patients with no physical disease whose symptoms are caused by stress, and that without psychotherapy, these people will suffer needlessly.

By now, more than 80 studies have looked at somatizing patients in various medical settings and geographical regions. The findings consistently show the benefits of psychotherapy in reducing these patients' stress, the physical symptoms it triggers, and the frequency of visits to physicians.

In one of the most recent studies, my colleagues and I followed Medicaid recipients in Hawaii, who were among the state's most extensive users of medical services. These people, who made up the top 15 percent of Medicaid recipients in their medical costs, accounted for a full 80 percent of all money paid out by Medicaid. Many of these people, though not all, appeared to be somatizers.

For the study, two-thirds of these patients were offered free, brief psychotherapy. The final third, the control group, were not. The study found that patients who received even brief therapy showed significant declines in their visits to doctors, days spent in the hospital, emergency room visits, diagnostic procedures, and drug prescriptions, and their overall health-care costs. For example, long-term Medicaid recipients averaged roughly a 10- to 20-percent drop in medical costs after therapy.

HOW THERAPY WORKS

Just how does psychotherapy break the somatizer's cycle of fruitless doctor visits? It is a characteristic of human beings that we prefer physical pain to a psychic pain that seems inescapable. The goal of psychotherapy is to help the person find alternatives to translating stress into a physical symptom and eventually to resolve the emotional problem that led to it.

Not all cases of somatization are as dramatic or complex as Lenore's and Ron's. Most will respond to a few sessions of counseling and do not require intensive psychotherapy. Bill's situation is typical.

For 20 years, Bill had been the controller of a small business. He and the owner had become close friends, and their two families spent many holidays together. When Bill was in his late fifties, the boss retired and the boss's son took over.

The son immediately set out to computerize the accounting department. Like many men his age, Bill was convinced he could never understand computers. His worries escalated from there: Because of his fear of computers, he was certain he would be fired and be unable to find another job. Too young to retire and too old for the job market, he felt trapped.

Bill began to complain regularly to his physician about a lack of energy, a loss of interest in his job, and a dwindling appetite. He either could not fall asleep or, if he did, would awaken within an hour or so and remain wide-eyed the rest of the night. Bill was manifesting many of the symptoms of depression—a direct result of his job stress—but his physician did not pick up on it. (Depression in its milder form usually goes unrecognized.) When the doctor could find no physical basis for Bill's complaints, he reassured him in the somewhat patronizing fashion often reserved for older Americans: "You are not as young as you used to be. You've got to slow down. Take a few days off, and if you don't feel better, come back."

Bill returned several times and received the usual reassurances. During one visit, Bill interjected, "You know, Doc, I have this new young boss who is really on my back." But the physician, with a full waiting room, did not have the time to listen to Bill's story. On a later visit, Bill said that his new boss was making him nervous. This earned him a tranquilizer, which helped a bit with his sleep, but it did not solve the fundamental problem.

On the eleventh visit, Bill complained of low-back pain. He had now translated his stress into a physical symptom. This time Bill was referred to an orthopedic surgeon, who finally concluded that there was nothing physically wrong with Bill and referred him to psychotherapy. Feeling angry and insulted, convinced that his problem was medical, Bill saw the psychotherapist only because he was afraid that his doctors would stop treating him if he didn't.

However, in just a few sessions, the therapist directly addressed Bill's underlying stress. At his therapist's urging, Bill took a brief course in computers and found to his surprise that he was able to understand them. Soon, Bill returned to work and set about taking more extensive computer training. Both his depression and his low-back pain disappeared.

Although people of any age can become somatizers, research has shown that psychotherapy is especially helpful in reducing doctors' visits among elderly people. Doctors often do not listen carefully to the complaints of an older patient, and may fear that they won't really know how to respond to the patient. But studies show that even a very brief course of therapy can alleviate much of the pain and suffering associated with old age.

One story that had a happy ending concerns Sarah, a 72-year-old widow who retired to Florida after the death of her husband. Her doctor could only attribute her aches and pains and frequent office visits to old age. And yet his examinations showed that she was extraordinarily healthy for a woman of any age, let alone one in her seventies. Sarah's doctor didn't know how to react to her relentless complaints and her sense of worthlessness and loneliness. In desperation, he prescribed a tranquilizer.

The medication made Sarah confused and disoriented (not infrequent side effects in the elderly), which led to a referral for a psychological examination. Her confusion cleared quickly when the psychotherapist discontinued the tranquilizer. During the examination, however, he realized that Sarah was a lonely woman whose physical complaints stemmed from feeling unwanted and unneeded. As the therapist listened, he heard Sarah say that she wanted to do something useful, but the only work readily available was at the local McDonald's. This was far beneath the socioeconomic level Sarah and her fellow widowed retirees had enjoyed, and she was afraid "the girls" would scoff if she took such a job.

The therapist heard Sarah's message and supported her wish to work. He helped her muster the courage to defy her friends and take the job at McDonald's, where she felt useful once again. The young people on staff there energized her and developed much affection for her, nicknaming her the "groovy old lady."

Several months later, Sarah's doctor became concerned when he realized he had not heard from her in a long time. Fearing the worst, he asked his nurse to check up on Sarah. The nurse reported back that Sarah was healthy and free of her aches and pains. In fact, she was having a ball.

KEEPING THERAPY BRIEF

Over the last decade, and especially in the last few years, researchers have made much progress in pinpointing which types of therapy work best for which conditions. One major advance that's particularly helpful in treating somatization is the rise in the use of brief psychotherapy. Rather than dissecting the patient's entire psychic make-up, a short-term, targeted intervention focuses on a specific problem and its consequences. It may employ techniques from all the schools of psychotherapy, ranging from the Freudian to the behavioral. Brief psychotherapy may take between 1 and 15 sessions, with about 6 sessions required on average.

Recent studies have demonstrated that brief psychotherapy is effective for about 85 percent of somatizers. It teaches them a greater repertoire of responses to stress so that they can stop translating emotional issues into physical symptoms. Thus, the cost of therapy is likely to be offset in the medical savings the treatment provides. On occasion, under extreme stress (such as after the death of a loved one) the patient may temporarily begin to somatize again. But one or two therapy sessions are usually sufficient to stop it.

Treating somatization can put an end to the suffering and pain of many patients who return time after time in futile visits to doctors. The more that physicians and psychotherapists work together, the more often somatization will be readily detected and successfully treated.

THE BOTTOM LINE

Research indicates that many of the patients in a doctor's waiting room do not really suffer from a medical problem but from emotional distress that they have translated into a physical symptom. Clinicians call such patients somatizers. Often, the maladies they complain of are those that are still somewhat mysterious to medical science and cannot be easily diagnosed; these days, they often include environmental allergies and chronic fatigue syndrome. In many cases, the complaints are linked to the patient's real physical vulnerabilities—for example, a somatizer who has a history of legitimate allergies may be susceptible to mysterious allergic reactions under stress.

Although these patients do not have a physical illness, their suffering is real. They often travel from doctor to doctor in search of a cure, but they are rarely helped unless an insightful physician refers them to a psychotherapist. Through therapy, patients can come to understand that their physical symptoms are an expression of their emotional conflicts. They learn to confront the stress and to develop a range of healthier strategies for coping with it. When they no longer "need" the physical symptom, their visits to doctors dwindle. Research shows that offering such patients brief psychotherapy can dramatically cut the number of their visits to doctors and the cost of their health care.

III

WHAT YOU CAN DO:
RELAXATION
AND BEYOND

14

THE RELAXATION RESPONSE

BY HERBERT BENSON, M.D.

EARLY IN MY CAREER AS A CARDIOLOGIST, I WAS INTRIGUED BY THE observation that patients had higher blood pressure during times of stress. That connection, in fact, was part of popular folklore: The notion that "you'll raise your blood pressure if you get upset" was common among physicians and lay people alike.

But while most people believed that stressful circumstances can elevate blood pressure, little was known about the nature of this link or how best to counteract it. If your doctor found that your blood pressure was elevated, you were likely to be treated with medication. That meant that people who had high blood pressure only during periods of stress might be needlessly taking drugs and subjecting themselves to possible adverse side effects and extra expense.

Fascinated by this link between mind and body and inspired by the possibility of simplifying the treatment for stress-induced high blood pressure, I decided to focus on this area after I finished my cardiology training at Harvard's Thorndike Memorial Laboratory. Working in the medical school's department of physiology, I undertook a series of studies between 1967 and 1969 in which I used biofeedback techniques to train monkeys to control their own blood pressure.

The approach was a simple application of biofeedback principles (described in Chapter 18), but it was surprisingly effective. My colleagues and I

HERBERT BENSON, M.D., is the Mind/Body Medical Institute Associate Professor of Medicine, Harvard Medical School; chief of the Division of Behavioral Medicine at the New England Deaconess Hospital; and the founding president of the Mind/Body Medical Institute.

monitored each animal's blood pressure, and whenever it began to go up, we flashed a white light for the animal to see. When the animal's blood pressure dropped, we flashed a blue light. Through the use of appropriate rewards, we were able to train the animals to change their blood pressure in either direction.

As the results of our work became known, some young people who were students of meditation approached me. "Why are you working with animals?" they asked. "Why don't you study humans? We think we can lower our blood pressure through transcendental meditation."

I thanked them for their interest, but I didn't want to get involved with anything as far from the mainstream as meditation was at that time. They were quite persistent, however, coming back day after day. Ultimately, they convinced me that it would be worthwhile to study meditation and its possible effect on blood pressure, and I designed an experiment to test their claim. My colleagues and I also decided to take a wide range of measurements to see if other physiological factors might change with meditation as well.

At about the same time, psychologist Robert Keith Wallace and physiologist Archie F. Wilson had started similar experiments in California on practitioners of transcendental meditation. By chance, our experimental designs were virtually identical. Later, Wallace decided to join us in Boston, and we were able to combine and expand our data on the bodily changes that occur during meditation.

In 1968, we took the meditators who had volunteered to be studied and fitted them with measurement devices—even placing catheters in their veins and arteries—to record changes in a number of physiological functions, from breath rate to brain waves. The volunteers sat quietly for some time, getting used to all the instrumentation.

After an hour or so, when the subjects were in a quiet, resting state, we took measurements for 20 minutes and then asked them to meditate. There was no change in their posture, no change in their activity; they simply changed the content of their thoughts. During this meditation period, which also lasted 20 minutes, the measurements continued.

Finally, the volunteers were asked to return to their normal way of thinking. Again, there were no visible changes in posture or other activity. Their minds simply shifted from a meditative focus back to everyday thoughts, as our measurements continued for a final 20 minutes. Thus, the experiment included a premeditation period, a meditation period, and a postmeditation period.

The results of our experiments were striking, with dramatic physiological changes as people shifted from everyday thinking into meditation. Several aspects of metabolism—the basic "maintenance functions" that keep the body operating—dropped significantly during meditation, even though they had already been operating at a low level as our volunteers rested quietly before meditating. Compared to the simple resting state, the volunteers consumed 17 percent less oxygen while meditating and produced less carbon dioxide as well. Breathing slowed down from a normal rate of 14 or 15 breaths per minute to approximately 10 or 11 breaths per minute. And there was a decrease in the total amount of air moving in and out of the lungs—a measure called *minute ventilation.*

We also noted a precipitous drop in the amount of a chemical called

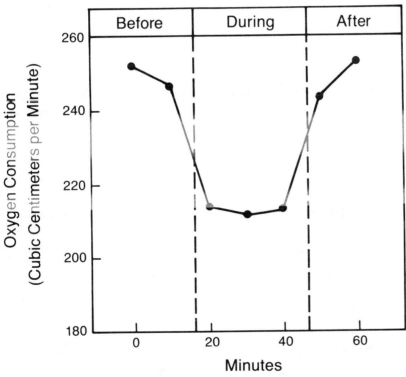

HOW METABOLISM CHANGES WITH THE RELAXATION RESPONSE
The body's metabolic rate, an overall measure of biochemical activity, is reflected in the amount of oxygen consumed. As this graph shows, oxygen consumption drops significantly in meditators when they switch from simply resting ("Before") to meditating ("During"), and rises when they stop meditating ("After").

lactate in the bloodstream. High levels of lactate have been associated in psychiatric studies with anxiety and disquietude; low levels, with peace and tranquility. We found some of the lowest levels ever recorded in human beings.

Finally, brain wave patterns during meditation were slower than those found in everyday thinking. There were more low-frequency alpha, theta, and delta waves in the meditative period—waves associated with rest and relaxation—and fewer of the high-frequency beta waves associated with normal waking activity.

Interestingly, one thing we did *not* observe in these experiments was a drop in blood pressure. But these meditators had low blood pressure to begin with. And as we will see later, the physiological state associated with meditation—which we were on the verge of discovering—does not lower blood pressure in everybody, although it can certainly do so for many people.

Our findings launched us on a 25-year journey that continues to absorb our attention today. It has led to the elucidation of one of the body's most remarkable means of regulating its own physiological machinery—a stress-reducing phenomenon we call the *relaxation response*.

In the fall of 1988, my colleagues and I founded a research, teaching, and training facility called the Mind/Body Medical Institute at the New England Deaconess Hospital and the Harvard Medical School. It was the first institute of its kind, devoted to the study of this response and other self-help measures—including exercise, nutrition, and cognitive therapies—and their potential role in the prevention and treatment of disease. In addition to research, we disseminate information to the lay public about these approaches and teach health-care professionals how to use them in practice. At the New England Deaconess Hospital, we now offer groups for people with a range of medical conditions, including high blood pressure and heart disease, cancer, and chronic pain, as well as offering professional training (see Resources).

We and others have found that the relaxation response can help in the treatment of many medical problems; in some cases, it can eliminate them entirely. It's important to remember that most diseases have many different possible causes and contributing factors, and the relaxation response targets only one: stress. But this is no small feat, because stress alone can precipitate a wide range of unhealthy conditions, as described in many places elsewhere in this book.

To the extent that any disorder is caused or made worse by stress, the relaxation response is useful. It is never a substitute for regular medical care.

However, it is a scientifically proven treatment that is totally compatible with other approaches of modern medicine.

A UNIQUE STATE OF RELAXATION

When we performed our first experiments in the late 1960s, there were just two conditions known to decrease metabolism below the resting state: sleep and hibernation. Early on, we asked whether the changes of the relaxation response could indicate that human beings had a hitherto unrecognized capacity to hibernate.

One accurate way to differentiate hibernation from sleep is by measuring rectal temperature. Rectal temperature decreases up to more than 60 degrees in a hibernating animal—40 times the temperature drop seen in a sleeping animal. But rectal temperature measurements taken during meditation revealed that there was virtually no temperature change, showing that meditation was not a hibernatory state.

But neither were meditators in a state of sleep. During sleep, decreases in metabolism occur over a period of one to five hours; during meditation, they occurred within three to five minutes. In addition, the brain wave patterns of sleep differ from those seen in meditation.

Almost immediately, a hypothesis came to me that would explain this apparent conundrum. I was performing the experiments in the very same laboratories that were used by physiologist Walter B. Cannon early in this century, and I was very well versed in his work and that of his contemporaries. Our hypothesis was based on an understanding of the so-called *fight-or-flight*, or *emergency, response*, which Cannon had described (see Chapter 2).

Cannon discovered that injecting an extract from the adrenal glands into experimental animals could trigger a set of physiological changes, including increases in blood pressure, heart rate, and breath rate, and a three- to four-fold increase in the amount of blood flowing to the muscles. The adrenal extract contained what was later called *adrenaline* (epinephrine) and *noradrenaline* (norepinephrine). Cannon reasoned that this set of changes was the animal's way of preparing to either fight or flee—hence the name fight-or-flight response.

I also remembered the work of the Swiss physiologist Walter R. Hess, a Nobel Prize winner. Hess's findings coupled with Cannon's gave us a key to understanding the relaxation response.

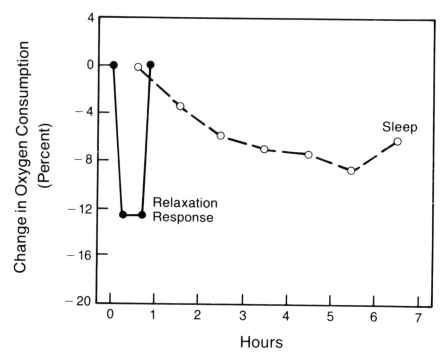

HOW THE RELAXATION RESPONSE DIFFERS FROM SLEEP
While both sleep and the relaxation response bring a decrease in oxygen consumption, the change occurs much more rapidly with the relaxation response. Although the relaxation response period shown in this graph was only 20 minutes, oxygen consumption remains low for as long as a person elicits the relaxation response.

In the 1930s and 1940s, Hess found that by stimulating certain areas of the brain in laboratory animals, he could bring about a response opposite to the fight-or-flight response, which he called, in translation, "a protective mechanism against overstress." This response was characterized by a state of tranquility, relaxed muscles, and decreased blood pressure and breathing rate.

We hypothesized that Hess's *protective mechanism* might be related to the changes that we had found during meditation. If this were true and we had discovered a basic physiological response in human beings, it seemed likely that approaches other than transcendental meditation would prove capable of bringing it forth.

MEDITATION AND PRAYER: UNIVERSAL PATTERNS

It seems that there are two basic components to transcendental meditation: First, the silent repetition of a sound, called a *mantra*, to minimize distracting thoughts; and second, the passive disregard of thoughts that do intrude, followed by a return to the repetition. (See "How to Elicit the Relaxation Response.")

Using this formula, we spent several years reviewing the secular and religious literatures of the world to see whether these basic steps had been described previously. We looked not only at traditions that used a sound like a mantra, but also at those that used the prolonged repetition of a word, prayer, phrase, or muscular activity as a point of focus for the attention. And in virtually every culture we examined that had a written history, the basic steps were present.

For example, in Judaism, at the time of the Second Temple—roughly from the fourth and fifth centuries B.C. to the first century A.D.—followers of a philosophy called *Merkabolism* would squat in a fetal-like posture and focus on their breathing. They would repeat the name of a magic seal on each exhalation and disregard other thoughts when they came to mind.

In Christianity, repetitive prayers dating back almost to the time of Christ evolved by word of mouth, appearing first among the Desert Fathers, who were ascetics living in northern Egypt in the second, third, and fourth centuries A.D. One of these prayers was ultimately codified in the 14th century on Mount Athos in Greece, where the technique is still practiced in Byzantine monasteries. The instructions were to pay attention to your breathing and on each exhalation repeat silently the prayer, "Lord Jesus Christ, have mercy on me." Should other thoughts come to mind, the instructions were to passively disregard them and return to the repetitive prayer. This prayer has survived to this day in many branches of Christianity and is currently called the *Jesus Prayer* or the *Prayer of the Heart*.

Very similar practices are found within Islam, Buddhism, Shintoism, Taoism, and Confucianism, with the only difference being in the words to be repeated. In Islam, where the process is called *Dhikr*, the repetitive focus is often a phrase from the Koran or the word *Allah*. In a ceremony of Shintoism, the focus is on counting in association with breathing. And in one prayer of Tibetan Buddhism, the phrase *Om Mani Padme Hum* (*Hail, Jewel of the Lotus*) is repeated.

HOW TO ELICIT THE RELAXATION RESPONSE

Some general advice on regular practice of the relaxation response:

- Try to find 10 to 20 minutes in your daily routine; before breakfast is a good time.
- Sit comfortably.
- For the period you will practice, try to arrange your life so you won't have distractions. Put the phone on the answering machine, and ask someone else to watch the kids.
- Time yourself by glancing periodically at a clock or watch (but don't set an alarm). Commit yourself to a specific length of practice, and try to stick to it.

There are several approaches to eliciting the relaxation response. Here is one standard set of instructions used at the Mind/Body Medical Institute:

Step 1. Pick a focus word or short phrase that's firmly rooted in your personal belief system. For example, a nonreligious individual might choose a neutral word like *one* or *peace* or *love*. A Christian person desiring to use a prayer could pick the opening words of Psalm 23, *The Lord is my shepherd*; a Jewish person could choose *Shalom*.

Step 2. Sit quietly in a comfortable position.

Step 3. Close your eyes.

Step 4. Relax your muscles.

Step 5. Breathe slowly and naturally, repeating your focus word or phrase silently as you exhale.

Step 6. Throughout, assume a passive attitude. Don't worry about how well you're doing. When other thoughts come to mind, simply say to yourself, "Oh, well," and gently return to the repetition.

Step 7. Continue for 10 to 20 minutes. You may open your eyes to check the time, but do not use an alarm. When you finish, sit quietly for a minute or so, at first with your eyes closed and later with your eyes open. Then do not stand for one or two minutes.

Step 8. Practice the technique once or twice a day.

Inspired by these findings, we expanded our experiments. We wanted to be sure that the physiological changes we had described could be evoked by any practice that included the basic two-step process, not only by transcendental meditation. We used the same instrumentation as we had in the initial meditation experiment. But rather than practicing transcendental meditation, individuals simply repeated the number *one* on each exhalation and passively disregarded any intrusive thoughts. As we predicted, we found changes that were indistinguishable from those of our earlier findings with transcendental meditation.

We also thought about the fact that many of the examples we had uncovered in our research had their roots in religious practice. For some people, we thought, a religious motivation might enhance their commitment to practicing these techniques.

To be sure that modern religious practices could evoke the relaxation response, we brought into our laboratory people who regularly prayed. We found that repetitive prayer—in Judaism, a *davening*-type prayer; in Catholicism, a rosary-type prayer; and in Protestantism, a "centering" prayer—produced the same physiological changes that we had originally noted in transcendental meditation. We now recommend that our religious patients consider using such a prayer when they elicit the relaxation response and that nonreligious patients use any sound, word, or phrase with which they are comfortable.

OTHER MEANS OF ELICITING THE RELAXATION RESPONSE

A wide array of techniques can elicit the relaxation response. At the Mind/Body Medical Institute and the Division of Behavioral Medicine, we offer a variety of techniques from which individuals make their choice. The techniques may be religiously based or have a secular focus. When people choose a technique that conforms to their own preferences, it is much more likely that they will adhere to the practice.

The relaxation response comprises an assortment of physiological changes: a decrease below resting levels in oxygen consumption, heart rate, breathing rate, and muscle tension—plus a decrease in blood pressure in some people—and a shift from normal waking brain wave patterns to a pattern in which slower brain waves predominate. As our research has continued, we have found that many of these same changes can be triggered by methods somewhat different from transcendental meditation and prayer. (See the table, "Physiological Changes with Different Techniques.")

One of these techniques is yoga, an ancient form of "active meditation" from the Hindu and Buddhist traditions. In *hatha yoga*, the form most commonly practiced in the United States, there is no central mental focus, no repetition of a mantra or prayer. Instead, practitioners concentrate on their breathing and on assuming a series of physical postures, moving between them slowly and with concentration. The practice is actually a form of *mindfulness meditation*, described in Chapter 15, which differs from approaches like transcendental meditation in some significant ways. Nevertheless, yoga has also been shown to evoke the physiological changes of the relaxation response.

We have also found that several Western secular techniques designed for stress management can elicit the changes seen in the relaxation response. Among them:

AUTOGENIC TRAINING

This technique, developed in Germany by the physician Johannes H. Schultz, was designed to bring forth the tranquil reaction that Hess described as counteracting the fight-or-flight response in animals. The standard exercises of autogenic training include focusing on feelings of heaviness and cultivating a sense of warmth in the limbs, combined with a passive focus on breathing. You are told that your attitude toward the exercises should be one of *passive concentration*—not intense or compulsive, but rather of a "let it happen" nature. (See "Autogenic Training: Basic Instructions.")

PROGRESSIVE MUSCLE RELAXATION

This technique was first described in the 1920s by the American physiologist Edmund Jacobson. To start, you lie down in a quiet room. A passive attitude, again, is essential. You are taught to recognize even the slightest muscle contractions so that you can release them and achieve a deep degree of muscular relaxation. (See "Progressive Muscle Relaxation: Basic Instructions.")

HYPNOSIS

To induce this state, which is characterized by increased suggestibility, a hypnotist begins with instructions to make you calm and relaxed while you re-

Technique	Oxygen consumption	Respiratory rate	Heart rate	Alpha waves	Blood pressure	Muscle tension
Transcendental meditation	Decreases	Decreases	Decreases	Increase	Decreases*	(Not measured)
Zen and yoga	Decreases	Decreases	Decreases	Increase	Decreases*	(Not measured)
Autogenic training	(Not measured)	Decreases	Decreases	Increase	Inconclusive results	Decreases
Progressive relaxation	(Not measured)	(Not measured)	(Not measured)	(Not measured)	Inconclusive results	Decreases
Hypnosis with suggested deep relaxation	Decreases	Decreases	Decreases	(Not measured)	Inconclusive results	(Not measured)

*In patients with elevated blood pressure.

PHYSIOLOGICAL CHANGES WITH DIFFERENT TECHNIQUES

Several techniques have now been shown to elicit a constellation of related changes, all part of what we have called the relaxation response. While not every change has been measured with every technique, the overall results suggest that these methods trigger the same natural physiological pattern.

cline or rest comfortably in a sitting position. These instructions are given before the hypnotic suggestions are presented. Indeed, as these instructions are followed, heart rate, breathing rate, and blood pressure all decrease and the brain waves become slower—physiological changes similar to those of the relaxation response. (See Chapter 16.)

THE RELAXATION RESPONSE AND HYPERTENSION

The use of the relaxation response in medicine is based on the recognition that stress can cause or exacerbate many different conditions, as described in other chapters of this book. But even for conditions where the relaxation response has clear clinical potential, its usefulness may vary greatly from person to person.

AUTOGENIC TRAINING: BASIC INSTRUCTIONS

This method uses simple phrases to cue your body to elicit the relaxation response. These phrases should theoretically elicit specific physiological responses; for example, the phrase, "My arms are heavy and warm," is meant to increase blood flow to the arms.

Get comfortable and have someone slowly read you these instructions, or make a tape recording to use until you get the hang of it:

Close your eyes and focus on the sensations of breathing. Imagine your breath rolling in and out like ocean waves. Think quietly to yourself, "My breath is calm and effortless . . . calm and effortless. . . ." Repeat the phrase to yourself as you imagine waves of relaxation flowing through your body: through your chest and shoulders, into your arms and back, into your hips and legs. Feel a sense of tranquility moving through your entire body. Continue for several minutes. . . .

Now focus on your arms and hands. Think to yourself, "My arms are heavy and warm. Warmth is flowing gently through my arms into my wrists, hands, and fingers. My arms and hands are heavy and warm." Stay with these thoughts and the feelings in your arms and hands for several minutes. . . .

Now bring your focus to your legs for a few minutes. Imagine warmth and heaviness flowing from your arms down into your legs. Think to yourself: "My legs are becoming heavy and warm. Warmth is flowing through my feet . . . down into my toes. My legs and feet are heavy and warm."

Now scan your body for any points of tension, and if you find some, let them go limp, your muscles relaxed. Notice how heavy, warm, and limp your body has become. Think to yourself: "All my muscles are letting go. I'm getting more and more relaxed."

Finally, take a deep breath, feeling the air fill your lungs and down into your abdomen. As you breathe out, think, "I am calm . . . I am calm. . . ." Do this for a few moments, feeling the peacefulness throughout your body.

Then, as your practice session ends, count to three, taking a deep breath and exhaling with each number. Open your eyes and get up slowly. Stretch before going back to everyday activities.

The case of hypertension (the medical term for high blood pressure) is a good example. For some people with hypertension, stress is the main cause and the relaxation response may solve the problem entirely. For others, stress is not a factor at all and medication may be the best approach to the problem. Hypertension has many possible causes, and the relaxation response should only be expected to help in cases when stress is at least a significant component.

We and others have accumulated considerable evidence that the relaxation response can indeed lower blood pressure in many people with hypertension. But the issue has become confusing, because some researchers have failed to find that relaxation has this effect. In one large-scale study published in 1992 in the *Journal of the American Medical Association*, patients who practiced "stress management" techniques failed to achieve lower blood pressures than those who did not practice the techniques. The study was quoted in the media as evidence that relaxation is not effective in treating hypertension.

Although it will take further work to sort out the results of that study, I believe they do not contradict or undermine previous findings. As we subsequently published in the same journal, this 1992 study made no effort to determine whether stress was affecting the subjects' blood pressure in the first place. In fact, subjects in this study did not have true hypertension at all, but blood pressure in the high normal range. The researchers also did not record the precise type of stress management techniques these people chose to use, nor did they keep track of how regularly the subjects practiced those techniques.

On average, our studies and others show that the relaxation response can lower blood pressure by about 5 to 10 millimeters of mercury in people with hypertension. The relative effect of the relaxation response will vary, depending on the degree to which an individual's high blood pressure is caused by stress. For example, an individual may have severely elevated blood pressure that requires treatment with antihypertensive medications. If stress is one of the contributing factors, the regular practice of the relaxation response would lower blood pressure to the extent that stress is elevating it. Although medications would still be required, the amount of medication necessary would be reduced and the likelihood of undesirable side effects from the medications would be lessened. At the present time, the only way I know to test the effectiveness of the relaxation response is to start practicing it and track the results.

PROGRESSIVE MUSCLE RELAXATION:
BASIC INSTRUCTIONS

In progressive muscle relaxation, you methodically sweep through your body, tensing and then relaxing each major muscle group. This attunes you to the difference in feeling when your muscles are tensed or relaxed and is another way to elicit the relaxation response.

This technique can be done in any large chair that supports your head and neck, but is best done lying on your back on a firm but soft surface, such as a thick carpet or workout mat. (A bed is too soft— you're more likely to glide off to sleep.) Lie on your back with your arms along your sides. Loosen any clothing that's uncomfortably tight, and take off your shoes.

You can have someone read you the instructions, or make a tape for yourself. These should be read at a slow, easygoing pace:

First, tense the muscles throughout your body, from head to toe. Tighten your feet and legs, tense your arms and hands, clench your jaw, and contract your stomach. Hold the tension while you sense the feelings of strain and tightness. Study the tension and notice the difference between how the muscle feels when it is tensed and when it is relaxed. Then take a deep breath, hold it, and exhale long and slowly as you relax all your muscles, letting go of the tension. Notice the sense of relief as you relax.

Now you're going to tense and relax individual groups of muscles, keeping the rest of your body as relaxed as you can. You'll hold the tension for a few seconds in each part of your body while you get a clear sense of what the tension feels like; then breathe deeply, hold the breath for a moment, and let go of the tension as you exhale.

Start by making your hands into tight fists. Feel the tension through your hands and arms. Relax and let go of the tension. Now press your arms down against the surface they're resting on. Feel the tension. Hold it . . . and let go. Let your arms and hands go limp.

Shrug your shoulders tight, up toward your head, feeling the tension through your neck and shoulders. Hold . . . then release, letting go. Drop your shoulders down, free of tension.

Now wrinkle your forehead, sensing the tightness. Hold . . . release, letting your forehead be smooth and relaxed. Shut your eyes as tight as you can. Hold . . . and let go. Now open your mouth as wide as you can. Hold it . . . and gently relax, letting your lips touch softly. Then clench your jaw, teeth tight together. Hold . . . and relax. Let the muscles of your face be soft and relaxed, at ease.

Take a few moments to sense the relaxation throughout your arms and shoulders, up through your face. Now take a deep breath, filling your lungs down through your abdomen. Hold your breath while you feel the tension through your chest. Then exhale and let your chest relax, your breath natural and easy. Suck in your stomach, holding the muscles tight . . . and relax. Arch your back . . . hold . . . and ease your back down gently, letting it relax. Feel the relaxation spreading through your whole upper body.

Now tense your hips and buttocks, pressing your legs and heels against the surface beneath you . . . hold . . . and relax. Curl your toes down, so they point away from your knees . . . hold . . . and let go of the tension, relaxing your legs and feet. Then bend your toes back up toward your knees . . . hold . . . and relax.

Now feel your whole body at rest, letting go of more tension with each breath . . . your face relaxed and soft . . . your arms and shoulders easy . . . stomach, chest, and back soft and relaxed . . . your legs and feet resting at ease . . . your whole body soft and relaxed.

Take time to enjoy this state of relaxation for several minutes, feeling the deep calm and peace. When you're ready to get up, move slowly, first sitting, and then gradually standing up.

Relaxation can be especially effective for people with "white-coat hypertension"—those whose blood pressure is high only when they are in the doctor's office or a similarly stressful setting. With national advertising campaigns characterizing high blood pressure as "a silent killer" and an "internal time bomb," the very act of having your blood pressure measured can stir self-fulfilling fears of being diagnosed with this potentially deadly condition.

itself. Recent studies suggest that 25 percent or more of patients diagnosed with high blood pressure actually have white-coat hypertension.

One patient of ours, a 55-year-old advertising executive, was told that he had slightly elevated blood pressure in a physical examination ten years ago. Worried about the potential for a stroke, he became quite anxious for days before every medical checkup—and then had very high blood pressure readings when he finally saw the doctor. Even when he took antihypertensive medication at higher and higher doses, there was little change in his physician's measurement of his blood pressure. Yet a monitor that tracked his blood pressure during normal daily activities showed his blood pressure was low the rest of the time. In fact, he often felt dizzy and weak during the day, suggesting that the medicine was lowering his blood pressure too much.

Suspecting that he might be suffering from white-coat hypertension, we taught this patient to use the relaxation response to control his anxiety in the physician's office. His feelings of fear gradually subsided, until he ultimately became comfortable in the doctor's office. From then on, his blood pressure was consistently normal. After roughly a year of practice, he was able to stop his medication completely, and he has not required blood pressure treatment for five years.

Although this patient's condition was a model of white-coat hypertension, the value of the relaxation response is not limited to such cases; it can be useful in the treatment of many kinds of hypertension. For example, the relaxation response can help people using other nondrug treatments for hypertension, such as dietary salt restriction, exercise, and weight loss. All of these approaches require behavioral changes that can be difficult and anxiety provoking, and using the relaxation response can make them less stressful and easier to follow.

OTHER MEDICAL APPLICATIONS

Over the past several years, many research groups have performed scientific studies to test the value of the relaxation response in the treatment of a wide range of medical conditions. At the New England Deaconess Hospital, we have taught the relaxation response to people with muscle tension pains (which can include some headaches), infertility, insomnia, psychological problems, cardiac arrhythmias, premenstrual syndrome, and several common symptoms related to cancer and AIDS. For these conditions, there is good evidence that the relaxation response can undo some or all of the damage caused by stress and have a significant clinical impact. We are also using the relaxation response experimentally for people with psoriasis, asthma, and hyperactivity.

The following are some of the conditions we treat most frequently at the New England Deaconess Hospital—those for which there is the most evidence that the relaxation response can be helpful.

PAIN

Stress and anxiety decrease the threshold for pain, making people more sensitive to the initial pain sensations and making some kinds of pain seem especially intense. This can set up a vicious circle: When pain strikes, the sufferer begins to worry about how bad it will get, and that anxiety makes the perception of pain worse (see Chapter 6).

The relaxation response, which can break this pattern, has proven to be useful in the therapy of many kinds of pain. For example, it is extremely useful in alleviating stress-related muscle aches and headaches and can bring some people with these problems complete relief, sometimes within just a few weeks.

With more severe chronic pain, the relaxation response may not bring total relief, but it may allow people to tolerate the pain more easily. Studies by physician and pain specialist Margaret A. Caudill and her associates at the Mind/Body Medical Institute have shown that when the relaxation response is utilized with other behavioral therapies, patients decrease their physician visits by 36 percent on average, with those who had previously made the most doctor visits showing the greatest reduction.

INFERTILITY

Couples dealing with infertility often feel they have lost control over a central part of their lives and become depressed, anxious, and angry. Treatments for infertility are expensive and can cause emotional stress. And high levels of stress, in turn, can contribute to infertility by causing irregular ovulation, hormonal changes, fallopian tube dysfunction, and perhaps a decrease in sperm production.

The studies of psychologist Alice D. Domar and her colleagues at the Mind/Body Medical Institute have shown that a program based upon the relaxation response can significantly decrease the stress of the experience of infertility. Furthermore, she and her colleagues have found that couples undergoing this stress reduction program are more likely to become pregnant (see Chapter 12).

INSOMNIA

About one in every six Americans has chronic insomnia. The problem can have both psychological and physiological components: Many people with insomnia have rapid brain wave patterns that are typical when a person is under stress. Recent studies at our institute by psychologist Gregg Jacobs and his colleagues have shown that insomnia patients taught the relaxation response, together with other behavioral techniques, can learn to fall asleep more easily. On average, these patients fell asleep four times more rapidly after treatment, and their brain wave patterns slowed as well. In both respects, these successfully treated patients resembled normal people who had never had insomnia.

The relaxation response may enable people with insomnia to give up sleeping pills—a transition that can be difficult, but that can also result in more restful sleep. One of our patients had been taking medication for sleep every night for more than three months, but she still required one to three hours to fall asleep and felt tired and irritable during the day. In preparing to try the relaxation response as an alternative, she first gradually stopped using all her sleeping pills; her insomnia worsened, and her sleep was quite poor for about two weeks. But within three weeks of being taught the relaxation response and other behavioral techniques, she was regularly able to fall asleep within 20 minutes. She also told us that she felt less irritable, more energetic, and much more "like her old self."

ANXIETY, ANGER, HOSTILITY, AND DEPRESSION

Stress leads to psychological changes that can, in turn, affect the body. Anxiety can cause nausea, vomiting, diarrhea, and panic attacks, while hostility and anger have been shown to be risk factors for heart disease. Many studies have now shown that in people who regularly elicit the relaxation response, there is a decrease in anxiety, anger, and hostility, as well as depression.

SYMPTOMS FROM TREATMENT FOR CANCER AND AIDS

The relaxation response has proven a useful adjunct in the treatment of cancer and AIDS, especially as a means of quelling the symptoms many patients develop in anticipation of chemotherapy. Approximately one-third of cancer patients undergoing chemotherapy develop anticipatory nausea and vomiting, a conditioned response to the nausea-inducing drugs that may begin up to 24 hours before the drug is actually administered. The symptoms escalate with repeated treatments, often becoming resistant to antinausea drugs and, in many cases, leading patients to refuse to continue chemotherapy.

Psychologist Ann Webster at the Mind/Body Medical Institute, like other investigators (see Chapter 5), has shown that anticipatory nausea and vomiting can be reduced significantly with behavioral techniques that incorporate the relaxation response. These include hypnosis; relaxation response training with guided imagery; biofeedback coupled with relaxation response training; and systematic desensitization, which uses the relaxation response to combat the anxiety patients have associated with chemotherapy.

One AIDS patient of ours had a long-standing asthma condition that worsened when he took a medication that was essential to his treatment. When he used an aerosol necessary to prevent pneumocystis pneumonia (an AIDS-related condition), he would have an asthma attack and suffer with asthma for many days, until he began to be afraid that he might die from the therapy.

This patient's intolerance to aerosols became even more critical when he stopped responding to his primary AIDS medication. In order to be eligible for an antiviral medication, he had to be able to take the aerosolized treatment as well. Through the use of an audiotape, he was trained to elicit the relaxation response. When he practiced the response immediately before receiving his aerosolized treatment, he found he could tolerate the medication without developing an asthma attack. Later, he was able to receive the antiviral treatment.

WHAT TO EXPECT FROM THE RELAXATION RESPONSE

If you want to try using the relaxation response to help treat a medical condition, first talk to your physician or other health-care provider. He or she should know what you plan to do because it may alter the amount of medication you require.

If you are wondering whether there might be any dangers in eliciting the relaxation response, the answer is that its side effects are essentially those of sitting quietly or praying twice a day. Although a very small minority of people find that practicing the relaxation response can be stress-inducing (see "When Relaxation Turns to Panic"), side effects for most people are essentially nonexistent.

As you elicit the relaxation response, you may notice that your rate of

---

WHEN RELAXATION TURNS TO PANIC

Occasionally, people who try relaxation methods for the first time find that they actually become *more* anxious. In our experience at the Mind/Body Medical Institute, this is extremely uncommon. In any case, it's usually easily corrected.

Some people feel fearful when they close their eyes. In this case, it is easy enough to practice the relaxation response with your eyes open, either gazing in a relaxed way at a picture or an object or getting up and practicing the walking or jogging technique described at the end of this chapter.

For others, focusing on breathing can make them overly conscious of the "effort" involved, causing a panicky feeling. Again, walking or jogging should provide a fine alternative.

---

breathing slows. You may even notice periods in which you feel as if you have stopped breathing for a short period of time. Furthermore, you may become aware of the fact that your heart rate has slowed. Your muscles will become relaxed, and you may become aware that a muscle ache or pain that you had at the beginning of the session is gone by the end. Other changes may include a slight welling of tears in your eyes or a sensation of warmth in your hands and feet. At the end of a period of sitting, most people report feeling peaceful and calm, yet also more alert and less fatigued than before.

Continued practice of the relaxation response can bring feelings of greater control over life. Instead of feeling like a "cork bobbing on the sea" (as one of our patients reported feeling before learning the relaxation response), regular practice leads to a sense that emotions—and the physiological reactions that go with them—can be brought under your control. One psychological benefit is a greater sense of self-assurance; the physical benefits are decreases in stress-related conditions and symptoms.

Do not expect these changes to occur immediately. Although a sense of peace and quiet occurs right after eliciting the relaxation response, long-term psychological and physiological changes may take several weeks or months.

Moreover, the changes do not appear all at once; on a day-to-day basis, they are sometimes imperceptible. Indeed, like many people, you may first become aware of the improvement when another person comments on how you have changed. But as more time elapses—generally after a month or so of regular practice—if you look back at your initial feelings and symptoms and compare them with your current state, you will recognize the positive changes that have occurred.

FUTURE DIRECTIONS

As we have expanded our research into the relaxation response, we have found increasing evidence that the relaxation response can serve not only as a "solo" means of reducing stress, but also as an "amplifier" of sorts to maximize the effects of other mind/body approaches, such as visualization and imagery (see Chapter 17). We distinguish between the relaxation response "for its own sake" and the relaxation response as a means of enhancing other strategies by referring to these two approaches as Phase I and Phase II of the relaxation response.

Phase I includes the basic physiological changes that occur as a result of eliciting the relaxation response, including decreased activity of the sympathetic nervous system. In Phase II, which occurs *immediately after* eliciting the relaxation response, we have observed that the mind is more receptive to new information: The relaxation response quiets the mind and tones down the "static" of cascading thoughts.

In that quiet space of mind, the potency of other mind/body approaches appears to be enhanced. You probably have experienced some difficulty in focusing your attention when you are very anxious or distracted. So it makes sense that when your mind is quietest, you are better able to concentrate, solve problems, and, if presented with visual imagery, make the most of that imagery's impact on the mind. Ongoing experimental work should tell us a lot about the therapeutic potential of this combined approach and its value as an adjunct to standard medical treatments.

We are also continuing to do research on other meditative traditions that suggest the potential of the relaxation response and related approaches may be even greater than we had realized. For example, we have been studying Tibetan Buddhist monks who are advanced practitioners of a form of meditation that has dramatic physiological effects. In an annual ritual, these monks shed almost all their clothes, wrap themselves in icy wet sheets on a near-

THE RELAXATION RESPONSE DURING EXERCISE

In 1978, we discovered that the relaxation response could also be elicited during exercise. We measured various physiological changes in volunteers as they pedaled on a stationary bicycle. Some were told simply to bicycle at a constant rate for 30 minutes, and, as expected, we found no changes in their metabolism during that time.

But some subjects, while riding their bicycles at exactly the same rate, were instructed to focus on a sound, a word, a phrase, or a prayer, and passively disregard other thoughts when they came to mind. Even though they worked just as hard as the other bicyclists, their metabolic rates—the speed at which they burned calories—decreased by 11 percent, a sign of the relaxation response.

More important for most people who do regular exercise is the psychological benefit of adding the relaxation response to a workout. Many joggers say that they experience a "high" after walking or running four to five miles (see Chapter 19). By using a relaxation response technique while you exercise, it is possible to experience this mild euphoria in the first or second mile.

The relaxation response can be elicited during walking or jogging by following these steps:

Step 1. Get into sufficiently good condition so that you can jog or walk without becoming excessively short of breath.

Step 2. Do your usual warm-up exercises before you jog or walk.

Step 3. As you exercise, keep your eyes fully open, but attend to your breathing. After you fall into a regular pattern of breathing, focus in particular on its in-and-out rhythm. As you breathe in, say to yourself, silently, "in"; when you exhale, say "out." In effect, the words *in* and *out* become your mental devices or focus words, in the same way that you would use your personal focus words or phrases with other relaxation response methods.

If this in/out rhythm is uncomfortable for you (you might feel that your breathing is too fast or too slow), you may focus on something else. For example, you can become aware of your feet hitting the ground, silently repeating, "One, two, one, two" or "Left, right, left, right."

There is, of course, nothing wrong with focusing on a faith-oriented word or phrase during exercise; in fact, it could make your exercise more satisfying. (One high-ranking U.S. Army chaplain, a Catholic, repeats the Jesus Prayer in rhythm to his footsteps as he runs each day.)

Step 4. Remember to maintain a passive attitude, simply disregarding disruptive thoughts. When they occur, think to yourself, "Oh, well," and return to your repetitive focus word or phrase.

Step 5. After you complete your exercise, return to your normal after-exercise routine.

Note: If you are over 40 or if you suffer from a physical ailment, ask your physician's advice before starting any exercise program.

---

freezing night, and proceed to enter a state of deep meditation in which they focus on specific mental images associated with generating heat. By doing this, they are able to raise their skin temperature to levels warm enough to dry the sheets—an observer can actually see the steam rising off them. Under these conditions of cold and wetness, physiological principles would predict that individuals would uncontrollably shiver and perhaps die.

In other monks, we have found that oxygen consumption and other metabolic functions decrease much lower than in people practicing conventional meditation. Whereas in conventional meditation oxygen consumption decreases 16 to 17 percent, these monks lower their oxygen consumption by up to 64 percent. The mechanisms responsible for these remarkable physiological alterations are not understood.

We are also doing further research to answer a key question: If the relaxation response is performed only once or twice a day for 10 to 20 minutes, how can its effects last long enough to influence a range of stress-related conditions? The late psychophysiologist John Hoffman and his associates at Harvard Medical School demonstrated that in people who regularly elicit the relaxation response, the body is less responsive to the stress hormone noradrenaline, even during times of the day when they are not specifically practicing the response. This means that it takes more noradrenaline to bring about an increase in heart rate and blood pressure in these people than it does in others.

Although the basis for this broad protective effect remains unclear, regular practice of the relaxation response does seem to block the ability of stress hormones to influence the brain and the body. In this respect, this function of the relaxation response resembles a class of drugs used to treat the symptoms of stress-related conditions: the alpha- and beta-blockers, which act by blocking the action of noradrenaline. The relaxation response may be a natural way of achieving the same kind of effect without the side effects of the drug.

Finally, we believe that the relaxation response can be used much more widely to help people, especially young people, to counter the stress in their lives. Many people seek relief from stress and anxiety through alcohol and drug abuse; others who cannot cope with the stress of modern life become violent or commit suicide. Because these problems often develop during adolescence, the Mind/Body Medical Institute is developing stress management curricula based on the relaxation response for use by high school students. It is our hope that these programs can help prevent violent or self-destructive behavior and give these young people coping skills that will serve them throughout their lives.

Modern medicine currently relies on two major therapeutic approaches: medications and procedures such as surgery. Until recently, little emphasis has been given to mind/body approaches, perhaps because of the traditional separation of mind and body that has characterized Western science since the time of Descartes. But as scientific evidence continues to establish the significance of mind/body interactions, a third major approach to medical treatment should evolve: one characterized by self-care through the mastery of mind/body interactions. The relaxation response should prove an important element of this very promising approach.

THE BOTTOM LINE

By practicing two basic steps—the repetition of a sound, word, phrase, prayer, or muscular activity; and a passive return to the repetition whenever distracting thoughts recur—you can trigger a series of physiological changes that offer protection against stress. These changes—which include lower heart rate, breathing rate, and, in some people, lower blood pressure—make up the natural relaxation response that is the opposite of the fight-or-flight response to stress. While the relaxation response was discovered in studies of people practicing meditation, other forms of relaxation offer similar benefits.

The relaxation response has been proven beneficial in many stress-related conditions, often as a supplement to conventional medical treatment. In cases that are not stress related, it cannot be expected to treat illness effectively by itself. But it can be very useful in enhancing both mental and physical health, and it may find even broader applications in conjunction with visualization and imagery and other mind/body techniques.

15

MINDFULNESS MEDITATION: HEALTH BENEFITS OF AN ANCIENT BUDDHIST PRACTICE

BY JON KABAT-ZINN, PH.D.

PICTURE THIS: SOME 25 OR 30 PEOPLE ARE SITTING ON STRAIGHT-BACKED chairs around the sides of a comfortable hospital room. Their eyes are closed. The room is silent. It may look like they aren't doing anything, and in a sense they are not—other than concentrating in total stillness on the sensation of air moving in and out of their bodies as they breathe.

This exercise, called *sitting meditation*, is part of the practice of mindfulness, an approach that offers a unique way to help people cope with stress, pain, and chronic illness. The patients in this room suffer from a broad range of medical conditions, including heart disease, cancer, diabetes, chronic pain, high blood pressure, and many stress-related disorders. They are enrolled in an eight-week course based on intensive training in mindfulness at the University of Massachusetts Medical Center's Stress Reduction Clinic.

Like other mind/body therapies, mindfulness meditation can induce deep states of relaxation, at times directly improve physical symptoms, and help patients lead full and satisfying lives. But while more familiar forms of meditation involve focusing on a sound, phrase, or prayer to minimize distracting thoughts (as described in Chapter 14), mindfulness does the opposite. In mindfulness meditation, you don't ignore distracting thoughts, sensations, or physical discomfort; instead, you focus on them. This form of meditation

JON KABAT-ZINN, PH.D., is director of the Stress Reduction Clinic at the University of Massachusetts Medical Center in Worcester, where he is an associate professor of medicine.

practice, which is roughly 2,500 years old, stems primarily from the Buddhist tradition and was developed as a means of cultivating greater awareness and wisdom, with the aim of helping people live each moment of their lives—even the painful ones—as fully as possible. In our clinic, we have found that mindfulness practice can be beneficial for people facing a broad range of serious physical illnesses.

In the 13 years since the Stress Reduction Clinic was founded, well over 6,000 medical patients have gone through the program. Almost all of them were referred by their physicians—doctors who may have been skeptical at first about meditation, but who have learned from experience the benefits this approach offers their patients.

The people we work with in our program come with an extraordinarily wide range of medical diagnoses, life circumstances, and problems. Yet all share the desire to learn to control stress more effectively and to utilize their inner resources to improve the quality of their lives. One typical class included a 25-year-old mother distraught because she and her two-year-old baby had tested positive for HIV, the AIDS virus; a 72-year-old woman with a serious cardiac arrhythmia, whose doctors were running out of medications they could try to keep her heartbeat stabilized in the normal range; a 70-year-old heart attack survivor who was now facing colon cancer; two people with diabetes who wanted to learn to control anxiety; several people who suffered from severe, recurrent panic attacks; and a number of other people who were experiencing health problems as a result of personal predicaments that caused them extreme stress and apprehension.

Unlike standard medical and psychological approaches, our clinic does not categorize and treat patients differently depending on their illnesses. Our eight-week course offers the same training program in mindfulness and stress reduction to everyone. We don't emphasize what is "wrong" with people, but rather what is "right" with them: their capacity for learning, for mobilizing their inner strengths, and for changing their behavior in new and imaginative ways.

The Stress Reduction Clinic functions as a *complement* to high-quality medical treatment, not an alternative to it. The program is not held out as some kind of magical cure when other approaches have failed. Rather, it is a sensible and straightforward way for people to experience and understand the mind/body connection firsthand and use it to deal better with their illnesses and their lives.

We do not yet know if mindfulness practice can actually slow or reverse certain disease processes. This is an area that is currently being studied. However, at this point, we do have good evidence that mindfulness helps the people we see deal more effectively with their life situations, including the diseases that bring them to our clinic—and that is our primary goal.

Our patients are ordinary working-class and middle-class adults, of all ages and occupations. They come with no particular knowledge of meditation or interest in it; most come simply because their doctors told them to. We present the program from the start as a challenge: What can you do to help *yourself* as a complement to what your doctors and other health-care providers are already doing for you?

Part of this challenge is a friendly cautioning that taking this stress reduction program might itself be stressful, especially at first, because it involves hard work and discipline, including a commitment to meditate for 45 minutes a day at least six days a week. This is a major life-style change for anyone. Moreover, because you are not really "doing" anything in meditation—at least, not in the conventional sense—it takes a certain commitment and discipline to get over the hump of suspecting that all this "nondoing" is just a colossal waste of time.

For some people, the inherent difficulty of meditation practice is made easier by the profound states of relaxation and pleasant feelings it frequently produces. But mindfulness is about far more than feeling relaxed or tension-free. Its true aim is to nurture an inner balance of mind that allows you to face all life situations with greater stability, clarity, understanding, and even wisdom, and to act or respond effectively and with dignity out of that clarity and understanding.

That means an integral part of mindfulness practice is to face, accept, and even welcome your tension, stress, and physical pain, as well as mind states such as fear, anger, frustration, disappointment, and feelings of insecurity and unworthiness when they are present. Why? Because acknowledging present-moment reality as it actually is, whether it is pleasant or unpleasant, is the first step towards transforming that reality and your relationship to it. If you do not face things in this way, you are likely to become stuck and have difficulty changing or growing.

At the outset, we tell prospective participants that they don't have to like the meditation practice; they just have to do it for the eight weeks of the program. We strongly recommend to them that they follow the program with no agenda and no expectation that something special will happen, not even relaxation or reduced stress. We just want them to practice with as alert and open a mind as possible and then see what happens.

WHAT IS MINDFULNESS?

When most people hear the word *meditation*, they often think of transcendental meditation or similar practices used to evoke the relaxation response. In these approaches, you focus attention on one thing, usually the sensation of breath leaving and entering your body or a mantra (a special sound or phrase you repeat silently to yourself). Anything else that comes up in your mind during meditation is seen as a distraction to be disregarded. These practices can give rise to very deep states of calmness and stability of attention. They are known as the concentration, or "one-pointed," type of meditation—what Buddhists call *shamatha* or *samadhi* practices.

Mindfulness is the other major classification of meditation practice, known as *vipassana*, or insight meditation. In the practice of mindfulness, you begin by utilizing one-pointed attention to cultivate calmness and stability, but then you move beyond that by introducing a wider scope to the observing, as well as an element of inquiry. When thoughts or feelings come up in your mind, you don't ignore them or suppress them, nor do you analyze or judge their content. Rather, you simply note any thoughts as they occur as best you can and observe them intentionally but nonjudgmentally, moment by moment, as events in the field of your awareness.

Paradoxically, this inclusive noting of thoughts that come and go in your mind can lead you to feel less caught up in them and give you a deeper perspective on your reactions to everyday stress and pressures. By observing your thoughts and emotions as if you had taken a step back from them, you can see much more clearly what is actually on your mind. You can see your thoughts arise and recede one after another. You can note the content of your thoughts, the feelings associated with them, and your reactions to them. You might become aware of agendas, attachments, likes and dislikes, and inaccuracies in your ideas. You can gain insight into what drives you, how you see the world, who you think you are—insight into your fears and aspirations.

The key to mindfulness is not so much *what* you choose to focus on but the quality of the awareness that you bring to each moment. It is very important that it be nonjudgmental—more of a silent witnessing, a dispassionate observing, than a running commentary on your inner experience. Observing without judging, moment by moment, helps you see what is on your mind without editing or censoring it, without intellectualizing it or getting lost in your own incessant thinking.

It is this investigative, discerning observation of whatever comes up in the present moment that is the hallmark of mindfulness and differentiates it most from other forms of meditation. The goal of mindfulness is for you to be more aware, more in touch with life and with whatever is happening in your own body and mind *at the time it is happening*—that is, in the present moment. If you are experiencing a distressing thought or feeling or actual physical pain in any moment, you resist the impulse to try to escape the unpleasantness; instead, you attempt to see it clearly as it is and accept it because it is *already* present in this moment.

Acceptance, of course, does not mean passivity or resignation. On the contrary, by fully accepting what each moment offers, you open yourself to experiencing life much more completely and make it more likely that you will be able to respond effectively to any situation that presents itself. Acceptance offers a way to navigate life's ups and downs—what Zorba the Greek called "the full catastrophe"—with grace, a sense of humor, and perhaps some understanding of the big picture, what I like to think of as wisdom.

One way to envision how mindfulness works is to think of the mind as the surface of a lake or ocean. There are always waves, sometimes big, sometimes small. Many people think the goal of meditation is to stop the waves so that the water will be flat, peaceful, and tranquil—but that is not so. The true spirit of mindfulness practice is illustrated by a poster someone once described to me of a 70-ish yogi, Swami Satchidananda, in full white beard and flowing robes, atop a surfboard and riding the waves off a Hawaiian beach. The caption read: "You can't stop the waves, but you can learn to surf."

HOW TO PRACTICE MINDFULNESS YOURSELF

There are two ways to practice mindfulness, both of which are necessary to make it an ongoing part of your life. The first is through formal meditation practice, which usually involves specific techniques to help you keep your focus on the present moment over an extended period of time. The other is what we call *informal practice*, in which you simply remind yourself to be in the present moment during daily activities and "check in" from time to time to see if you are in fact being mindful. Ultimately, mindfulness is best thought of as a way of being, rather than as a technique. Fundamentally, it is a question of whether and to what extent you are willing to be fully awake in your own life as it unfolds.

FORMAL PRACTICES

The three most basic formal meditation practices used in our clinic include a technique called the *body scan; sitting meditation*; and various sequences of *hatha yoga* postures done slowly, gently, and mindfully. These three approaches are in many ways different doors into the same room. We encourage people to determine which one suits them best after trying all three over a period of weeks. Mindfulness of breathing is an integral part of all three of these techniques.

Each of these formal methods gives you a focus, or a series of different focal points, on which to concentrate your awareness. Whatever the object of attention, it usually doesn't take long before the mind wanders off, even though you fully intended to keep it in one place. Each time this occurs, before refocusing your attention, you first observe as nonjudgmentally as possible where the mind went off to—noting, for example, a memory, a thought about the future, a preoccupation with a sensation in the body, or a feeling such as boredom, impatience, or anxiety. You then gently bring your mind back to the object of your attention in the meditation.

Although this resembles one-pointed meditation in that you are bringing your mind back to a particular focus, whether it is the breath or something else, there is an important extra feature: You are also noting where your mind wandered off to. It is this noting of the changing quality of moment-to-moment experience that is the hallmark of mindfulness practice.

In the *body scan*, you slowly and systematically move your attention through the various regions of your body, from your feet to the top of your head, noting any physical sensations as you go along. This exercise is usually done lying on your back, which makes it easier than other approaches for people with chronic pain or other physical problems. (See "The Body Scan: Basic Instructions," at the end of this chapter.)

Sitting meditation is the best-known mindfulness practice, depicted in countless statues of cross-legged Buddhas. These statues really represent in the Buddhist tradition the embodiment of a fully awakened mind.

In sitting meditation, it is important to sit in a dignified position in which your head, neck, and back are erect but not stiff. Most of our patients choose to sit on straight-backed chairs rather than cross-legged on the floor on a cushion. In either case, the posture should reflect an inner attitude of wakefulness and dignity.

You usually begin by choosing a single object of focus—for example, your breathing. More specifically, you can concentrate on one aspect of your breathing, such as the feeling of the air as it passes in and out of your nostrils or the gentle expanding and deflating of your belly with each in-breath and out-breath. Once you have developed some concentration in this way, you can then extend your awareness into mindfulness by attending to changing qualities of the breath and to sounds, sensations, thoughts, and the like as they enter into your awareness. All the while, you maintain a nonreactive calmness and stability of attention as best you can, using the breath as an anchor.

A complete description of *hatha yoga* and its uses in mindfulness training goes beyond the scope of this chapter. Suffice it to say that, done properly, it is a gentle but powerful form of body-oriented meditation in its own right, and a way of cultivating musculoskeletal strength, flexibility, and balance as well as inner stillness and mindfulness. During yoga, you can practice mindfulness by attending to your breathing and to the various physical sensations of lifting, stretching, and balancing in a wide range of postures.

It is not easy to maintain the motivation to begin a formal meditation practice or to learn these techniques on your own from a book. For that reason, it can be very helpful to find a group of like-minded people who are also committed to regular practice. The Resources appendix has information on locating groups that may provide support for cultivating and deepening mindfulness practice, as well as on our guided meditation tapes, which can help you in your efforts to practice on your own.

INFORMAL PRACTICES

The time and energy you devote to formal mindfulness practice will support and strengthen your ability to be mindful in your daily life. In theory, it should be easy to engage in mindfulness right through your day just by reminding yourself to be in the present moment. Although it is that simple, in actuality it's not so easy to do. We tend to live a good portion of our lives on "automatic pilot," caught up in our own thoughts and feelings, our moods and our reactions to things, with little perspective on them. It's difficult to break out of that habit.

Because mindfulness is simply moment-to-moment awareness, any activ-

MINDFUL EATING: A TASTE OF MINDFULNESS

Try this exercise with any meal, a part of a meal, or even one mouthful. You'll find there are many occasions for practicing mindful eating. The idea is to eat with awareness, focusing moment by moment on seeing the food, taking it in, chewing, tasting, and swallowing. It is easier to practice mindful eating if you eat in silence than if you converse with other people. However, even in a group you can eat mindfully if you concentrate on doing so.

• First, look at what you are about to eat. What is it? How does it look? Where does it come from? How do you feel about putting this food into your body right now? How does your body feel anticipating eating in this moment?

• Tune in to your breathing as you look at the food, knowing you are about to take it into your mouth and body.

• Feel the food in your mouth. Chew slowly and focus your energy on the food's taste and texture. You might try chewing longer than you normally do to fully experience the process of chewing and tasting.

• Note any impulse you have to rush through this mouthful so that you can go on to the next. Let such impulses remind you that you already have food in your mouth, so you needn't go on to the next bite to have a complete experience of eating. Stay in the present moment with *this* mouthful, rather than rushing on to the next one.

• Before swallowing, be aware of the intention to swallow. Then feel the actual process of swallowing so that you become more conscious of this action as well.

• Approach each mouthful in the same way. Bring awareness to how much you are eating, how fast, how your body feels during and after the meal, and whether you are eating in reaction to various events in your life and to the feelings, especially anxiety or depression, that may result from them.

ity can become an occasion for practicing it: eating, showering, shaving, walking, driving, working, exercising, playing tennis, washing dishes, running errands, housecleaning, talking, playing with children, making love, or coping with a wide range of situations. (See "Mindful Eating: A Taste of Mindfulness.") The beauty of informal mindfulness practice is that it takes no extra time. All that is required is a "rotation in consciousness" from the automatic pilot mode to being fully awake.

A NOTE ON THE MEANING OF PRACTICE

Although we use the word *practice* to describe the cultivation of mindfulness, it is not meant in the usual sense of rehearsing to get better and better at something in preparation for some big event. Practice here means that you commit fully to being present in each moment. You are not trying to improve or to get anywhere in particular. You are not pursuing special insights or visions, and are not indulging in self-centeredness or self-consciousness. Practice simply means inviting yourself to embody calmness, mindfulness, and equanimity right here, right now, in this moment, as best you can.

Of course, with continued practice and the right kind of effort, calmness, mindfulness, and equanimity do deepen. Realizations, insights, and even profound experiences of stillness and joy do come. But it would be incorrect to say that the goal of practice is to make these experiences happen. The spirit of mindfulness is to practice for its own sake and just to take each moment as it comes, pleasant or unpleasant, good, bad, or ugly, and then work with that. With this attitude, everyday living becomes practice, and life itself becomes your meditation teacher and your guide.

MIND/BODY BENEFITS

Most patients who take our stress reduction program report that they enjoy it a great deal and feel it is a turning point in their lives. We have documented the program's short- and long-term effects by monitoring the health status of patients at the beginning and end of the program and by following up on them periodically afterward. In general, we find a sharp drop over the eight weeks in the number of medical symptoms patients report, as well as in such psychological problems as anxiety, depression, and hostility. These improvements occur reproducibly in the majority of patients in every class. They also occur regardless of diagnosis, suggesting that the program is relevant to people with a wide range of medical disorders and life situations.

In addition to having fewer symptoms, people experience improvements in health-related attitudes and behaviors and in how they view themselves and the world. They report feeling more self-confident, assertive, and motivated to take better care of themselves and more confident of their ability to respond effectively in stressful circumstances. They also feel a greater sense of control in their lives, an increased willingness to look at stressful events as challenges rather than threats, and a greater sense of meaning in life. Our follow-up studies show that the majority keep up their mindfulness meditation practice in one way or another (formally and informally) for up to four years, and report continuing benefits from what they learned in the program.

In one recent study, we found dramatic improvements in medical patients who also suffered from panic attacks. A common fear during a panic attack is that one is having a medical crisis, like a heart attack, that will be fatal. We find that people who can bring a mindful awareness to their breathing and to their thinking early in their experience of panic-related symptoms—like a tightness in the chest or shortness of breath—are less likely to go on to have a full panic attack.

Mindfulness is also being studied at our medical center as part of the rehabilitation program for people suffering from emphysema and chronic obstructive pulmonary disease (COPD), who must learn to function with a diminishing lung capacity. A mindfulness approach centered on breathing has been valuable in helping people with COPD keep from panicking when they experience shortness of breath from psychological stress or physical exertion. In preliminary studies, patients have reported that practicing mindfulness on a daily basis reduced the frequency and severity of their episodes of shortness of breath, increased their sense of confidence in controlling such episodes, and reduced their visits to the emergency room.

While studies of this kind do not prove the benefit of mindfulness, they do provide a strong foundation for further research. We are currently engaged in a number of controlled studies on the potential influences of mindfulness meditation on health and healing in people with specific diseases.

One such study, in collaboration with the University of Massachusetts Medical Center's Division of Dermatology, is exploring the effects of mindfulness meditation on skin clearing in patients with psoriasis—a skin disease known to have a stress-related component—who are also undergoing phototherapy (ultraviolet radiation), a standard treatment. We are measuring how fast skin clearing occurs in patients who meditate while receiving the ultraviolet light treatment, compared to similar patients who receive phototherapy without practicing mindfulness. The results from an initial study suggest that the meditators heal more quickly than those receiving only the light treatments.

HOW MINDFULNESS WORKS

Because mindfulness is a complex discipline involving a wide range of formal and informal practices, there are probably a number of different pathways by which it might have a positive influence on both your mental state and your physical health. Relaxation and changes in awareness may play different but complementary roles. A prime example is the use of mindfulness as a way to cope with a chronic pain condition that has not responded completely to traditional medical treatments (including drugs and surgery).

For some patients, notably people with muscle tension headaches, relaxation itself may be able to eliminate the problem. But for other patients—those with conditions such as chronic back pain, conditions involving nerve damage, and so on—regular relaxation usually offers only partial pain relief. However, in many such cases, the regular practice of mindfulness meditation seems to convey additional benefits by reducing the degree of *suffering* associated with a chronic pain condition. There is a certain kind of learning that goes on when you move in close to the pain with the intention to watch it, to breathe with it, even to relax into it by simply attending to the pain sensations without immediately running from them. This is not easy to do, but over time we have found that systematic mindfulness practice can help people come to see their discomfort as physical sensations that are separate and distinguishable from the negative emotions, thoughts, and interpretations those sensations often generate. This change in perception can lead to a more neutral and accepting perspective on the experience of the pain itself. Through mindfulness, you become directly aware of the reactive thoughts and feelings frequently associated with intense discomfort, such as "This pain is killing me," or "I can't go on if this keeps up." Such reactions unconsciously intensify the total pain experience, but they are potentially under our conscious control.

When people stop and ask themselves, "Right in this moment, is the pain really killing me?" the answer is usually "No." In other words, mindfulness helps patients understand that the depth of pain may come from the fear that it will continue unabated and uncontrolled, rather than from the bare physical sensation itself. This knowledge is usually enough to help people go on to develop effective practical strategies for living with significant chronic pain and the limitations it imposes, so that the pain need not totally dominate their existence and erode the quality of their lives. This is particularly useful for people who get inadequate pain relief from drugs or who are reluctant to use narcotics.

Regular mindfulness practice may also benefit physical health by increasing your sense of connection with other people and with your environment. Many people report that mindfulness meditation enhances the feeling of being part of the greater flow of life, a feeling many describe as a sense of oneness with the world, of being whole and being part of a larger whole.

Some studies have tentatively linked this psychological sense of connectedness, or oneness, with positive changes in immune function. We have collaborated with psychologists Joel Weinberger at Adelphi University and David McClelland at Boston University, who have done research on the human need for affiliation and closeness, to confirm that mindfulness really does foster a trusting sense of connectedness with others. Text analysis of stories written by patients in our program showed that they experienced more of these positive psychological changes than a control group of people who were still waiting to enter the program.

Increased trust and "oneness," along with other positive psychological changes we have observed in people in the clinic, imply that mindfulness practice can catalyze a profound change in people's outlook on themselves in relationship to the world. This degree of psychological change has been shown to endure for periods of up to three years in our follow-up studies, and it may last even longer.

It should be clear by now that mindfulness practice is not just a skill to help you handle a particular health problem; rather, it is a *way of being* that may allow you to appreciate more fully each moment of your life. However, mindfulness can only be of value if you have the discipline to practice regularly, as well as the motivation to try to be mindful in daily life. While it may not be for everybody, we have found that mainstream Americans in large numbers actually enjoy this relatively disciplined and demanding work of meditation over an eight-week period, enough to keep practicing in one way or another for years afterward. We also find that many of the people who drop out of our program, or who enroll but never attend, return a year or two later saying that they now feel ready to make the commitment to themselves.

It is important for you to know that if you try to meditate once or twice and don't feel relaxed, that is not a problem. This is one fundamental difference between relaxation exercises and meditation, especially mindfulness meditation. In exercises in which a state of relaxation is the acknowledged goal, if you don't feel relaxed at the end of it, then you can easily feel that you have failed, that either you are "no good at it" or the technique "doesn't work." So it is possible to fail in your attempts at relaxation.

In terms of formal mindfulness practices, failure is not an issue. There is no way to fail, because you are not trying to get anywhere or feel anything particular in the first place. As long as you are willing to breathe and be in the state you are already in, you are practicing mindfulness. If you stay with it, you will no doubt notice that the mind changes, the body changes, everything changes. Meanwhile, you just sit, or do the body scan, or practice yoga. In time, both mindfulness and concentration deepen, and with this deepening comes more reliable access to relaxation, inner calmness, and sustained awareness. This can be accompanied by new insights concerning who you are and how you relate to the world.

In addition, you might try to keep mindfulness alive in your daily life by asking yourself from time to time, "Am I awake now?" or "Am I fully here now?" Checking in with your breathing and with sensations in your body can be a useful anchor to keep your level of mindfulness high as you go through your day.

Mindfulness is here, in the present moment, whenever you want it. Nothing special is required. As the 15th-century poet Kabir put it:

Just throw away all thoughts of imaginary things
And stand firm in that which you are.

THE BOTTOM LINE

There is nothing magical or mystical about meditation. Basically, it is about paying attention, purposely, in the only time you have to live, namely this present moment. Mindfulness meditation can improve your ability to cope with medical and emotional challenges; its range extends well beyond that of one-pointed forms of meditation, where the goal is to focus your attention on one object and to bring your mind back to this focal point when it inevitably wanders.

In mindfulness meditation, you also begin by focusing your attention. But when your mind wanders, you observe where it has gone before you rein it in. This practice of observing thoughts, feelings, and sensations can help you achieve a calmer and broader perspective on them, one that sees and understands the mind and its activities more clearly. Mindfulness can be practiced anywhere, in any situation, but certain exercises—meditative sitting, the body scan, and yoga—are important to practice on a regular basis to deepen insight and self-understanding and to lessen your tendency to react automatically to stressful events or circumstances.

Like many mind/body techniques, mindfulness has only just begun to be explored scientifically. Preliminary clinical studies suggest that an eight-week mindfulness training program can improve a range of physical symptoms; reduce pain, depression, and anxiety; enhance feelings of trust and connectedness; and help motivate patients to take better care of their health. Generally, these benefits last for years beyond the actual mindfulness training sessions. Controlled studies are just beginning to investigate whether mindfulness can influence the healing process and help in the treatment of a number of diseases.

Mindfulness meditation involves a significant commitment to oneself. More than a technique, it is really a way of life. Many of those who practice it find that it can deeply enhance their mental and physical well-being. As one patient who is HIV-positive put it, "Mindfulness gave my life back to me."

THE BODY SCAN: BASIC INSTRUCTIONS

In this exercise, you lie on your back and move your attention slowly and systematically through the body, with moment-to-moment awareness of what you are feeling. Lying down is a wonderful way to meditate if you can stay awake in that position (which is no mean feat). To avoid being lulled to sleep, don't lie casually, but keep your legs uncrossed and your arms alongside your body with your palms up. To be of most value, the body scan should be practiced daily over a period of weeks. (For advice on using the body scan to work with pain and anxiety, see the book *Full Catastrophe Living,* listed in Resources.)

People's responses to the body scan vary greatly. Some experience calmness and a sense of well-being, which often includes a feeling of appreciating their body (sometimes for the first time in many years), a feeling of lightness or floating, or a sense of being energized. However, others sometimes feel increased tension, pain, anxiety, boredom, impatience, or other unpleasant feelings. These feelings often go away after a few days or weeks of practicing.

Ultimately, neither the pleasant nor the unpleasant feelings you may encounter are that important. What is important is a willingness to hold your feelings in awareness, whether they are pleasant, unpleasant, or neutral.

Don't be surprised if the sensations you are tuning in to change from moment to moment or from one region of the body to another. Notice that you may find some sensations pleasant, some neutral, and some extremely uncomfortable. See if you can observe your impulses—including the tendency to reject disagreeable thoughts or physical feelings—rather than automatically being carried away by them.

You can have someone read you these instructions at a slow, leisurely pace. Or you can make a tape for yourself to play while you do this exercise. (You can also order a prerecorded tape of the body scan; see Resources.) In either case, make sure the instructions leave you ample time to pay full attention to each part of the body in succession. The entire exercise can take 30 to 45 minutes, or it can be done more quickly.

• Bring your awareness to your breathing and just feel it move in and out of your body. When you are in touch with the flow of the breath—meaning you can feel a movement associated with it someplace in your body, such as at your nostrils or in the chest or abdomen—direct your attention to the toes of your left foot. Tune in to any sensations (or lack of sensations) in this region of your body. Try to remain aware of your breathing and your toes at the same time. Sometimes it helps to imagine that each in-breath travels all the way to your toes and each out-breath travels out from your toes.

- Keep this focus for a minimum of one to two minutes. If your mind wanders, gently bring it back to the feelings in your toes.
- When you feel ready, on an out-breath, purposefully let go of the toes and move your attention to the bottom of the left foot, including the heel touching the floor or the bed. Bring your attention and breathing to this region in the same way you just did with your toes. There is no "right" way to feel. The idea here is just to be in touch with your body, not to judge it or yourself.
- When you are ready (say, after a minute or two), move on to the top of your left foot—and the ankle, as well, if you choose. In this way, move through every region of your body. Systematically scan, as follows.

The left ankle . . . lower leg . . . knee . . . thigh . . . hip.

The toes of the right foot . . . bottom of the right foot and right heel . . . upper foot . . . ankle . . . lower leg . . . knee . . . thigh . . . hip.

The whole pelvis, including both hips . . . the genitals . . . buttocks . . . and rectum.

The lower back and abdomen.

The upper back, rib cage, and chest.

The shoulder blades and the shoulders.

- From here, you can go to the fingers and hands, doing left and right together, tuning in to the fingers . . . thumbs . . . palms . . . backs of the hands . . . wrists . . . forearms . . . elbows . . . upper arms and shoulders. Rather than letting go of each of these regions, expand your awareness from one region to the next until it includes the entire length of both arms, from the fingers to the shoulders. Then let go of the whole of the arms on one out-breath.
- Next, move on to the neck and throat. After breathing out and letting go there, too, move on to the head and face.

In scanning the face, start with the jaw and chin, then let the awareness gradually spread out to include, in sequence, the lips . . . teeth and gums . . . roof of the mouth . . . tongue . . . back of the throat . . . cheeks . . . nose (feel the air moving in and out of the nostrils) . . . ears (and hearing) . . . eyes . . . eyelids . . . area around the eyes . . . eyebrows . . . forehead . . . temples . . . scalp . . . and the entire cranium.

- Dwell for a while at the very top of your head. Imagine that you can exhale right through it like a whale or dolphin. See if you can feel yourself breathing in through the bottom of your feet and out through the top of your head, and vice versa. Keep this up for a few minutes and then let go of the body altogether. Just stay in the present moment with a sense of the breath flowing with no particular location.

- At this point, you can let go of your focus on your breath and simply be awake to whatever arises and predominates in your field of awareness at any given moment. This may include thoughts, feelings, sensations, sounds, the breath, stillness, silence. Be with whatever comes up in the same way you were "with" your toes and other body parts during the scan. In other words, see how you may tend to react to impulses, thoughts, memories, worries, and so on—but, instead, let yourself purposely observe them without rejecting or pursuing them or letting yourself be bored by any of them. Practice simply seeing them and letting them go, seeing them, letting go, seeing them, letting go, moment by moment, just lying here with no agenda other than to be present, to be awake.

16

HYPNOSIS: THE POWER OF ATTENTION

BY KAREN OLNESS, M.D.

IN 1987, AFTER INJURING MY THUMB IN A SKIING ACCIDENT, I DECIDED TO undergo surgery using self-hypnosis instead of chemical anesthesia. Although my surgeon was understandably dubious, he finally agreed—as long as medication was readily available, just in case. The injury presented an extraordinary opportunity to apply professional knowledge to personal circumstances: I had spent the previous 20 years teaching hypnotherapy—the therapeutic use of hypnosis—to patients and health-care professionals, as well as conducting research in the field.

The essence of self-hypnosis is to focus your attention intently. On the operating table, I put myself into a deeply relaxed state. I then concentrated deeply on a favorite memory: living on a farm as a child. In my mind, I felt what it was like to lie in the grass, gaze up at the heavens, and see a bit of the barn out of the corner of my eye. As the surgeon cut into the base of my thumb, I reassured him that I felt no pain. Throughout the operation, I kept my focus on that happy image of the farm and remained comfortable. Although I was perfectly aware that I was undergoing surgery, I just wasn't very interested in it. Colleagues experienced in hypnosis were present during the 45-minute procedure, which we videotaped. Afterward, I walked out of the operating room and had lunch with a friend. I felt great!

Though few people will make such extensive use of self-hypnosis, the technique clearly has immense potential. In fact, research is documenting its

KAREN OLNESS, M.D., is a professor in the Departments of Pediatrics, Family Medicine, and International Health at Case Western Reserve University, and is director of the Division of General Academic Pediatrics at Rainbow Babies and Children's Hospital, Cleveland.

usefulness in everything from managing chronic disease to changing poor health habits to coping with dental procedures. My colleagues and I have performed some of this research at Rainbow Babies and Children's Hospital in Cleveland. Although we have primarily studied children, many of our findings apply to adults as well.

BEYOND HOCUS-POCUS

Despite the popular stereotypes of swinging pocket watches and beady-eyed Svengalis, there is nothing magical or sinister about hypnosis. It is simply a form of self-induced, focused attention that can make it easier for you to relax or to learn to control your body's functions. The use of hypnosis for entertainment has been unfortunate because it has trivialized a serious therapeutic tool, promoted misconceptions, and led to unsuccessful applications.

In fact, people are usually led into hypnosis—a process called *hypnotic induction*—simply by listening to a voice giving them suggestions that help them become more and more deeply relaxed and focus their attention. You can enter a hypnotic state either by listening to a professional hypnotherapist or by listening to instructions on a tape. If you learn hypnosis to deal with a specific problem, as many people do, you will need to practice entering this special mental state on your own—the process of self-hypnosis. In addition, you will learn to use that state to give yourself specific suggestions to help you meet your goal.

Although hypnosis is now considered a worthy subject for scientific investigation, there is still much debate about whether it elicits a unique physiological state. At one extreme are detractors who claim that hypnosis is a sham, whose only effect is to motivate the patient psychologically to please the therapist. On the other side are researchers who believe hypnosis leads to measurable changes in brain activity that separate it from all other states of awareness.

In fact, recent brain wave experiments suggest that *something* is happening during hypnosis. A decade ago, my colleagues and I performed a study in which we coached children into a hypnotic state, had them listen to a series of sounds, and suggested to them that those sounds were getting softer. Even though the actual volume of the sounds remained constant, measurements with an electroencephalograph (EEG) showed that the children's brain waves changed in the same way that they would have if the sound level had really changed.

In another study, David Spiegel, a psychiatrist at Stanford Medical School, used an EEG to measure the brain wave patterns of people as they watched images flashed onto a television screen. Such visual stimulation creates high peaks in EEG recordings. Spiegel then coached these volunteers into a hypnotic state and had them imagine that a cardboard box was blocking the TV screen. Their EEG spikes became less steep, suggesting a drop in brain stimulation, as if the TV screen really were blocked.

In a later experiment on hypnosis and pain control, Spiegel measured the brain wave patterns of highly hypnotizable volunteers in response to a mild electric shock. When they were given the hypnotic suggestion that a local anesthetic had numbed their arms, their brain wave activity showed a lower reaction to the electric shock than they had experienced before hypnosis.

This type of evidence suggests that hypnosis does have measurable effects on the brain. However, research indicates that many brain wave changes associated with hypnosis can also be triggered by other methods of deep concentration, such as the relaxation response (Chapter 14). It seems that a hypnotic state can also occur spontaneously while reading a book, watching television, driving a car, listening to music, dancing, or doing t'ai chi. During most of these activities, people often recognize that they are in a different, but pleasant, state of focused awareness.

What separates hypnotherapy from the above activities is how you use the hypnotic state. Theodore Barber, a research psychologist who has studied hypnosis in great detail, sees hypnosis as a state of high suggestibility. Hypnotherapy makes use of this quality by having you deliberately offer yourself suggestions that can improve some aspect of your mental or physical functioning. Almost invariably, these suggestions come in the guise of imagery—you imagine seeing, hearing, smelling, tasting, or touching something. Without the focusing of attention that a hypnotic state offers, suggestions alone are unlikely to help you break bad habits or control pain, for example. And without the suggestions, a hypnotic state is unlikely to lead to behavior change. (For more on imagery and its use in healing, see Chapter 17.)

Here is an example of how hypnotherapy works:

Ann, age 9, had a habitual cough that began during a bout of viral pneumonia but continued for a year after she recovered. The cough was so disruptive that she was forced to leave school and be tutored at home, which left her depressed and lonely. Once doctors had concluded there was no anatomical explanation for the cough, Ann was referred to a pediatrician for hypnotherapy. The doctor told her that people could learn to "be the boss" of their reflexes, and Ann agreed to learn to control the cough.

The pediatrician found out as much as she could about Ann's interests and dislikes and then tailored a relaxation exercise using hypnosis especially for her. Because Ann loved music, the pediatrician had her imagine she was listening to a favorite instrumental piece to induce a hypnotic state. Ann was told that she could become as deeply relaxed as she needed to be by increasing her sense of tranquility with each new musical phrase. Ann used a biofeedback machine (see Chapter 18) to alert her to her level of relaxation, so that she could identify what deep relaxation felt like and could duplicate the sensation at home. Ann also noticed that whenever she coughed, the biofeedback machine registered that her body was less relaxed.

Ann practiced relaxation through self-hypnosis at home three times a day. Within a week, her coughing episodes had dropped by about 25 percent.

During the second visit, the pediatrician helped Ann design her own mental control system for the cough reflex to be used while under hypnosis. Ann envisioned that her nervous system was controlled by a complicated system of light switches that she could turn on and off at will. Then she practiced turning off the switch that triggered the cough reflex. She also focused on imagining how pleasant life in school would be without the cough. Over the next week, the frequency of Ann's coughs dropped by 75 percent, and during the third week they disappeared entirely. When she was evaluated one year later, the cough had not returned.

HYPNOSIS: FACT AND FICTION

As the above example shows, hypnosis is not at all a mysterious force but a form of concentration that can be put to work to benefit your health. To further clarify what hypnotherapy can and can't do, consider some myths:

While in a hypnotic state, you're under the hypnotist's control. Nonsense. All hypnosis is self-hypnosis. It is important to have a knowledgeable person teach you in the beginning, but you must reinforce the teaching yourself in order to be successful. Hence, you learn what you choose to learn. A hypnotist cannot make you do something against your will; no one can force you to rob a bank through hypnotic suggestion. In fact, the act of imagining, so important in hypnotherapy, is not a passive experience but a goal-directed, purposeful "doing."

Hypnotists use the same methods with all their patients. Wrong again. Hypnotic suggestions are based on *your* imagination, not the hypnotist's. For that reason, the imagery used varies from person to person and can make use of any of the body's senses. Children especially make use of vivid visual imagery. Many people have excellent auditory imagery: they can imagine favorite songs and symphonies in their heads. Others have strong kinesthetic imagery and can imagine the pleasant feeling of a whirlpool bath or petting a cat. Before designing a teaching plan, a good hypnotherapist will take pains to understand your preferred images, ways of thinking, and likes and dislikes. After all, you're more apt to practice self-hypnosis if the induction method is natural and pleasant.

During hypnosis, you'll be unconscious, in a trance. Actually, you'll be perfectly aware of what is going on around you, but you may choose not to focus on it. Hypnosis works best when you concentrate on your internal images and avoid being distracted by outside noises and activities. One child said, "It's like daydreaming, only you decide what you'll daydream about and how long and how come." However, if a life-threatening event like a fire were to occur, you'd immediately become alert and be ready to flee with everyone else.

You can't get out of hypnosis without going through a special ritual. Elaborate rituals, such as counting forward or backward, are unnecessary. You can leave your changed state of awareness rapidly whenever you choose.

Only some people can undergo hypnosis. Many scientific studies have assessed hypnotic responsiveness, and a number of scales have been devised for this purpose. However, clinical studies have not found them to be useful. In general, any person with normal learning skills can learn self-hypnosis for specific purposes that are in her or his best interest. Although some people have a greater natural ability to focus their attention in using hypnosis, others can learn to increase this ability through practice.

HYPNOTHERAPY IN MEDICINE

Depending on the individual's situation, hypnotherapy can be used as a complement to medical care or as a primary treatment. Many people find that hypnotherapy's benefits are enhanced by using biofeedback, a system that gives you almost instant progress reports on your attempts to induce physiological changes. Biofeedback helps patients see that they can indeed control certain bodily functions simply by altering their thoughts, and the added confidence helps them improve more rapidly.

Before beginning any course of hypnotherapy, be sure the clinician is knowledgeable, not only about hypnosis, but about the particular problem you need to have treated. (For guidance in assessing a therapist's skills, see "How to Find Good Instruction.") If you have not had a careful diagnostic assessment, you may end up using self-hypnosis for an illness that requires a different sort of therapy. For example, in a review of 80 children referred to our clinic specifically for hypnosis, 25 percent turned out to have an unrecognized biological problem for which hypnosis was not the proper primary treatment (though in some of those cases, it was a helpful addition).

Here are the most common medical uses of hypnotherapy.

MANAGEMENT OF CHRONIC ILLNESSES

There is little doubt that the regular practice of self-hypnosis is helpful to people with chronic disease. The benefits include reduction of anxiety and fear, decreased requirements for analgesics, increased comfort during medical procedures, and greater stability of functions controlled by the autonomic nervous system, such as blood pressure. Training in self-hypnosis also enhances the patient's sense of control, which is often battered by chronic illness. Finally, hypnotherapy may have direct clinical effects on certain chronic diseases, such as reducing bleeding in hemophiliacs, stabilizing blood sugar in diabetics, and reducing the severity of asthma attacks.

PAIN MANAGEMENT

Nearly every normal adult and child can use self-hypnosis to reduce the fear and anxiety that accompany pain and that can heighten it (see Chapter 6). With sufficient practice, many adults can learn to tolerate various painful procedures without medication. In a review of 18 clinical trials, Robert P. Blankfield, a specialist in family medicine at Case Western Reserve University School of Medicine, found that hypnotherapy was useful for patients undergoing a wide range of procedures—including hysterectomy, coronary bypass surgery, hemorrhoid surgery, and abdominal surgery. Among the benefits of hypnotherapy were shorter hospital stays, decreased nausea and pain, and more rapid healing.

Spinal anesthesia illusion, a technique widely used for surgery in people who have little or no tolerance for chemical anesthesia, was developed by

HOW TO FIND GOOD INSTRUCTION

Probably the least expensive way to learn self-hypnosis is through a book, audiotape, or videotape. However, these aids are not as useful as they claim to be. Hypnosis is a very individual experience: The images that work best for one person may hardly work at all for another. Hence, you're unlikely to find an ideal audiotape for you.

Beware especially of products that make unsubstantiated claims, such as subliminal learning tapes that can supposedly teach you to lose weight, improve your attitude, or sharpen your memory. Research has not supported such claims. In general, anything that seems too easy should be suspect. Making the best use of hypnosis requires weeks and months of practice—and your goal has to be realistic.

For all of these reasons, there are great advantages to learning self-hypnosis through individualized sessions with a coach or teacher. Like any skill, hypnosis is learned more rapidly with guidance. You're more apt to see improvements if there's someone available to correct your errors, give advice, and encourage you to practice.

Hypnosis should be taught only by professionals in the health sciences, including medicine, dentistry, and psychology. Seek out a person who is not only well trained in hypnotherapy but also knowledgeable about your specific problem. For example, if you want to use hypnosis for pain control during dentistry, find a dentist who specializes in the technique rather than a general hypnotherapist. Such a person would know whether an adequate diagnostic assessment has been done and could recommend further tests if necessary.

Make sure the clinician gets to know something about you before giving instructions. You aren't looking for a "cookbook" procedure but a hypnotic method tailored to your needs. For one person, imagery-based relaxation exercises may be the best route for inducing hypnosis; for another, progressive muscle relaxation may work best.

To find a qualified hypnotherapist in your area, contact the American Society of Clinical Hypnosis or the Society for Clinical and Experimental Hypnosis (see Resources).

Philip Ament, a dentist and psychologist in Buffalo, New York. In this method, the hypnotherapist helps induce a state of deep relaxation by having the patient count mentally or focus on a favorite image. The coach then suggests that the patient will feel a growing numbness spread from the navel to the toes as she or he counts to a higher and higher number. Once the patient feels numb, surgery can proceed. Afterward, the hypnotherapist gives the patient suggestions that lead to the gradual return of normal sensations.

Self-hypnosis can also be an effective means of headache control. Twelve controlled experiments have found it to be the preferred method for reducing migraine attacks in children and teenagers. In a study at Minneapolis Children's Medical Center, 30 schoolchildren with migraines were randomly assigned to receive one of three treatments: propranolol (a drug for high blood pressure commonly used to prevent migraines), a placebo in the form of a pill, and self-hypnosis. Only the group that learned self-hypnosis experienced a significant drop in the frequency and severity of their headaches.

Other clinical studies have reported similar findings. (In some of these studies, but not all, self-hypnosis included the use of biofeedback.) Research also suggests that hypnotherapy benefits adults suffering from migraine headaches as well.

It takes the average adult two months of daily practice to learn pain control. However, if you have an immediate need, you may achieve some benefit quickly.

HYPNOSIS AND DENTISTRY

Some adults have learned to tolerate drilling, extraction, and periodontal surgery using hypnosis as the sole anesthesia. In one case, a 44-year-old man who required periodontal surgery but physically could not tolerate local anesthesia was trained in self-hypnosis for a week. At the beginning of the surgery, he gave himself the suggestion that his mouth and jaw felt comfortable, even though he was aware of the procedure and of his environment. Then, for the remainder of the operation, he imagined himself on a mountain overlooking the Caribbean. At the end of the surgery, he gave himself suggestions to minimize bleeding and speed healing. He was comfortable throughout the procedure and was able to eat dinner that evening. He underwent two subsequent surgeries with similar results.

Hypnosis is beneficial during dental procedures even if chemical anesthesia is also used. Research shows that it reduces anxiety and fear; helps control bleeding, salivation, and gagging; and lessens postoperative discomfort. In children, too, it can decrease the chances of developing a dental phobia.

PREGNANCY AND DELIVERY

Lamaze and other popular breathing techniques during labor and delivery may actually work by inducing a hypnotic state. Some pregnant women choose to go even further in controlling the pain by learning formal self-hypnosis techniques. Studies have demonstrated that women who learn self-hypnosis prior to delivery have shorter labors and more comfortable deliveries than other pregnant women. There are even reports of cesarean sections performed with hypnosis as the sole anesthesia. (In one documentary film of such a procedure, the mother, an opera singer, sang throughout the incision and delivery!)

Self-hypnosis can be taught with great success to expectant parents in groups. Husbands can be taught how to coach their wives—because most women appreciate having a trusted person working with them during labor and delivery—and can rehearse their coaching in the group setting. With this training, most husbands are able to help their wives during the actual labor and delivery.

ANXIETY

Performance anxiety, better known as stage fright, is a psychological problem, not a medical one, but it is common, potentially disabling, and often treated with drug therapy. Hypnosis offers an alternative. Typically, the therapist helps the performer undo a conditioned physiological response to performing, such as hyperventilation or nausea. This method can be used to help calm children and adolescents preparing for such activities as ice skating tournaments, basketball free throws, piano recitals, tennis tournaments, ski slalom races, and swimming meets. Because such children are highly motivated and accustomed to practice routines, they usually do well with self-hypnosis.

Hypnotherapy can also be used to quell the fear associated with exams, writing tasks, and public speaking. But in order to have a rapid, automatic response when faced with the fearful situation, an adult must be willing to devote sufficient practice time (usually 30 minutes daily) for a few months before the event. Children require less practice.

ESPECIALLY FOR CHILDREN

Young people have far greater success with hypnosis for medical purposes than do adults, perhaps because using imagination comes so easily to the young. In the course of their daily play, children move in and out of various states of awareness without closing their eyes or sitting still to concentrate. Through hypnotherapy, children can develop pain control strategies in just a few practice sessions; adults often require many sessions. Children can also quickly learn to control the various responses measured by biofeedback machines as signs of relaxation, such as fingertip temperature or heart rate.

Breaking bad health habits is also easier for children, perhaps because they have had less time to reinforce them and can imagine life without them more easily than adults can. Numerous studies document the effectiveness of hypnotherapy to resolve thumb sucking, hair pulling, bed-wetting, tics, and habitual coughs. In a study of more than 500 children with habit problems, 80 percent began to improve significantly after just three or four self-hypnosis training sessions.

Once children solve an immediate problem through hypnotherapy, they often naturally use self-hypnosis in other areas of their lives. Parents will report, for example, that a child who learned self-hypnosis in preparation for dental surgery later used hypnotic suggestion to prepare for a swim meet.

For hypnotherapy to work for children, there must be no underlying biological problem, and the child should be well motivated and willing to assume the primary responsibility for change. Be sure to find a good hypnotherapist: People who teach children self-hypnosis must be knowledgeable about child development and proceed only after a careful assessment of the child's medical situation, understanding of the habit and of the motivation of the child and family members. The Society for Behavioral Pediatrics provides information on hypnosis in children (see Resources).

Under the right circumstances, hypnotherapy is less expensive, time-consuming, and dangerous than some other tactics that may be used for pediatric problems, such as medications to thwart bed-wetting. An additional benefit is the enhanced self-esteem and sense of competence that children gain from resolving a problem on their own.

HYPNOSIS AND THE IMMUNE SYSTEM

During the past 20 years, many published studies have linked stress or de-pression with immunological changes in both animals and humans. There have been a few large leaps from these findings to attempts to treat immune-system-mediated diseases with mind/body therapies. Perhaps best known is the use of imagery to mobilize positive immune responses in cancer patients (see Chapters 5 and 17). Such procedures may induce an altered state of awareness, perhaps similar to hypnosis; but for the most part, research has not yet shown them to be therapeutic.

However, a few controlled studies involving healthy people have now shown that it is indeed possible to alter certain immune system responses through such mind/body techniques as hypnosis. At Minneapolis Children's Medical Center, we conducted the first study in this area specifically related to children.

At the outset, we measured the levels of certain immune system sub-stances called *salivary immunoglobulins* in the saliva of 57 children, ages 6 to 12. The children were then split into three groups. The first group learned a simple form of self-hypnosis, using imagery to relax deeply. The second group learned the same exercise with additional hypnotic suggestions to increase salivary immunoglobulin. (We had shown them a videotape on how the im-mune system works and then simply asked them to increase the immune substances in their saliva.) The third group spent the time engaged in ordi-nary conversation.

Afterward, the children's saliva was measured again. The second group, which had learned the specific suggestions, showed a striking increase in their levels of one of the salivary immunoglobulins, called *IgA*. The other two groups showed no change.

In a recent study with adolescents, we found that self-hypnosis training led to significant changes in the activity of white blood cells. These cells are key components of the immune system.

Although such studies raise intriguing possibilities, more research is nec-essary to determine how extensive such voluntary changes can be, how much training is required to trigger them, and what the clinical significance and applications may be, if any.

One well-documented medical use of self-hypnosis that probably works by training the immune system is the treatment of warts (see Chapter 8).

Preliminary studies have suggested that hypnotherapy can make warts shrink and disappear. A multi-institutional study is now comparing the standard topical treatment of warts with the self-hypnosis method.

HABIT CONTROL

There is a common misconception that hypnosis works wonders for people who want to kick poor health habits. In fact, this is the area in which hypnosis is probably least helpful. Hypnosis works by harnessing your imagination. If you can't imagine giving up a habit—which is often the case if the habit is entrenched—hypnosis can't help you do it. For example, in a study of adolescent girls who were obese because they overate, the only ones who were able to lose pounds *and* keep them off long-term were the small minority who, from the start, were able to imagine and describe vividly how their lives would change when they lost weight.

Quitting smoking is one of the most popular applications for hypnotherapy. But none of the many one-session individual or group hypnosis programs to help smokers break the habit are likely to have long-term effects. Typically, these sessions have you focus on the negative outcomes of smoking (yellow nails, black lungs, and so on) or on positive images of what life would be like without cigarettes (for example, how fresh your clothes would smell). The glitch: For many people, smoking is so intrinsic to their lives that they can't fully envision their world without the habit.

These people may understand intellectually why they should stop. They may say that they wish to quit and may even invest time and money in various methods. But countless images of yellow nails or fresh-smelling sweaters won't help them until they can fully imagine their lives without smoking, a process that may require lengthy reflection and self-assessment.

THE BOTTOM LINE

In hypnotherapy, you enter a hypnotic state—a relaxed state of intense, focused concentration—and offer yourself suggestions aimed at improving your mental or physical health. Almost always, these suggestions are made in the form of imagery—using your ability to see, hear, touch, smell, and taste things in your mind.

Virtually anyone can be coached into hypnosis. And despite the myths,

---

IS HYPNOSIS FOR YOU?

Your honest answers to the following questions can help you determine whether self-hypnosis is likely to work for you.

☐ *Do you like to take personal responsibility for your health?* If you'd rather have your problem solved with a pill, hypnosis is not for you. Without a desire to take charge of your health, you'll be unlikely to stick to a hypnotherapy program.

☐ *Do you have a good imagination—either visual, auditory, or kinesthetic?* Almost everyone does. However, if you *believe* that you do not, you are probably less likely to benefit from hypnotherapy because all the strategies for using it work by harnessing your imagination.

☐ *Do you have a clear outcome in mind?* For hypnotherapy to work, you must know what you wish to accomplish—and believe that you can do it. Hypnotherapy is often unsuccessful in helping people kick entrenched habits like smoking because they can't really imagine life without the habit, even though they want to quit. If you're having trouble in this area, ongoing help from a coach or therapist may be necessary.

☐ *Are you willing to put in the time to acquire this skill?* Hypnotherapy is rarely effective overnight—although some gains may come quickly.

---

you will not be "out of it" while you are under hypnosis and will not need to perform some special sort of ritual to return to a normal state.

Hypnotherapy can be used for medical and emotional problems as a primary or additional treatment, depending on the particular circumstances. Among the medical uses of hypnotherapy are controlling pain (including pain at the dentist or during labor and delivery) and the management of chronic illnesses. Preliminary evidence suggests that hypnotic suggestion may influence the immune system, but the practical applicability of these changes is still unknown.

Although hypnotherapy is often used in efforts to break such bad habits as smoking, this approach has a low success rate in adults. However, hypnotherapy is especially effective for habit control and other uses in children, in part because of their great powers of imagination and openness to suggestion.

Hypnosis can be learned on your own, but it is easier to master with the help of expert guidance. It is essential that the coach or teacher be a health-care professional who is thoroughly knowledgeable about the problem you want addressed. You must also be carefully diagnosed for medical problems before embarking on hypnotherapy.

Perhaps the greatest general drawback to hypnotherapy is that it takes time and effort to learn. True, an injured person undergoing treatment in an emergency room can quickly master some self-hypnotic skills to help control pain and anxiety. But that is a rare situation in which the patient is highly motivated to learn very quickly. Most of the problems that hypnosis tackles, whether poor health habits or chronic physical problems, have developed over months or years, and time is required to eliminate them.

But although self-hypnosis demands a long-term commitment, the benefits can be well worth it. We live in a society that has become dependent on pharmacological interventions to solve medical problems. Imagine the difference it would make if nearly everyone, beginning in childhood, were to learn and practice self-regulation methods like hypnosis, and thus develop a greater sense of mastery over their own lives.

17

IMAGERY: LEARNING TO USE THE MIND'S EYE

BY MARTIN L. ROSSMAN, M.D.

WHEN HE FIRST CAME TO SEE ME FOR TREATMENT, 24-YEAR-OLD JASON wanted to manage his asthma better and perhaps reduce his need for medication. With that goal, I taught him a simple relaxation technique. First, he relaxed the muscles in his body, one at a time, and imagined himself in one of his favorite places. Next, he used a more specific kind of mental imagery: envisioning his lung passages opening wide and air moving through them freely. By practicing this imagery exercise for about 20 minutes twice a day, he was able to lower his drug dosage and even went for long periods without an asthma attack.

Then, suddenly, the method stopped working. In fact, sometimes imagery made it *harder* for him to breathe. Because imagery had once helped him control his asthma so successfully, I suggested that we try a different type of imagery exercise to help him understand what had gone wrong.

After Jason lulled himself into a relaxed state, I advised him to allow an image to enter his mind that would offer a clue to the mystery. He began to see an agitated dwarf dressed like a Roman soldier patrolling the entrance to a tunnel. The dwarf, who called himself Romeo, said he was guarding the roads to Jason's heart. If anyone started to get too close, he would close off the tunnel entrance. Jason thought the tunnel reminded him of a bronchial tube. He also pictured many such guards at the "outposts" of his bronchial tubes

MARTIN L. ROSSMAN, M.D., is a clinical associate in the Department of Medicine at the University of California, San Francisco, and codirector of the Academy for Guided Imagery in Mill Valley, California.

and saw the tubes all contract and close down in response to a threatened "invasion."

After this exercise, Jason realized that the resurgence of his asthma coincided with the onset of a new romance. His intense feelings for his girlfriend so frightened him that he had been unknowingly using the asthma to keep her away. Because of his illness, he often canceled their dates. And when they were together, she spent much of the time taking care of him, though he really wanted a relationship based on mutual caring. With frustration and embarrassment, he recalled previous budding romances that had been sabotaged by flare-ups of his asthma.

Similarly, he now saw that he had unconsciously used his condition for emotional purposes during childhood. Back then, having an attack meant getting extra care from his mother and the chance to skip activities he disliked, such as gym class and trips to visit relatives.

To break the cycle, I encouraged Jason to tell Romeo that he appreciated being protected from emotional pain, but that this vigilance was, in itself, causing pain and physical illness. In his mind, he told the dwarf that he felt ready to risk more intimate relationships, though he still wanted some protection. He began to imagine a series of checkpoints at different distances along the "roads" to his heart and how it felt to allow various people closer. He even envisioned issuing "security clearances" to certain individuals, including his girlfriend. This helped him experience how it felt to allow different levels of intimacy.

After that session, Jason was better able to relax and regulate his breathing. Over the next several months, his asthma did occasionally worsen, but he took those episodes as a sign to pay closer attention to his feelings, especially about his deepening romantic relationship. Within a year, his flare-ups again became rare occurrences.

Jason's case demonstrates two major ways in which guided imagery, as this approach is called, is now used in health care. It can be used *actively* to help alleviate symptoms, as Jason did by envisioning his bronchial tubes widening. And it can be used *receptively*—"allowing" images to come to mind— to help us understand the emotional meaning our symptoms may have.

The use of inner visions to help the healing process is hardly a new concept. Tibetan Buddhists have been using images in this way since the 13th century, if not earlier. The Buddhist approach typically involves meditating on the image of a deity in the act of healing a symptom. Shamanistic practices in cultures throughout the world have employed a similar approach. Only recently, however, has imagery been used by Western physicians and health-care providers.

As a primary-care physician treating mostly patients with chronic conditions, I became interested in imagery first as a way to help alleviate my patients' suffering. Since 1972, I have taught imagery techniques to thousands of people. I have seen many people recover from their illnesses after using imagery and others who have been helped by imagery to lead rewarding lives in spite of their disease.

There are still only a few carefully controlled, scientific studies to show precisely how great an impact imagery by itself can have on the body. Such studies are difficult to design and carry out, for several reasons. For one thing, imagery is often used in conjunction with other mind/body techniques, such as hypnosis and simple relaxation, making it difficult to separate out the effects of the imagery alone. In addition, the "receptive" imagery techniques are so extremely individualized that it is hard to quantify their effects.

Nevertheless, a small but growing body of clinical evidence strongly suggests that imagery can help people with a wide range of physical illnesses. And some sophisticated physiological studies are pointing the way to understanding just how imagery exerts its effects.

HOW DOES IMAGERY WORK?

The modern use of therapeutic imagery usually entails a 20- to 25-minute session that begins with a relaxation exercise to help focus attention and "center" your mind. If this doesn't adequately ward off distractions, you can also start by inducing a hypnotic state.

Although imagery is often used together with hypnosis (described in Chapter 16), the two techniques are independent and complementary. Put simply, hypnosis is the induction of a particular state of mind, while imagery is an activity. It's perfectly possible to have one without the other, though the combination may be most effective.

In hypnotherapy, specific suggestions are used to relieve physical symptoms, and imagery is generally the most powerful and effective way to provide such suggestions. Rather than simply saying "Your pain is diminishing," for example, a hypnotist may ask you to imagine a painful part of your body feeling warm or going numb. (Imagery itself can also be used to induce a hypnotic state in the first place.)

During a typical session of imagery, you focus on a predetermined image designed to help you control a particular symptom (active imagery) or you allow your mind to conjure up images that give you insight into a particular problem (receptive imagery). Depending on your needs, imagery can be explored on your own, with the help of a book or audiotape, or with a therapist's guidance (see Resources).

Although science has not found a precise basis for imagery's healing abilities, we know enough to make some reasonable speculations about how it works. Visual, auditory, and tactile imagery seem to arise from the brain's cerebral cortex, the seat of higher mental functions, such as language, thinking, and problem solving. (Imagery having to do with smell or emotional experiences may arise from more primitive brain centers.)

When researchers have used a sophisticated technique called *positron emission tomography* (PET) to monitor the brain during imagery exercises, they have found that the same parts of the cerebral cortex are activated whether people imagine something or actually experience it. This suggests that picturing visual images activates the optic cortex, imagining that you are listening to music arouses the auditory cortex, and conjuring up tactile sensations stimulates the sensory cortex. Thus, vivid imagery can send a message from the cerebral cortex to the lower brain centers, including the limbic system, the emotional center of the brain. From there, the message is relayed to the endocrine system and the autonomic nervous system, which can affect a range of bodily functions, including heart rate, perspiration, and blood pressure (see Chapter 2).

Many clinicians believe that the more fully you imagine something, the more "real" it seems to the brain and the greater the amount of information sent to the nervous system. This is one reason it's helpful to use as many senses as possible during guided imagery sessions. (For example, you might imagine lying on the beach, feeling the warm sand, listening to the ocean, and smelling the sea air.) While visualization is certainly the most common form of imagery—and, for most people, the easiest—it's not the only one. People who have trouble visualizing may be able to relax by imagining the warmth of the sun, recalling a favorite tune, or conjuring up the aroma of brewing coffee or the taste of freshly baked bread.

THE VALUE OF IMAGERY

Three major qualities of imagery make it particularly valuable in mind/body medicine and healing: It can bring about physiological changes, provide psychological insight, and enhance emotional awareness.

PHYSIOLOGICAL CHANGES

Imagery has great potential to affect physiology directly. If you were consciously to try to salivate right now, you probably wouldn't be able to. But notice what happens if you imagine the following. (This exercise is particularly effective if you close your eyes and have a friend read aloud the next two paragraphs.)

> You are standing in your kitchen in front of a cutting board. Next to it is a good, sharp knife. Take a few moments to imagine the kitchen: the color of the countertops, the appliances, the cupboards, windows, and so on. Also notice any kitchen smells or sounds—the running of a dishwasher or the hum of a refrigerator.
>
> Now imagine that on the board sits a plump, fresh, juicy lemon. In your mind, hold the lemon in one hand, feeling its weight and texture. Then place it back on the board and carefully cut it in half with the knife. Feel the resistance to the knife and how it gives way as the lemon splits. Notice the pale yellow of the pulp, the whiteness of the inner peel, and see whether you have cut through a seed or two. Carefully cut one of the halves in two. See where a drop or two of juice has pearled on the surface of one of the quarters. Imagine lifting this lemon wedge to your mouth, smelling the sharp fresh scent. Now bite into the sour, juicy pulp.

At the end of this exercise, most people will salivate, especially from the back of the jaws—a simple illustration of imagery's ability to trigger a physiological response. But imagery can also trigger physical reactions that are more subtle than salivation and more important for health. There is preliminary evidence that imagery can have specific effects on the immune system, although the explanation for these findings remains unclear. In several experiments, researchers have looked at the physical effects of imagery combined with other relaxation and stress management techniques, such as the relaxation response, biofeedback, and progressive muscle relaxation. Although these studies did not focus narrowly on imagery, they do suggest it can contribute to a wide range of changes in such physiological functions as heart rate, blood pressure, breathing patterns, brain wave rhythms, blood flow, gastrointestinal activity, sexual arousal, and the release of various hormones and neurotransmitters.

PSYCHOLOGICAL INSIGHT

Imagery can also help illuminate the connections between stressful circumstances and physical symptoms, where such connections exist. It does this by helping you see the big picture.

When you perceive the world as most people usually do, through logical, linear thinking, you attempt to break it down into small pieces and find the sequences that lead from one piece to the other. Logical thinking is similar to watching a train round the bend: You see one car at a time, with maybe just a little bit of the car that went before it. But imagery puts you in a balloon hundreds of feet above the track, high enough to see the entire train and several miles of track, as well as the town it came from and the city it's going to, the fields through which the train runs, and the mountain range in the distance. You grasp the whole picture and see how each of its parts is related to the rest. In much the same way, imagery can help you perceive connections between physical symptoms and emotional or stressful situations you wouldn't otherwise realize.

Here's an example. Two years ago I treated a woman who suffered from chronic arm pain that defied medical diagnosis. During an imagery exercise, she saw the pain as angle irons in her shoulders and metal bars in her arms. She said the images were hard, rigid, cold, and unyielding. When asked for other associations, she immediately thought of her grandfather, whom she had nursed for two years until he died some months before. She wept as she told me she had loved him a great deal, but hadn't been able to have the relationship she wanted with him because he was emotionally hard, cold, and rigid—the very qualities represented in the image of her pain.

I had her use imagery to create a dialogue with her grandfather. In her mind, she expressed all of her feelings to him, and he seemed to soften and thank her for the loving care. He told her he loved her but wasn't able to express it. They embraced, and a warm feeling began to run through her arms. She had a few follow-up sessions and has been pain-free ever since. The imagery exercises helped her make the connection between her physical pain and its psychological cause, and she was finally able to heal.

EMOTIONAL AWARENESS

The third significant attribute of imagery is its close relationship to the emotions. You can think of the emotions as the means by which thoughts create changes in the body: Fear makes our hearts pound, grief makes us shed tears, and joy leads to laughter. But the natural ways of demonstrating emotions—especially negative ones, such as anger and sadness—are often socially unacceptable and are suppressed. People may then find unhealthful outlets for such emotions, such as physical symptoms or behaviors (smoking, drinking, workaholism, and so on) that lead to health problems. Imagery is one of the quickest and most direct ways to become aware of one's emotional state and its potential effects on health.

Here's a brief exercise to illustrate the emotional power of imagery:

Close your eyes. Take a couple of deep, slow breaths, letting yourself relax as you exhale. Begin to focus inside, and recall a room from your childhood. Notice what you see there and any sounds you might hear in the room. Is there an aroma? What else do you notice? Do any feelings come up as you imagine this? Just notice them and let them be there. Then let that image fade, and imagine that you are looking at a very close friend, smiling at you. Notice your friend's smile and his or her eyes. What does this person seem to be communicating?

Take a few minutes to think about this experience, perhaps writing down some notes about it. How did you feel as you contemplated these two simple images? How much did you write? Notice that it was all communicated to you in a second or two through each image. These mental pictures (in whatever sensory mode they appear) are very often worth thousands of words and are a very efficient form of information storage and recall.

HEALING THROUGH IMAGERY

Although there is little careful, well-controlled research on the medical benefits of imagery, clinical reports suggest that the technique may help treat a wide range of conditions, including chronic pain, allergies, high blood pressure, irregular heartbeats, autoimmune diseases, cold and flu symptoms, and stress-related gastrointestinal, reproductive, and urinary complaints. Imagery may also help speed healing after an injury, such as a sprain, strain, or broken bone.

Many of these benefits stem directly from the relaxing effects of imagery. In fact, the most common, most useful, and easiest application of imagery in health care is its use in relaxation and stress reduction. Many people find guided imagery the simplest, most natural way to relax.

To get a taste of how relaxing imagery can be, try a simple, quick exercise:

Keep your eyes closed while you take a few deep, easy breaths, and imagine yourself in the most peaceful, beautiful, serene place you can conjure up. Think of a time when you felt relaxed and peaceful—perhaps a walk in the park, a day on a sunny beach, or an evening at a concert—and focus intently on the sights, smells, and physical sensations associated with that event. Focus on this image for about five minutes.

When you return to everyday reality, you're likely to feel calmer, more alert, and refreshed—as if you'd had a much longer rest. This sort of imagery is common to most relaxation techniques, from progressive muscle relaxation to various forms of meditation (see Chapter 14).

Beyond relaxation, however, active imagery is used—often together with hypnosis—to conjure up positive images designed to alleviate physical symptoms directly. In some cases, these images may have a direct physiological effect. When Jason, the man with asthma, visualized his bronchial tubes opening, he probably began breathing more slowly and deeply without quite being aware of it—changes that would be particularly beneficial for his asthma.

In other cases, imagery may have a beneficial effect on patients even though its effect on their disease can't be determined. The use of imagery in cancer therapy is a good example. In the early 1970s, radiation oncologist O. Carl Simonton and psychologist Stephanie Simonton taught active imagery to cancer patients in the hope that it would help them fight off the disease. (A typical exercise was to imagine the immune system's cells devouring the cancer cells.) Their work received a great deal of publicity and sparked a lot of interest in imagery in general.

In the two decades since the Simontons developed their approach, no definitive, well-controlled study has been done to show whether this kind of imagery improves the overall prognosis for people with cancer (see Chapter 5). But many people find this kind of imagery helpful, even if it doesn't cure their disease. They report such benefits as relief from anxiety and pain, greater tolerance of chemotherapy or radiation therapy, and a heightened ability to cope with the illness. Imagery helps them to relax and to feel less helpless.

People with cancer or any other illness should not rely on imagery as their sole means of treatment when other, proven methods are available. Still, imagery can be a powerful aid in increasing the effectiveness of medical treatments or helping people to endure them. Combined with relaxation techniques, imagery has helped people to tolerate such diagnostic and therapeutic procedures as magnetic resonance imaging examinations, bone marrow biopsies, and cancer chemotherapy and radiation. It can also help people prepare for surgery and recover from it.

Another role imagery plays in medical care is to put you in touch with your feelings about your illness. Imagery can be helpful in almost any medical situation that requires problem solving or decision making. By using receptive imagery to explore your emotional reactions to your medical circumstances, you may emerge with a clearer sense of how best to treat an illness or live well in spite of it. You may also better understand how your life-style choices may be affecting your health. If your illness is fulfilling some emotional need, coming to terms with that need may ease your physical symptoms.

Receptive imagery treatment may involve a dialogue with images representing symptoms or the illness, such as Jason's encounter with Romeo. During receptive imagery sessions you may also wish to develop an image of your "inner adviser"—an embodiment of your inner wisdom—who can help you understand the emotional meaning of body sensations and symptoms. In my experience, this two-way use of imagery to spur communication between mind and body yields the most profound healing responses.

THE BOTTOM LINE

Depending on the severity of your problem, you may want to try using imagery on your own or with professional help. (For advice on finding help, see Resources.) Since imagery may change the body's requirements for medications, it may be best for you to use it under the guidance of your physician, depending on your medical condition. In any case, if you plan to begin an imagery program, it's best to set relatively small goals at first, perhaps aiming simply to learn to relax. Most people can experience relaxation with imagery in a very short time, even during the first session. Once you've mastered that, you can go on to try more complex forms of imagery.

For chronic symptoms, such as pain, you may want to begin by practicing 15 to 20 minutes twice a day for three weeks. This is usually enough to see if the imagery is helpful. For receptive imagery, it often takes two or three sessions with an experienced therapist or instructor to get initial results. It may take longer if you are working on your own or with self-help tapes.

If you use active imagery, keep a daily journal in which you estimate your symptoms' severity day to day. Over several weeks, this will help you determine whether the imagery is having an effect. Similarly, if you are using receptive imagery, it can be helpful to keep a journal of your experiences with imagery, as well as your dreams and emotional reactions.

Until more careful research is done, we don't really know imagery's potential or limitations as a healing tool. Some people seem to respond to it remarkably well, while others don't. Many factors, from your physical condition to your inner resolve, may affect the treatment's success. Experimenting with imagery, however, is easy, safe, and inexpensive. All it takes is the time and willingness to unlock the power of your imagination.

18

BIOFEEDBACK: USING THE BODY'S SIGNALS

BY MARK S. SCHWARTZ, PH.D., AND NANCY M. SCHWARTZ, M.A.

THE STUDENT WAS SKEPTICAL, BUT THE INSTRUCTIONS WERE CLEAR: TO earn an A in the biofeedback course, she would have to learn how to bring the temperature of her hands up to 92 degrees from their present level of 72 degrees. Success would mean she had mastered an important goal: to exercise control over the autonomic nervous system—the part of the nervous system that regulates bodily functions such as blood flow, skin temperature, and heart rate.

The tool her college professor offered was a simple electronic device with a temperature sensor taped to the tip of her finger. A high-pitched tone reflected the coldness of her hand. If she succeeded in warming that hand, the pitch would drop. The task was to learn how to raise her temperature using the device as her guide and then duplicate the hand-warming on her own.

For two weeks, she tried various strategies to lower the tone. First, she tried telling herself repeatedly that her skin temperature was going up. No luck—the pitch stayed high. Next, she tried to picture her hands feeling warmer and warmer by imagining herself at the beach. This lowered the

MARK S. SCHWARTZ, PH.D., past president of the Biofeedback Society of America, is a staff psychologist at the Mayo Clinic in Jacksonville, Florida. NANCY M. SCHWARTZ, M.A., is a licensed mental health counselor and a certified biofeedback therapist in private practice in Orange Park, Florida.

pitch, but only slightly. Finally, she concentrated on actually feeling the warm blood pulsing in her fingertips. At last, the tone dropped from soprano to alto.

This was only the first step. For her final exam, she would have to warm her skin temperature without guidance from the instrument. For weeks, she practiced at home. She thought about her pulse, imagining the blood right under her fingertips warming her skin. By exam day, she was warming her hands regularly and earned the A.

The story would end there if the student had not discovered an unexpected dividend in all those weeks of training: The weekly migraine headaches that had plagued her for years had all but disappeared. The hand-warming process was a way of calming the activity of the autonomic nervous system, and thus easing the migraines.

The experience changed the woman's life. Inspired by her experience and her new ability to make positive changes in her health, she developed a career in biofeedback.

The woman is Nancy Schwartz, coauthor of this chapter and now a certified biofeedback therapist in Orange Park, Florida. She met coauthor Mark S. Schwartz in 1987 because of her career: He was president of the Biofeedback Society of America, and she was studying for her certification from his recently published book on biofeedback. They are now a team in writing and in life.

THE EVOLUTION OF BIOFEEDBACK

Biofeedback therapies emerged in the 1970s, when advances in psychological and medical research converged with developments in biomedical technology. Improved electronic instruments could convey information to patients about their autonomic nervous systems and their muscles in the form of audio and visual signals that patients could understand. The word *biofeedback* became the shorthand term for the procedures and treatments that make use of these instruments, and biofeedback came into widespread use.

Biofeedback means living (*bio*, as in biology) feedback. It uses special instruments and methods to expand the body's natural internal feedback systems. All of us are constantly receiving feedback from our bodies and responding to it. Your arm feels pain from carrying a package or suitcase too long, so you put it down or switch arms. Your heart pounds too rapidly while jogging, and you know to slow down. However, many of the body's systems produce subtle changes of which people are not aware. Scientists and practitioners reasoned that amplifying and transforming the body's signals into useful information would put us on our way toward increasing our voluntary control over these systems.

Today, computers give more detailed and more interesting information than the early biofeedback instruments could. A therapist can help you understand how to relate the external signals to bodily changes. With biofeedback, you learn more about the relationships among thoughts, posture, breathing, and these internal changes.

A therapist can then give suggestions and instructions to help you make the changes needed to learn more control of your body. As you learn, feedback signals reflect your progress. Biofeedback shows you and your therapist which strategies work for reaching your treatment goals.

Biofeedback is successful in helping people learn to regulate many physical conditions partly because it puts them in better contact with specific parts of their bodies. Any bodily process and change that we can measure accurately, we can use as biofeedback. For example, biofeedback can help teach people to tighten muscles at the neck of the bladder to better control their impaired bladder function. It can help postoperative patients learn to reuse muscles of the legs and arms. It can help teach stroke patients to use alternate muscles to move a limb if the primary ones can no longer do the job. Biofeedback is also helpful in training patients to use artificial limbs after amputation.

While some people can learn these skills without the help of electronic instruments, biofeedback is useful clinically for many people who are unable to learn them by other means. It is now part of the treatment of many disorders, including headaches, anxiety, Raynaud's disease, high blood pressure, teeth clenching and grinding, asthma, chronic pain, incontinence, and muscle disorders.

Researchers are also experimenting with biofeedback treatments for conditions believed to stem from irregular brain wave patterns, such as epilepsy and attention deficit hyperactivity disorder (ADHD) in children. When one attaches patients to an electroencephalograph (EEG), which displays brain wave patterns, the patients see which brain waves they are producing and in what quantity. In ADHD, for example, there are not enough of the specific waves needed for concentration and focusing. Children learn how to change their brain waves and then learn to produce the same effect without the EEG instrument and feedback. Results with this method are promising.

Professionals who use biofeedback believe it provides new, logical approaches to solving some health problems. When you use the information to make changes that can help reduce or stop symptoms, you replace feelings of helplessness with knowledge and the feeling that self-regulation is possible. In some cases, people learn faster and more reliably with biofeedback than with other approaches.

FIVE COMMON TYPES OF BIOFEEDBACK

Any bodily process or change that therapists can monitor accurately can be used for biofeedback. Here are the most frequent measurements used and the disorders they help treat.

ELECTROMYOGRAPHIC (EMG) BIOFEEDBACK
What it measures: Muscle tension.
Method: Sensors attached to the skin detect electrical activity related to muscle tension in that area. The biofeedback instrument amplifies and converts this activity into useful information. The feedback displays degrees of muscle tension and guides you toward relaxing the muscles or tensing them, depending on your goal.
Often used for: Tension headaches, physical rehabilitation, chronic muscle pain, incontinence, general relaxation.

THERMAL BIOFEEDBACK
What it measures: Temperature of the skin, as an index of blood flow changes from constriction and dilation of blood vessels. Low skin temperature usually means decreased blood flow in that area. Cold hands or feet may mean arousal of parts of the autonomic nervous system.

Method: Therapists tape a temperature-sensitive probe (sometimes called a *thermistor*) to the skin, often on a finger. The instruments convert this information into feedback you can see and hear. Temperature feedback can help you learn to reduce constriction of blood vessels in hands and feet.

Often used for: Raynaud's disease, migraine headaches, hypertension, anxiety, general relaxation.

ELECTRODERMAL ACTIVITY (EDA)

What it measures: Changes in sweat activity too small to feel.

Method: Two sensors attached to the palm side of the fingers or hand measure sweat. They produce a tiny electrical current that measures skin conductance based on the amount of moisture present. Increased sweat can mean arousal of part of the autonomic nervous system. Stressful thoughts, rapid deep breathing, and feeling startled can increase sweat output.

Often used for: Anxiety, hyperhidrosis (a condition characterized by overactive sweat glands).

FINGER PULSE

What it measures: Pulse rate and force (the amount of blood in each pulse).

Method: A sensor attached to a finger helps measure heart activity as a sign of arousal of part of the autonomic nervous system.

Often used for: Hypertension, anxiety, some cardiac arrhythmias.

BREATHING

What it measures: Breath rate, volume, rhythm, and location (chest and abdomen).

Method: Some therapists place sensors around the chest and abdomen. Another method measures air flow from the mouth and nose. The feedback is usually visual. You learn to take deeper, slower, lower, and more regular breaths using abdominal muscles.

Often used for: Asthma, hyperventilation, anxiety, general relaxation.

THE RELAXATION CONNECTION

Biofeedback is often part of relaxation treatments for lowering physical tension and arousal that cause and worsen many disorders. These include migraine and tension headaches, high blood pressure, chronic pain, and anxiety. Some researchers attribute biofeedback's success in treating various health problems to the relaxation it promotes.

A general goal of relaxation treatments is to lower body tension and change faulty breathing patterns in order to reduce symptoms. Specific relaxation goals include reducing the number of times you become tense and the intensity and duration of that tension. Other goals include relaxing deeply enough and doing it often enough and long enough each time to help.

Many people can and do reach these goals of relaxation without biofeedback. The question is not whether biofeedback is always necessary—it isn't—but whether it would add something useful to your treatment.

For example, you might subjectively feel relaxed, but measurements might show that you are not relaxing your body. Biofeedback either gives you assurance that physical changes are occurring or indicates that they are not. For many people, the benefits of healing relaxation depend on actual bodily relaxation; the subjective sense of feeling relaxed is not enough.

If you are not relaxing enough, biofeedback gives you information to let you know when you are heading in the right direction. It lets you and your therapist know which techniques are helpful and which ones are not.

Another asset is its ability to help people focus on tension and relaxation within the body. One can use biofeedback to target a specific body part—say, the muscles in your neck or the blood vessels in your hand—making relaxation treatment more specific and effective.

For others—those who already can relax their muscles and the body's systems—biofeedback increases awareness and confidence in relaxation skills. Such confidence can be a wonderful part of the healing process: It can increase motivation and positive expectations and help people relax more consistently in their daily lives.

EXAMPLES OF APPLICATIONS

Although biofeedback is used in the treatment of many problems, some applications may be especially useful. The treatment of headaches and Raynaud's disease are two examples of biofeedback therapy with more well-controlled studies and well-documented positive effects of biofeedback than in most other treatment applications.

HEADACHES

Preventing and treating headaches is a common use for biofeedback. For headaches caused or increased by muscle tension, therapists place biofeedback sensors on your head and sometimes other places, such as your neck. This is electromyographic (EMG) biofeedback. The instruments feed back electrical activity from muscle tension. You become more aware of your tension and relaxation, learn rapidly to decrease the excess tension, and gain confidence that you can do so.

Research results are variable. Overall, one can expect that at least 50 percent of patients treated will improve by about 50 to 80 percent. Biofeedback clinics usually report better results than controlled research studies; the clinics often report that at least 70 percent of patients are about 50 to 85 percent improved. It is possible that these higher numbers are due to the experience of clinic staffs, different selection of patients, and their focus on tailoring therapy to each individual patient. Treatment may also involve other procedures for some patients.

About the same percentage of headache patients improve when treated by relaxation without biofeedback. One possible conclusion is that biofeedback and relaxation are similarly effective. However, this comparison is misleading, because one strategy may be much more effective than another for a given individual. For example, some research suggests that some headache patients who do not respond to a muscle relaxation treatment will find relief with EMG biofeedback.

Warming the hands, and sometimes the feet, is a type of biofeedback commonly used for migraine headaches. Many practitioners combine this *thermal biofeedback* with relaxation methods. Some combine it with EMG biofeedback to reduce the muscle tension often found in migraine patients. The relaxation, hand-warming, or both may reduce or prevent the constriction of blood vessels linked to migraines.

There is still debate over whether hand-warming is necessary for successful treatment of migraines, and how much warmth one needs to get the best results. Clinicians cannot yet predict for whom these methods will work or exactly how high the hand temperature must become. Some report good results with temperatures in the mid-90s, while other studies find improvement unrelated to hand-warming. (For more on headache treatment, see Chapter 6.)

RAYNAUD'S DISEASE

This disorder involves constriction of blood vessels in the fingers and toes, leading to very cold skin. In biofeedback treatment, a therapist places temperature sensors on the fingers and sometimes the toes. The temperature information fed back to you helps you learn to warm your fingers and toes and stop the constriction of the blood vessels.

Research using thermal biofeedback for this condition often shows that most patients can reduce their symptoms by at least two-thirds. These results often remain strong in follow-up reports years later. Using thermal biofeedback is probably better than using relaxation alone.

A few studies have used a *cold stress* challenge, in which the temperature around you or on the skin surface becomes slowly colder as you receive thermal biofeedback to help you warm your skin. This experimental procedure results in greater improvement, with one well-controlled study reporting a 92 percent drop in Raynaud's symptoms and good results after two years. Although this experimental method holds even more promise than thermal biofeedback alone, the method is not yet widely available.

A BIOFEEDBACK SESSION

Although biofeedback treatments differ depending on the problem, the type of setting, the therapist, and the instruments used, some general principles apply. Many sessions start with a brief period to allow you to adapt to the skin sensors and recording procedure and to test the instruments. For later comparison, the therapist will probably take some baseline recordings of how your body responds without feedback or specific treatment suggestions.

The therapist may then ask you to relax on your own. This will show your present ability to regulate your body processes without external feedback. Some people are already skillful at this, so biofeedback serves mostly to confirm their abilities.

SELECTING THE RIGHT THERAPIST

Assessing the qualifications of a biofeedback therapist need not be a discouraging task.

First, find out the therapist's academic degrees. Most biofeedback providers are psychologists or have graduate degrees in psychology, counseling, or a related area. Many physicians, nurses, physical therapists, occupational therapists, social workers, and other health-care professionals also provide biofeedback therapies. However, we suggest you limit your selection to therapists with a license to practice independently without supervision, or to those supervised by a state-licensed and qualified professional.

One good sign of a therapist's capabilities is certification by the Biofeedback Certification Institute of America. This organization administers the national certification program for biofeedback—it started certifying professionals in 1981. To qualify, therapists must meet specific standards for education, training, experience, and continuing education. The absence of that certificate does not mean lack of qualification, but its presence is a useful sign.

Look for a practitioner who has experience with other patients with your disorder. Less experienced therapists can be competent, but they should be honest with you about their limitations. If they have good training and are well supervised, they can still be the right choice for you.

A good therapist willingly educates you about biofeedback's role in your treatment. Ask questions until you understand the reasons for the treatment and the procedures. They should make sense to you.

Observe the therapist's skills with the instruments and procedures. Then consider your comfort level, trust, and overall satisfaction. If you are ill at ease, discuss your concerns. If you feel unable to discuss them, consider seeking help elsewhere.

For organizations that can help you find a biofeedback therapist, see Resources.

To get a clearer picture of the problem you're trying to manage, the therapist may see how certain tasks affect your body. For example, if your problem is anxiety, your therapist may ask you to hyperventilate or imagine yourself in a stressful situation. If standing aggravates your back pain, the therapist may ask you to stand for several minutes and measure the tension in your back muscles. The instruments also will record what happens to your body after the task. Does it return to its normal condition, and if so, after how long?

You are then ready for the feedback portion of the session. You may receive the information directly through audio and visual signals, or the therapist may tell you what is happening in your body. This portion usually lasts from 30 to 60 minutes. For uncomplicated situations and follow-up visits, shorter sessions are also useful.

The therapist may alternate feedback segments with periods when you practice without feedback, to help you gauge how well you are learning self-regulation. Treatment usually includes home practice.

Of paramount importance is finding a competent therapist, one you like and trust. (For advice on how to do this, see "Selecting the Right Therapist.") It is also important to know the therapist's strategy. Here are questions to ask:

WILL THE THERAPIST OBSERVE AND HELP ME IN MOST SESSIONS?
Biofeedback therapists should be present to operate and adjust instruments, observe, guide, and record information. However, being alone during part of some sessions can be a plus—as long as the therapist is still recording your physiological information. It gives you a chance to practice and improve on your own.

WILL THE THERAPIST TAILOR TREATMENT TO MY NEEDS?
Some professionals work within a set or minimum number of sessions. Others expect you to master skills in a specific sequence. Although such rigid programs can work, they are not for everyone. Therapy should be flexible enough to take your particular situation, symptoms, and skills into account.

WHAT TYPES OF INSTRUMENTS WILL THE THERAPIST USE?
In some cases, therapists work with computer displays. For other conditions, a simpler device may suffice. Either way, the therapist should explain the choice and treatment plans to you.

If you need to see two or more feedback signals, a computer display is easier to understand. A computer is also a good choice if the therapist wants to record several channels of feedback for more detailed review later. Computer displays can make biofeedback more informative and interesting. Fancy equipment may be helpful, but is not always necessary.

Your treatment may also include using a portable feedback device for a few weeks. These devices, which can be simple to use and inexpensive, are helpful if you need extra practice during real-life activities. Avoid buying portable devices from catalogs or through advertisements, however, unless you have professional instruction and guidance in selecting and using the device.

HOW LONG WILL TREATMENT TAKE?

Be sure the therapist explains the length of treatment to your satisfaction. Often it isn't necessary to achieve mastery to reduce your symptoms. If you have doubts about the treatment length proposed, get another opinion.

It usually takes 6 to 20 office sessions to achieve relaxation goals. Some people may need more. Treatment of chronic pain, for example, often requires dozens of sessions. For other conditions, a few office sessions can be enough. Even a single session can be helpful occasionally. Making treatment a priority in your life and practicing faithfully can often shorten the length of treatment.

WHAT WILL IT COST?

Fees range from about $75 to $150 per hour—on a par with the rates health professionals charge for similar or related forms of therapy. The exact fee depends on the type of biofeedback, the area of the country, and the professional's field and degrees. Billing is usually by the session or by 15-minute units.

Many (but not all) insurance carriers reimburse for biofeedback. There may be restrictions on which disorders a company will pay for or the type of biofeedback and therapists it recognizes. Check with your insurance company before embarking on treatment.

WORRIES AND DRAWBACKS

Although a few patients are uneasy about biofeedback devices, very few have negative reactions to treatments. Patients rarely remain anxious about the technology or about the recordings of their bodily activity, although some find feedback signals distracting.

Biofeedback instruments are safe. No electricity goes through you from any feedback instruments, except the very tiny amount from some that measure the output of sweat glands. They cannot shock you. If you have an artificial cardiac pacemaker, some other implanted electrical device, or a serious heart disorder, the Association for Applied Psychophysiology and Biofeedback (AAPB) does recommend that you check with your physician before using biofeedback devices that measure sweat. This is a very cautious statement, however; we know of no cases of problems that have been published or reported at meetings of the AAPB.

Some people do become anxious when they practice deep relaxation, whether achieved with biofeedback or another method (see Chapter 14). But this is primarily true for people who are already prone to anxiety reactions.

Relaxation treatments may reduce the dosage of certain medications that some people need. Examples are thyroid replacement, insulin, blood pressure medicine, and seizure pills. This change in the necessary dosage can be a positive result of treatment (do not attempt to decrease your medication without consulting your physician). However, if you are unaware of the possible decreased need, then biofeedback could result in your taking more medication than you need. Be sure to inform your biofeedback therapist about any medications you take, and alert your physician that you are using biofeedback relaxation treatments.

Therapists are often unable to predict which patients will do well with biofeedback (although we know much more now than a few years ago). Although questions remain, biofeedback can be an important tool for patients who want to play an active role in their treatment. By putting you in touch with your body's systems, biofeedback is a unique and useful addition to mind/body medicine.

THE BOTTOM LINE

Biofeedback is a group of techniques and treatments that help you to use your body's own signals and abilities to improve your health. Biofeedback instruments detect and amplify signals from your body's physiological processes—signals of which you would normally be unaware. The instruments transform these very small bodily signals into audio and visual signals, such as displays on a computer screen. The feedback instruments are sources of useful information that can help guide you.

By increasing their awareness of bodily processes, many patients learn to control them better and develop confidence in their control. Research and clinical experience support the use of biofeedback procedures and treatments as primary or partial treatments for many symptoms and disorders. With very few exceptions, biofeedback is a noninvasive and very low risk treatment.

Research on exactly *how* biofeedback works is inconclusive. Some studies link its benefits directly to physiological changes that the patient learns to make voluntarily. Other experiments find benefits even for patients who do not make the desired changes in the physiological measures. Biofeedback may help some patients to increase their sense of control, heighten their optimism, and lessen the feelings of helplessness triggered by chronic health problems.

Biofeedback gives therapists information to help them plan and guide a patient's therapy. Some therapists can treat you successfully without biofeedback. However, the proper question is not whether biofeedback is always necessary; a better question is, would some form of biofeedback *add* something useful to your treatment?

Doctors and therapists will help you decide whether biofeedback can be of value to you. Choose a well-qualified therapist—an essential factor in success with biofeedback—and ask questions about anything you do not understand. Your caregivers should willingly discuss your questions.

Your view of treatment affects what you do, how you do it, and your chances for success. Your participation, increased knowledge, confidence, positive expectations, and compliance with your therapist's recommendations are all important. Biofeedback fits well into the current views that focus on patients' active participation in their own health care.

19

EXERCISE FOR STRESS CONTROL

BY MICHAEL H. SACKS, M.D.

THERE IS A HILL AT THE NORTHERN END OF CENTRAL PARK IN NEW YORK City that I have been running for 25 years. I have had moments of running it effortlessly, invincible as I reached the crest; also moments of pain and gasping for breath, when I wondered why I was punishing myself. Now when I go for a run at age 52, partially hobbled by bad knees, I often walk more than I actually run—but I always make the effort on that hill. The hill is a magic space where I put things in perspective—not only the joys, sadness, anger, and boredom of my daily life, but those special occasions of celebration or tragedy. It is a place of exhilaration, discipline, challenge, escape, mortification, and, at rare moments, of transcendence. It is part of the rhythm of my life.

I am committed to exercise, and I have been for years. Although I will try to give an objective picture of the potential benefits of exercise, I speak from the perspective of a dedicated runner. In my heart, I believe everyone should exercise. As many people find, regular exercise often triggers a previously undiscovered need to proselytize.

The gospel of exercise spread through the 1980s, and it is spreading still—so much so that the fitness-obsessed runner and the Nautilus-muscled model have become stereotypes of popular culture. But while the passion for exercise is familiar, it's often misunderstood. People don't exercise simply to improve their physical well-being or in an attempt to stay thin or stave off the

MICHAEL H. SACKS, M.D., is a professor of psychiatry at Cornell University Medical College and an attending psychiatrist at the Payne Whitney Psychiatric Clinic in New York City.

effects of aging. They become dedicated to exercise because they find it helps them feel good, emotionally as well as physically.

Exercise can be a powerful method of relaxation, and it can help people deal effectively with the stress of daily life. In various studies, researchers have found that exercise can decrease anxiety and depression, improve an individual's self-image, and buffer people from the effects of stress. Not every study has shown the precise benefits the investigators were looking for; but taken as a whole, the research strongly supports the common experience that exercise can elevate mood and reduce anxiety and stress. Some early studies even suggest that the stress-reducing effect of exercise—not just its cardio-vascular benefits—may help improve physical health.

Although the scientific studies of exercise have focused largely on running, it's hardly the only form of exercise that can have these benefits. Exercise comes in a wide variety of types: aerobic and nonaerobic, solitary and group activities, competitive and noncompetitive sports, endurance activities and those that are based on skill (see "What Kind of Exercise Is Right for You?"). Any of these activities, even fencing or table tennis, can help you feel more focused and relaxed, as long as you pick an activity that fits your personality and physical abilities—and one that you enjoy.

Research on the psychological benefits of exercise has focused on three main areas: stress reduction, antianxiety effects, and antidepressant effects.

EXERCISE AS A BUFFER AGAINST STRESS

Your high school coach who said that exercise and sport build character may have been on to something. Regular exercise does seem to affect one aspect of character in particular: the ability to withstand stress. Exercise and physical fitness can act as a buffer against stress, so that stressful events have a less negative impact on psychological and physical health.

In one experimental study of stress, for example, researchers asked a group of runners and a sedentary control group to unscramble a list of ana-grams, without telling them that these "anagrams" were actually nonsense combinations of letters and were unsolvable. When the subjects were unable to find solutions to these puzzles, they were callously told that their performances were "well below average." Both the exercisers and the nonexercisers had significant increases in muscle tension and anxiety when they were told of their supposedly poor performance, but the increases for the sedentary control group were significantly higher. In addition, people in the sedentary group had a significant increase in blood pressure when they were told they'd done badly. The exercisers did not.

Findings like these pose a conundrum. It's not clear whether the exercisers' blood pressure remained normal because fitness had improved the health of their cardiovascular system or whether the psychological effects of exercise made it easier for them to shrug off a stressful experience. Because exercise has a direct impact on physical health, it's hard to tell whether it helps prevent stress-related illness through its physical effects, its psychological effects, or both. Exercisers may also be more likely to avoid unhealthy ways of dealing with stress, such as smoking, drinking, or overeating—what has been described as the "granola effect" of exercise.

Whatever the reason, however, there is now a growing body of evidence that regular exercise can help people stay healthy under stress. In this regard, exercise can work together with social support, positive attitudes, personality, and other factors that improve stress resistance.

In research with business executives, psychologist Suzanne Kobasa of the City University of New York has found that both a personality style she calls *hardiness* and exercise can complement each other as buffers against stress. Hardy individuals are defined by characteristics that Kobasa calls the "three Cs": They are *committed* to their work; they see change as a *challenge* rather than a threat; and they feel in *control* of their lives. Kobasa has found that hardy people are less likely than others to get sick when they are under stress, as are people who exercise regularly. But people who exercise *and* have a hardy personality style are more resistant to illness than those who have only one of these stress-buffering characteristics.

Other studies have found similar results. At the University of Washington, psychologist Jonathon Brown rated college men and women by the amount of stress in their lives, their exercise level (as they reported it), and their aerobic conditioning—an objective measure of physical fitness related to exercise. The amount of stress did have an effect: The greater the stress, the more likely the students were to experience a range of medical problems. But when Brown looked at the students with high stress levels in more detail, he found that those who did enough exercise to be aerobically fit had fewer visits to the university health center than did people who were less fit.

There's also some evidence that regular exercise can improve the functioning of the immune system (although excessive exercise can actually *de-*

WHAT KIND OF EXERCISE IS RIGHT FOR YOU?

There are three major components of recreational exercise: aerobic, nonaerobic, and skill development. Most exercise activities include more than one.

Aerobic exercise, such as walking or jogging, quickens the heart for sustained periods and can be continued for 20 to 45 minutes without being exhausting. It is called *aerobic* because it is done at a pace that allows an adequate supply of oxygen to reach your muscles as you work out. You are probably exercising aerobically if you can hum to yourself or carry on a conversation as you work out.

Anaerobic exercise involves intense or explosive spurts of strenuous activity that leave you gasping for breath—for example, weight lifting or sprinting full speed for 100 meters. This kind of exercise develops speed, strength, and power. It can only be done for a minute or two at a time, because it depends on a limited store of glycogen—a sugar stored in the muscles that is rapidly depleted, resulting in intense muscle fatigue.

Skill development includes flexibility, balance, and coordination—elements developed by yoga and by sports like tennis and golf.

Each kind of exercise produces different physiological effects. Aerobic exercise makes the cardiovascular and respiratory systems more efficient; anaerobic exercise builds muscle mass; and skill development affects muscular coordination, flexibility, balance, and tone. But despite these differences, all these types of exercise can produce psychological benefits and help combat stress.

To obtain the psychological benefit of exercise, the key is to choose an exercise you enjoy, one that fits your personality. Do you prefer competitive sports or a noncompetitive activity? Do you like repetitive, predictable exercise that allows you to let your mind wander, or exercise that requires more concentration and skill? Would you rather play a team sport or work out on your own? Think back: When you were a child or teenager, did you have a favorite activity or an athletic ideal?

Here are some basic tips on starting an exercise program:

Make the activity as playful as possible. It won't always be fun, and you may have to pass through a period when you just don't feel like exercising. But if it's generally more enjoyable than burdensome, you'll stick with it.

Consider getting lessons and joining a group at first. Encouragement, direction, and group support can be very helpful at the beginning. Most YMCAs and health clubs offer beginner groups, and most communities have groups of hikers, bikers, tennis players, and the like who are glad to share their experiences with interested newcomers.

Exercise often. Although you should exercise three or four times a week for the physical benefits, slightly more frequent exercise—four or five times a week—seems to maximize the psychological effects.

Start slowly. Depending on your condition, you may not be able to exercise as intensely as you'd like to at first. Many former athletes become very discouraged when they find they can't easily do what they did 5, 10, or 15 years ago. Don't be in a hurry, and don't compete with an image of yourself from the past. Listen to your body.

crease immune function). Research has consistently shown that white blood cells increase for a period of time after exercise, although this increase may be too short-lived to have a major impact on immunity. In a recent study, however, researchers at the University of Miami found that a regular exercise program had beneficial effects on immunity in men infected with HIV, the virus that causes AIDS.

The psychological benefits of exercise may have contributed to this improvement in immune function: The HIV-infected men who exercised were less depressed and anxious than HIV-infected men who did not exercise. In fact, the effects of exercise on both mood and immunity were similar to those of a stress management program, tested in a parallel study of HIV-positive men by the same group of investigators (see Chapter 23). But here, as in many studies, more work is needed to sort out the physical from the psychological effects of exercise.

Although much remains to be learned, studies like these suggest that people who exercise regularly show a healthier response to emotional stress than sedentary people. Most research in this area has focused on aerobic exercise, which improves heart and lung capacity. However, any kind of exercise can help buffer the effects of stress if it helps build a person's feelings of control, confidence, effectiveness, and mastery over life.

EXERCISE AND ANXIETY

Everyone experiences anxiety from time to time: You recognize it through the sensations of tightness in the chest, heart palpitations, and sweaty palms, accompanied by a general feeling of fearfulness, difficulty concentrating, and frightening thoughts. Since the 1970s, studies of normal volunteers have consistently shown that regular exercise has a "tranquilizer effect" that decreases anxiety.

Paradoxically, many people find that their anxiety level actually increases when they first begin to work out—say, at the start of a run. But their anxiety then stabilizes as they continue to exercise; and 5 to 30 minutes after they finish exercising, they're less anxious than they were before they started. This decrease in anxiety, which has been correlated with reductions in muscle tension, has actually been shown to be greater than the effects of the tranquilizing drug meprobamate.

Exercise is only a short-term fix for anxiety, however. The postexercise period of relaxation lasts for only four hours or so, and anxiety generally returns to its previous level within 24 hours after a workout. So someone with chronic anxiety may have to exercise every day to see an effect. The timing of the tranquilizer effect also suggests that someone who becomes particularly anxious during the day—at a stressful job, for example—might do best to exercise first thing in the morning. In contrast, someone with insomnia might want to exercise in the late afternoon—although exercising *too* late in the day may make it difficult to fall asleep.

Some studies suggest that exercise should be fairly intense, but not exhausting, to best elicit the tranquilizer effect. In one study, college women runners who jogged 24 miles per week were significantly less tense than those who ran either 15 or 52 miles per week. But other researchers have found that light exercise, such as walking or swimming, decreases anxiety just as effectively as vigorous jogging does. And many people claim that golf, tennis, handball, biking, and other sports help them relax, although there is little

WHEN EXERCISE BECOMES STRESSFUL

Although exercise generally has positive psychological effects, under some circumstances it can actually lead to psychological problems.

One kind of problem occurs in committed exercisers when an injury prevents them from working out. This interference in their exercise plans can make them anxious or depressed, especially if they have a well-established, daily routine. In some cases, the reaction may be so severe that they seek psychological or psychiatric help.

The other problem comes from exercising too much. Overexertion can lead to a state of fatigue characterized by anxiety or depression, insomnia, and a loss of interest in one's personal life. Competitive endurance athletes, such as swimmers and distance runners, often suffer from this kind of cumulative exhaustion; so do some recreational athletes who try too hard to improve their performance. If you're exercising at a high level and are feeling down, think about easing up on the exercise; such a change usually brings a rapid recovery

formal research on the tranquilizer effect of such activities. If you want to try using exercise to relax, you may need to experiment to find the type and the level of exercise that work best for you.

One interesting approach has been to separate anxiety into its two major components—the cognitive (or mental) and the somatic (or physical)—and to recommend different activities for people with different types of anxiety. Thus, people who suffer from physical symptoms of anxiety—gastrointestinal problems, sweating, palpitations, pacing back and forth, and so on—may be especially likely to benefit from exercise. In contrast, those whose main problem is worrying, difficulty concentrating, or intrusive thoughts may find more relief from meditation or some other form of mental relaxation. (See "What's Your Stress Style?") Of course, it's possible to combine these approaches; some Zen monks run as a form of meditation, and Herbert Benson has developed guidelines for using the relaxation response during exercise (see Chapter 14). Although the difference between cognitive and somatic anxiety is still

WHAT'S YOUR STRESS STYLE?

People experience stress in different ways, and those differences sometimes determine which relaxation techniques are most effective for them. Some people react to stress mostly in their body, while others have primarily mental reactions. And about a third of people experience stress both mentally and physically. The following short quiz can give you a rough idea of your tendency.

When you're feeling anxious, what do you typically experience? Check all that apply.

☐ 1. My heart beats faster.
☐ 2. I find it difficult to concentrate because of distracting thoughts.
☐ 3. I worry too much about things that don't really matter.
☐ 4. I feel jittery.
☐ 5. I get diarrhea.
☐ 6. I imagine terrifying scenes.
☐ 7. I can't keep anxiety-provoking pictures and images out of my mind.
☐ 8. My stomach gets tense.
☐ 9. I pace up and down nervously.
☐ 10. I'm bothered by unimportant thoughts running through my head.
☐ 11. I become immobilized.
☐ 12. I feel I'm losing out on things because I can't make decisions fast enough.
☐ 13. I perspire.
☐ 14. I can't keep worrisome thoughts out of my mind.

Scoring: Give yourself a "body" point for each of these: 1, 4, 5, 8, 9, 11, 13.

Give yourself a "mind" point for each of the following: 2, 3, 6, 7, 10, 12, 14.

If you have more mind than body points, you tend to have mental reactions to stress. If you have more body than mind points, your stress-reaction style tends to be physical. And if you have about the same number of each, you're a mixed reactor, experiencing stress both physically and mentally.

These are only rough guidelines. But if you are seeking a way to handle stress, they may help you find an approach that works for you more quickly.

Vigorous exercise, such as jogging or swimming, may be especially helpful for people who mostly react physically. They can also be helped by methods of deep muscle relaxation or yoga, which also break up the physical pattern of stress.

Those who mainly experience stress as a mental reaction, through worrisome thoughts and the like, tend to find relaxation in activities that engage the mind completely, like meditation, reading an absorbing book, or playing a challenging game like chess.

Those who experience stress both ways do well with physically involving activities that also demand full mental engagement: competitive sports like tennis, racquetball, or volleyball, for instance, or some of the physical exercises of mindfulness meditation (see Chapter 15).

under study, it can be a useful concept in helping you find a form of relaxation that best suits you personally.

EXERCISE AND DEPRESSION

Exercisers tend to be less depressed than people who don't exercise. That much is known. What's not clear is whether people are able to stave off depression by exercising, or whether less depressed, more energetic people are more likely to exercise in the first place.

At Purdue University, psychologists D. D. Lobstein and A. H. Ismail found that middle-aged professors who got a good deal of exercise were much less depressed than the most sedentary of their colleagues. But when the sedentary professors were put on a fitness program and followed it over four years, their depression didn't lift—suggesting that their depressed mood may have led to their inactivity, rather than the other way around. Exercise alone probably won't do much for someone who has been depressed for a long time. Nor will it help a person gripped by an acute episode of severe depression. Such people are often so immobilized that they can barely get out of bed, let alone go for a jog in the park.

However, exercise can be helpful—perhaps as helpful as psychotherapy, in some cases—for people with more moderate forms of depression that are nevertheless persistent and intense enough to require professional help. In a well-known study, psychiatrist John Griest and his associates at the University of Wisconsin assigned 24 clinic patients with moderate depression to either an exercise program or one of two widely used forms of treatment: time-limited psychotherapy (limited to 12 weeks) or long-term psychotherapy. In the two standard treatment groups, therapists met with the patients once a week; in the exercise group, patients went jogging with a trainer three times a week for 45 to 60 minutes at a time.

After 12 weeks, about three-quarters of the patients in each of the three treatment groups had gotten over their depression. That by itself may not mean much; depression often lifts within a few months even if the depressed person receives no treatment at all. But one year later, the people who had been treated with running therapy were still running on their own and were free of depression, while half of those who received either the time-limited or long-term psychotherapy had returned for treatment.

A second study found similar results with 60 subjects divided between exercise (walking and jogging), meditation training, and group psychotherapy. Although all treatments were equally effective at first, a follow-up three months after the end of treatment showed the exercisers and meditators had made further gains, while those in group psychotherapy had a tendency to relapse.

Those two studies were small and were not flawless. Griest noted that many patients who expected traditional therapy were very reluctant to try exercise instead. But the research does suggest that exercise is as good as or better than standard medical treatment for moderate depression—and with depression on the rise in the population, that's a finding worth further study.

Several studies have shown that exercise is also good for the mild, transient kinds of depression most people experience from time to time, such as acute feelings of sadness, discouragement, and self-deprecation. In one typical study, undergraduate women taking a psychology course were enlisted to participate in an experiment on "stress management." Forty-three of the women were identified as having a mild depression and were randomly assigned to either a jogging program, relaxation training, or no treatment at all (they were told they were on a waiting list). After ten weeks, women in all the groups became less depressed, but the exercise group improved the most.

HOW DOES EXERCISE HELP THE PSYCHE?

Although there is good evidence that exercise can improve mood, exactly how it does so is still unclear. In general, there are two kinds of possible explanations: the psychological and the physiological.

In the psychological view, the effects of exercise are not unique. Instead, exercise is similar to many other activities—such as reading a book, going to a movie, or watching a sporting event—that can relieve anxiety or depression somewhat, simply by offering a diversion. In some studies, people who rested in a recliner or ate lunch with friends had the same reduction in anxiety as people who exercised; apparently the "time out" by itself had a beneficial effect. The antianxiety effect of exercise could be due to the "time out" or distraction it provides. The busy executive who finds relief in a mid-day workout and attributes it to exercise might simply be finding relief in the distractions it offers from the pressures of work.

Furthermore, many of the physiological changes produced by exercise, from deep breathing to an elevated heart rate, are very similar to those that occur in anxiety or other states of physical arousal. The arousal produces a state of heightened awareness—nothing more. But the feelings that accompany that arousal will be determined by its context. Running on a track can be boring or fun; running from a mugger is terrifying. It's the psychological setting of the physical activity that determines its effect on mood.

Physiologists see the brain as a complex arrangement of neurons, and they see anxiety and depression as the results of electrical and biochemical processes in those neurons. Exercise clearly affects those processes. It increases blood flow to the brain, releases hormones, stimulates the nervous system, and increases levels of morphinelike substances found in the body (such as beta-endorphin) that can have a positive effect on mood. Exercise may trigger a neurophysiological high—a shot of adrenaline or endorphins—

that produces an antidepressant effect in some, an antianxiety effect in others, and a general sense of "feeling better" in most.

An integrated approach, which is the one I favor, holds that both psychology and physiology help account for the beneficial effects of exercise on mood. The benefits can come from many factors: the decision to take up exercise, the symbolic meaning of the activity, the distraction from worries, the acquisition of mastery over a sport, the effects on self-image, and the biochemical and physiological changes that accompany the activity. I have found that patients and friends who are depressed usually feel better immediately after their first exercise session; the simple decision to do something positive about the depression may help. But further benefit accrues over time as they learn athletic skills, become aerobically conditioned, and improve their body image.

IMAGERY, FANTASY, AND THE ILLUSIONS OF EXERCISE

Physical activity often seems to promote fantasies, daydreams, and the imagination, which play a vital role in the psychological benefits of exercise.

One friend of mine, a runner, has used the same daydream for years. As he runs, he imagines that he is breaking away from his main competitor in the last two miles of the marathon to win an Olympic gold medal in world-record time. As he crosses the imaginary finish line in the Olympic stadium (at which point he is actually at the end of a four-mile jog in front of his house), he stops and waits for his competitor. As his rival crosses the finish line, they embrace in a display of great sportsmanship. Afterward they become friends and foster world peace.

This friend of mine is not a daydreamer by nature, but a hard-working, extremely aggressive advertising director. He regards his fantasy as an escape, a B movie in which he is the scriptwriter, director, and star. In his exercise fantasy, he is able to balance the ruthless, unforgiving competition of his job with an image of a more cooperative way of life. Through such internal scripts, or "dramas of exercise," an exerciser can creatively express aspirations and resolve conflicts in a playful way.

Many exercisers don't have such specific fantasies but experience a free-floating sense of well-being that has been called a "blank daydream"—a satisfying absence of mental content. Related to this state is the focused sense of "being on," "having flow," "rhythm," and so on, that competitive athletes value highly and that can bring on an intense feeling of elation.

The "feel-better phenomenon" of exercise may stem largely from the kinds of mental images, feelings, and thoughts associated with exercise. Of special importance is the interplay between images of ourselves as we are, flawed and mortal, and the images of ourselves as we once thought we were or wanted to be. Many children aspire to be superheroes, to challenge human limits, to run like an Olympian or to soar like Superman. Although our mature adult selves abandon such dreams as we grow older, the dreams still remain part of the child deep within us, seeking expression.

When you exercise, the possibilities open to you in your imagination can remain infinite. It doesn't matter that you jog a mile in 10 or even 15 minutes; your imaginary clock can read 3 minutes, 40 seconds. This playful suspension of the real world, together with the expression of the physical exuberance of childhood, is at the psychological core of exercise.

We all enjoy stories of extraordinary physical accomplishment: the 70-year-old marathoner, the two young adults who ran 2,000 miles across the foothills of the Himalayas with only their anoraks, or the 50-year-old mountain climber who finally attained the summit of Everest. Rationally, we may regard these as stories of somewhat absurd endeavors. But as exercisers, we imagine that we could do what these athletes did and see their feats as wondrous triumphs over age, over physical limitations—even, in our imaginations, over death itself.

THE BOTTOM LINE

Regular exercise has a variety of psychological benefits that, in turn, can help improve physical health. It acts as a buffer against stress and may thus help protect the cardiovascular and immune systems from the consequences of stressful events. Frequent exercise is an effective treatment for anxiety and, according to some research, is as effective as psychotherapy in treating mild or moderate depression.

Exercise seems to elevate mood both through its physiological effects on the nervous system and through its direct psychological effects: It provides a distraction from everyday concerns and offers an opportunity for positive fantasy. Although aerobic exercise offers the greatest cardiovascular benefit, any form of enjoyable exercise can give you a psychological lift and help counteract the effects of stress in your life.

IV

WHAT YOU CAN DO: FRIENDS, ATTITUDES, AND COPING

20

Social Support: How Friends, Family, and Groups Can Help

By David Spiegel, M.D.

More than a decade ago, I began organizing support groups for women with advanced breast cancer because I wanted to learn how to help the dying. I learned a good deal more about living.

As a psychiatrist leading weekly 90-minute sessions, I watched the women cry together over the deaths of group members, cheer small victories, and plot strategies for coping with recalcitrant husbands, stubborn children, and difficult friends. I was struck then, and continue to be impressed, by the almost instant rapport these women shared, the often unspoken sense of understanding that grew out of their similar circumstances.

The groups were part of a study my colleagues and I were conducting at Stanford University on the health benefits of social support. When we followed up on the women later on, it did not surprise me to discover that the groups had helped the women emotionally. I was far less prepared, however, for another finding that would change the direction of my research: These women ultimately lived an average of 18 months longer than did women with comparable breast cancer and medical care who did not go to such groups. That meant the women who went to groups lived twice as long from the time we first saw them.

The added survival time was longer than any medication or other known medical treatment could be expected to provide for women with breast cancer

DAVID SPIEGEL, M.D., is a professor of psychiatry and behavioral sciences and director of the Psychosocial Treatment Laboratory, Stanford University School of Medicine.

so far advanced. Something about the intense social support the women experienced in these sessions appeared to influence the way their bodies coped with the illness. Living better also seemed to mean living longer.

In some ways, it is hardly astonishing that the women's close relationships with each other should have prolonged their lives. From the day we are born, social support is essential to our survival. Human beings have a more prolonged period of helplessness and dependency than any other mammals. For years, we must rely fully on the physical and social skills of our parents.

Since primitive times, we have also formed alliances beyond the family unit to increase survival odds even more. Many other animals are stronger, faster, and have keener sensory perception than do humans. But the human brain has allowed us to think, remember, plan, talk, and interact with each other in very complex ways. As a result, we have been able to form tribes, clans, towns, cities, states, and nations—all in an effort to protect ourselves from predators (whether animal or human) and to provide stable sources of food, clothing, and shelter.

Today, it is obvious that one way social support keeps us alive is by creating institutions, like hospitals, that help us survive. But does the human talent for bonding also have direct biological benefits for individuals? Could our advanced brains be the route through which our skill at social relations and lapses in that skill affect the way our bodies cope with disease and deterioration? Since the surprising results of our study on breast cancer support groups, such questions have fueled my research on the ways relationships and community influence our health.

WHAT THE STUDIES SHOW

Evidence of a link between social support and physical well-being has grown in recent years, thanks to a number of large-scale studies. This research shows that having a good number of close social relationships is associated with a lower risk of dying at any given age. The classic example is research on residents of Alameda County, California. Scientists looked at the social networks of thousands of people in relation to their odds of dying. As part of this research, epidemiologist Lisa Berkman, now at Yale, and Leonard Syme, a professor of epidemiology at the University of California, Berkeley, studied the relationship between death rate and four types of social support: marital status, contact with extended family and friends, church membership, and other group affiliations. They found that a measure of each type of relationship, and measures of all of them put together, predicted mortality over the ensuing nine years. Specifically, those individuals who were least socially connected were twice as likely to die as those with the strongest social ties, even when health habits such as smoking, alcohol use, physical activity, obesity, and use of preventive health programs were taken into account.

Similar studies in Georgia and Michigan, and abroad in Sweden and Finland, have obtained comparable results. For example, sociologist James House, of the University of Michigan, gathered data on social connections from 2,754 adults who were interviewed during visits to their doctors. House found that the most socially active men were two to three times less likely to die within 9 to 12 years than those of a similar age who were most isolated. The risk for socially isolated women was one-and-a-half to two times as great. These studies make it clear that daily contact with people may help to prolong life.

Research that has looked specifically at sick people shows that once serious illness strikes, social support continues to affect their chances of staying alive. In 1990, epidemiologists Peggy Reynolds and George Kaplan at the University of California, Berkeley, studied the number of social contacts that cancer patients had each day. Women with the least amount of social contact were 2.2 times more likely to die of cancer over a 17-year period than were the most socially connected. The link between social support and cancer was strongest for smoking-related cancers in men and hormone-related cancers, such as breast cancer, in women.

Along similar lines, in 1987 internist James Goodwin at the Medical College of Wisconsin and his colleagues published the results of a study on cancer survival in several thousand patients. The married cancer patients did better medically and had lower mortality rates than the unmarried. Similarly, in a study of 1,368 patients with coronary artery disease, Redford Williams and colleagues at Duke University (see Chapter 4) found that having a spouse or other close confidant tripled the chances that a patient would be alive five years later. (For more such findings, see "Marriage and Health.")

Of course, many social factors other than how much support people receive can account for why one patient survives longer than another. For that reason, most studies like this have been careful to eliminate the obvious confounding variables, such as smoking and alcohol abuse, differences in socioeconomic status, and access to health care. But by and large, the studies still consistently show that more and better social support from family and friends is associated with lower odds of dying at any given age.

MARRIAGE AND HEALTH

Marriage—at least a good marriage—is good for health. By the same token, a troubled marriage or a divorce may be physically harmful.

Married people live longer on average than do those who are single, whether widowed, divorced, or never married. In a study of more than 7,500 adults, epidemiologist Maradee Davis at the University of California, San Francisco, found that single men between 45 and 54 were twice as likely to die in a period of ten years as were married men of the same age.

Similar results were found in a study of death rates dating back to 1940: Single, widowed, or divorced men had a death rate twice that of married men; single women had a death rate 50 percent higher than that of married women. The divorced and widowed fared worst of all, especially among men in their 20s and 30s. Divorced men and widowers in that group had a death rate up to 10 times that of married men their age.

Perhaps because of its emotional toll, divorce seems to pose a particular health hazard. Several epidemiological studies, involving thousands of men and women, have found that men and women who are separated or divorced have poorer physical health than do comparable widowed, married, or single adults. Of all these groups, the divorced have the highest rates of acute medical complaints and chronic medical conditions that limit their activity and have more overall disability, even when age, race, and income are taken into account. They also have higher death rates from certain infectious diseases, including up to six times as many deaths from pneumonia.

A good marriage offers much more—and seems to have greater health benefits—than simple companionship. Maradee Davis found that even when single men lived with a family member or friend, their death rate was twice that of married men. While no one knows just why this is so, Davis conjectures that poor diet or other poor health habits put single men at greater risk. It may be that having a spouse to share your turmoil in stressful times helps keep you healthy.

Another possibility is suggested in a study by immunologist Ronald Glaser and psychologist Janice Kiecolt-Glaser at Ohio State University College of Medicine. As part of their ongoing research on the effects of psychological states on immune function (described in Chapter 3), they compared 38 women who had separated from their husbands up to six years previously with 38 similar married women. The married women had better immune function overall. And among the divorced women, the more strongly they still yearned to be reunited with the divorced spouse, the poorer their immune function—and the stronger their feelings of depression and loneliness.

But marriage is by no means a panacea. Data from six national surveys show that men and women who are unhappy with their marriages also report poorer health than do those who are content with their marriages. And a detailed study of the physiological effects of an unhappy marriage suggests that marital conflict has a corrosive impact on health. In that study, conducted at Indiana University by psychologists Robert Levenson and John Gottman, married couples had their heart rate and other autonomic responses measured—first while they talked for 15 minutes about how they spent their day, and then as they focused for another 15 minutes on some point of conflict, like in-laws or money.

Those couples who were least satisfied with their marriages over the following three years showed the greatest physiological arousal during the discussions and reported the poorest health. One thing that set these couples apart was that simply being in each other's presence triggered a higher level of arousal; for more happily married couples, that did not occur until they started talking about a disagreement. To put it simply, the less satisfied couples apparently got on each other's nerves. In the view of the Glasers, the study suggests that in a disturbed marriage consistent physiological arousal translates to persistent hormonal changes that could, over time, diminish the effectiveness of the partners' immune systems.

In an overview of research in the journal *Science* a few years ago, James House observed that the relationship between social isolation and early death is as strong, statistically, as the relationship between dying and smoking or having high serum cholesterol. So from a numerical standpoint, at least, the data suggest that it may be as important to your health to be socially integrated as it is to stop smoking or to reduce your cholesterol level. Whether developing new relationships will actually have such a strong benefit remains an open question. Nonetheless, for a factor so strongly related to health outcome, social support has been greatly underestimated by medical science.

WHY SUPPORT MAKES A DIFFERENCE

It is not hard to imagine how social support can aid people emotionally, especially when they are dealing with a serious illness: It helps them feel less alone and frightened and more competent in dealing with the disease. But how does this translate into an effect on the *body*?

One set of theories holds that social support leads to physical consequences by influencing behavior. For example, people who feel that others care about them are more likely to take the basic steps any grandmother would recommend for staying healthy or coping with illness: eating well, getting plenty of sleep, and exercising regularly. Similarly, social support helps people avoid bad habits—such as smoking, drug use, and excessive drinking—that can compromise the cardiovascular, immune, and nervous systems, making it harder for the body to handle physical distress.

Further, people who interact well with friends and family also tend to have positive relationships with physicians and other health-care providers. They present themselves as independent, active, valuable people who deserve and need the most vigorous kind of medical treatment. When seriously ill, such patients may survive longer than others because, encouraging their doctors to "go the extra mile" in treating them, they thereby receive more extensive and more attentive medical care.

Some researchers have looked beyond these behavioral explanations, however, and done studies that suggest a sense of connection with others may offer *direct* physical benefits by mitigating the degree of stress people experience. During times of stress, certain "stress hormones" are pumped into the bloodstream, potentially leading to a number of harmful physical and mental changes, including elevated heart rate, poor metabolism of sugar, suppression of immune function, depression, and anxiety (see Chapter 2). When stress becomes chronic, these hormones no longer ebb and flow normally; instead they remain consistently high, potentially impairing the body's ability to heal. Because illness is itself stressful, one theory holds, a disease can set off a damaging feedback loop, in which the illness and the high levels of stress hormones it triggers continually reinforce each other.

Feeling supported by others may serve as a buffer that mitigates the output of stress hormones during traumatic situations. Evidence comes from animal studies conducted by psychologist Seymour Levine at Stanford University. In one series of experiments, Levine conditioned a squirrel monkey to react with the stress response when a particular light flashed. First, the animal was given a mild shock during each flash; when the shock was eventually discontinued, the light flash still elicited a fearful response. The animal's stress reaction included a sharp rise in blood levels of the hormone cortisol, which often surges shortly after exposure to an acute stressor, such as a physical threat. However, Levine and his colleagues found that if the monkey had another monkey for company when the light flashed, the amount of blood cortisol the stressed monkey produced was only half as great. In another experiment, the monkey had five companions, and showed *no* increase in blood cortisol when the light flashed.

These results suggest that the presence of friends may shield the body from the consequences of stress—and the more friends, the better. Consider how different you might feel walking through a dangerous neighborhood after dark if you were alone, with one friend, or with five. Whether or not you were actually much safer in a group, you would certainly feel more secure.

In the past decade, the explosion of research into psychoneuroimmunology—the new field that explores the links between our thoughts, emotions, nervous system, and immune system—has included many studies on whether social support can directly affect the various cells that make up the body's immune defenses. For example, research on medical students by immunologist Ronald Glaser and psychologist Janice Kiecolt-Glaser at Ohio State University College of Medicine showed that certain cells in the students' immune systems became less effective during the stress of exams (see Chapter 3). However, medical students who felt connected to friends and family showed a

THE HEALING POWER OF PETS

Humans aren't the only source of a healing friendship: Pets, too, can be good for your health. Indeed, pets have been found to act as a kind of sedative, actually lowering the blood pressure of their owners simply by offering affection and good company. To be sure, the effect may be specific to animal lovers; those who see pets as more of a nuisance than a pleasure do not seem to benefit much from the company of animals.

But for pet lovers, the health benefits are striking. For example, a 1980 study of 96 people with heart disease, just released from a coronary care unit, found a higher survival rate one year later among pet owners, compared to petless patients with comparable disease. Indeed, psychiatrist Erika Friedmann of the University of Pennsylvania, who conducted the study, found that pet ownership proved an even stronger predictor of survival than having a spouse or extensive family support.

Furthermore, a 1990 study of 345 elderly pet owners found that they went to physicians fewer times in the course of a year than did a comparable group of elderly people who had no pets. UCLA psychologist Judith Siegel found that the pet owners in the study said they got great comfort from their pets during stressful times. In her study, dogs offered the most potent comfort.

Indeed, dogs can have a powerfully soothing effect on their owners' reactions to stress, according to findings by psychologists Karen Allen and James Blascovich of the State University of New York at Buffalo. They measured blood pressure and other indicators of a stress reaction in 45 women—all self-described dog lovers—while they did a series of stressful mental tasks, such as having to count rapidly backward from a four-digit number. When they worked only in the company of the researcher, or even with a friend nearby, their stress reactivity was high. But when they did such tasks with their dogs beside them, they showed no stress reaction. The dogs, it seems, took the bite out of stress.

much less pronounced immunological change than those who described themselves as lonely.

Such laboratory studies don't prove that social support increases resistance to disease or inhibits its progression. But they do provide evidence that psychosocial support may have positive effects on the activity of the immune system.

THE CASE FOR SUPPORT GROUPS

The 19th-century French author Alexis de Tocqueville called America "a nation of joiners," and fortunately the medically ill are now no exception. It is increasingly popular for patients with cancer, heart disease, arthritis, abdominal surgery, neurological illnesses, and a number of other disorders to meet regularly among themselves in groups, just like the women in our breast cancer study. Research is showing that these groups offer patients advantages similar to the social support they naturally receive from loved ones—namely, better emotional and physical health.

Why are these groups necessary? One of the costs of our highly technological society has been a fragmentation of the family. Many of our social institutions perform functions that previously were handled by a network of relatives—in particular, nursing and other care for the sick. Today, even someone who has close friends and relatives may find that this group isn't fully up to the task of coping with the crisis of a serious physical illness.

Life-threatening illness in particular is a frightening, even terrifying experience, but we often isolate people with such illnesses despite their desperate need to feel the support of others. Put yourself in the shoes of the VIP who checked into a New York hospital for a diagnostic biopsy. He was given the red carpet treatment, with visits from every prominent hospital official and a variety of concerned doctors, nurses, and friends. The day after the biopsy, he suddenly noticed that the only person still talking to him was the cleaning lady. She was also the only one who didn't know that the biopsy had shown a serious malignancy.

Terminally ill patients quickly come to feel excluded from the flow of everyday life. One cancer patient, who ate with difficulty because of radiation burns to her throat, looked around a restaurant and felt alienated from the other diners. She thought, "How lucky these people are to be able to *eat*." Sometimes patients withdraw from the world of the healthy, just as healthy people avoid the sick because they don't know how to react appropriately or are frightened by serious illness.

The support group program for women with breast cancer that we developed at Stanford (and continue to offer), called *supportive/expressive group therapy*, is a good example of how support groups can mitigate the emotional problems patients face. We began our research in 1976 with 86 women. Fifty of them were randomly assigned to support groups along with standard medical treatment; the other 36 did not attend groups.

The support groups we formed offered far more than hand-holding and good wishes. The sessions became a time and place for the women to express some of their deepest fears, what one called "that sense of waking up at three in the morning with an elephant sitting on your chest." She added, "I wonder if I will live to see my son graduate from high school or my daughter get married. I have to keep up a front everywhere else—that's so hard."

There was a good deal of crying in these groups, as well as laughter. One of the concerns about getting patients with a similar illness together is that they will become demoralized if members get sicker or die. To find out if this is so, we compared those group sessions in which there was bad news about a member to those in which the group was doing well. We found that the women were not scared by each other's medical problems because the risk of dying was something that each one worried about anyway. Rather, the groups provided a setting in which they could deal with their fears.

One member compared it to "looking down into the Grand Canyon when you are afraid of heights. You know that falling would be the end. Nonetheless, you feel better about yourself because you are able to look. That's the way I feel about death in the group. I can't say I feel serene, but I can look at it." The group offered a kind of focus for these fears. By venting their emotions, the women prevented the fear from taking over the other hours of their lives. (Groups that emphasize expressing painful emotions often work best if they are led by experienced health professionals, as ours were.)

The agenda of these groups became broad as many patients faced the reality that their lives would be shortened by the disease. Rather than banish the illness from their thoughts, they came to take it into account and reorder their life priorities. Poems were published, acts of kindness acknowledged, jobs changed, children nurtured. Many left relationships that seemed unproductive and enriched those that were important to them. As one husband of a patient put it, "I would give anything to have this disease go away, but I have to say that the time since my wife got cancer has been the best time in our marriage."

The groups also addressed the best ways to communicate with doctors. Seriously ill patients tend to both revere and fear their physicians. On the one hand, they do not want to trouble them; on the other, they are often afraid of asking too much for fear of learning more than they want to know. So they often leave the doctor's office haunted by unanswered questions. In our groups, patients encouraged one another to write down their questions and to insist on getting them answered. Some even accompanied their friends on doctors' visits.

Through all of this, the women came to care deeply and personally about one another, visiting each other in the hospital, writing and calling between group meetings. They shared their victories and defeats in fighting their illnesses.

At the end of the year, we compared the status of women who had attended the sessions to those who had received only standard medical care. We found that the group members were less anxious and depressed and were coping more effectively with their breast cancer. In addition, patients in the support groups actually became more emotionally stable, whereas those in the control sample showed increasingly disturbed moods. The group patients who were trained in self-hypnosis to combat pain also reported half as much pain as the control patients. (For more on self-hypnosis, see Chapter 16.) Thus, the support group seemed to help patients live better, with less anxiety, depression, and pain.

On a fundamental level, support groups may work for two reasons. First, they simply counter isolation. But second, and maybe even more important, they allow people to feel they can help *each other*, which makes them feel not only less helpless in the face of their illness, but competent and effective. After all, getting cancer or having a heart attack is in many ways a meaningless tragedy that hampers and diminishes life. But learning how to cope with it is a skill that lets you be of genuine help to another patient. By assisting each other in support groups, the physically ill can also enhance their own sense of self-worth.

SUPPORT AND SURVIVAL

The most striking finding of our study was the one that only became apparent a decade after the groups had ended. When we followed up on the patients to see what had become of them, we found that those in the support groups had lived an average of 18 months longer than those in the control sample. Considering their stage of cancer when the study began, that added year and a half represented a virtual *doubling* of survival from the time they entered our study.

Looked at another way, the statistics show that after four years, none of the control patients was still alive, but a third of the women in our support groups were. Indeed, two patients who were in the treatment group are still alive some 15 years later. The groups were no cure for cancer; most women did eventually die of the disease. But these data show that something had happened to the course of the cancer among women assigned to the support groups. The therapy seemed to influence their bodies' ability to fight back physically.

We never expected to find such an effect. In fact, I initially followed up on the women in our groups because I thought I could *disprove* the notion, popular in the mid-1980s, that psychological factors could affect the course of cancer. I assumed that the women in our groups, though they benefited emotionally, would have died at just the same rate as any other women with breast cancer so advanced. The fact that they lived so much longer came as a complete surprise, and we spent four years analyzing and reanalyzing the data—with the help of many colleagues—to make sure the effect was real.

Today, I still believe that popular claims about the mind's power to cure cancer are unfounded, and if these claims lead a patient to give up conventional treatment, they can be dangerous. Visualizing your immune system cells attacking your tumors is no substitute for chemotherapy. But for whatever reason, support from a group of caring people—a simple approach that addresses a basic human need—seems to have a powerful effect.

Since we published our findings in 1989, several other studies have demonstrated comparable effects on cancer patients. Psychologist Jean Richardson and colleagues at the University of Southern California randomly assigned patients with lymphoma or leukemia either to routine care for their illness or to a series of educational sessions and home visits. They found that the patients who received this extra support lived significantly longer than the others.

Psychiatrist Fawzy I. Fawzy and his colleagues at the UCLA Neuropsychiatric Institute took 40 patients with malignant melanoma and offered them an intensive six-week group program that emphasized education and emotional expression. These patients showed positive changes in the functioning of their immune systems six months later, compared with people in a control group who were given routine care but no group support. The researchers measured the functioning of natural killer (NK) cells, which seem to be involved in resistance to cancer. Patients who were in the support groups also seem to have more favorable survival odds. Preliminary data show that they went a longer time before they relapsed and had a lower death rate.

It isn't only cancer patients who profit from group support. Similar results are beginning to emerge from studies of patients with other illnesses as well. Often, social support is combined with education to good effect. For example, patients with rheumatoid arthritis who attend educational support groups not only cope better with their illness but show reduced swelling and better joint mobility, according to research by rheumatologist Halsted Holman at Stanford University (see Chapter 10). Other researchers have found that programs incorporating group support can lower the risk of heart attack for people with high heart-disease risk (see Chapter 4).

In one well-publicized, ongoing study of heart patients, internist Dean Ornish of the University of California, San Francisco, has shown that a program of group support, relaxation training, and a strict, low-fat vegetarian diet can begin to reverse the blockage of coronary arteries among people who have suffered heart attacks. Ornish believes that the social support component has been a leading factor in the patients' physical improvement.

TYPES OF SUPPORT GROUPS

Group therapy is available for people with virtually every kind of chronic illness. Colostomy clubs help patients who have recently had gastrointestinal surgery cope with the experience of having to wear a bag to empty their intestines. Groups such as Mended Hearts help patients who have had bypass surgery to regain confidence in their bodies. There are groups for people infected with the AIDS virus. And there are innumerable groups for cancer patients, many of them organized for patients in similar circumstances, such as those who have been newly diagnosed or have metastasized disease of a particular type, such as breast, colon, or lymphatic cancer.

Support groups usually combine a variety of approaches. The four most common are social support and venting emotions (both of which form the basis for our breast cancer support groups at Stanford), plus cognitive restructuring and education.

SOCIAL SUPPORT

Many groups provide social support either as a primary goal or as a welcome side effect. As a matter of course, regular contact with people who are facing similar problems lets members know that what they are going through is normal for people facing the same disease. Patients who feel they somehow caused their disease or failed to detect it early enough draw comfort from knowing others feel the same way. This connection can be especially helpful for people who suffer from illnesses that have a social stigma, such as cancer or AIDS.

Having the disease, the very thing that makes some people feel excluded from relationships with others, is the ticket of admission to the support group. Members often visit one another in the hospital, phone each other, share food and presents, and in various ways build a new social support network that complements the support provided by their own friends and family. Illness is an occasion for redefining personal values, and the demonstration of caring that often occurs in groups provides a vivid example of the importance of empathy with others.

EMOTIONAL VENTILATION

Some support groups—especially those led by health professionals—focus on helping members vent strong emotions about their situation. Many patients feel that they have to put on a front during their daily lives in order to avoid upsetting the people around them. Groups can provide an opportunity to express fears, pain, anxiety, sadness, and other difficult emotions in a sympathetic environment. The meeting becomes the place to deal with difficult problems, leaving members free to handle other issues outside of the group. A strong sense of acceptance and control comes from facing your worst fears and moving beyond them.

COGNITIVE RESTRUCTURING

In this approach, the goal is to help members change their perspective on their situation and their response to it. Those with medical disabilities are taught to view others as temporarily able-bodied—rather than seeing themselves as handicapped—and to learn how to elicit the physical help they need from others. Members give one another examples of ways to develop and use a new point of view about their illness. This strategy can also be used to battle poor health habits that can interefere with recovery. For example, smokers may be encouraged to concentrate on making a broad commitment to protect their body rather than focusing intently on trying to quit smoking, which can be self-defeating.

EDUCATION

Simply imparting information about a disease and its treatment can have a major effect. Support groups that are wholly educational are structured as a time-limited series of lectures—usually five to ten weekly or monthly meetings with doctors, nurses, and other health-care professionals—on the nature of the illness, its course and prognosis, and the variety of available treatments.

FINDING GOOD SUPPORT

The best place to begin a search for a support group is with your physician. He or she may know of one or even be sponsoring a group for people coping with your illness. Many hospitals and clinics provide such groups for their patients. Similarly, volunteer organizations such as the American Cancer Society and the American Heart Association sponsor some support groups and maintain referral services for such groups. Finally, there is no substitute for word of mouth. Chat with the people sitting next to you in the waiting room and see if they can refer you to any groups that have been helpful to them.

Support groups are often conducted by a health-care professional—a social worker, nurse, physician, or psychologist—frequently in conjunction with experienced patients. Some participate in programs for patients when they are hospitalized, and others convene meetings in homes or public meeting areas. Usually there is no charge, although there may be a modest fee to defray the expenses of renting the meeting place and paying for the professional's time. As a rule, avoid profit-making groups with advertising budgets, slick brochures, and hefty fees.

You will probably benefit from participating in a good group if you are curious about your illness and want to learn how to cope better. Meetings are less effective for people who dislike sharing their thoughts and feelings or are not terribly interested in how others cope. However, people who would fall into this latter category under normal circumstances sometimes find that in the face of illness they are suddenly quite interested in other people's responses.

Of course, the best way to judge whether a support group is right for you is to attend a meeting. View this visit as an experiment, an opportunity to learn something new about the illness from people who are expert at having it and treating it. Be prepared for open discussions of issues that you may consider very personal and embarrassing, such as fears that others can smell a colostomy bag, the agonizing and seemingly endless wait for the results of an MRI scan, or the painful reluctance to ask a doctor whether she or he recommends further treatment and who will be the one to provide it.

Try to be open about your feelings regarding your illness, but remember that you are free to choose how much to reveal about yourself. Think through your own ground rules: Are you worried that information about you will wind up in the wrong places? Are you afraid the group will tell you about consequences of the illness that you are not yet prepared to hear? Do you see attending a group as an admission that you have an illness you've been trying to deny?

Even if you find some of the thoughts expressed in the group upsetting or threatening, you should leave with a sense of having been helped and guided. If you emerge feeling attacked or belittled, the group is doing something wrong. Find another one.

One limitation of some support groups is their desire to maintain an optimistic atmosphere by not confronting the risks and problems associated with many medical illnesses. In some cancer support groups, for example, a member who suffers a recurrence can be made to feel unwelcome, as a "bad example" to the others. This is doubly unfortunate: It makes the ill member feel excluded at a time of great need and conveys an unfortunate message to the other members, namely that recurrence of the disease is too terrible to face. The exclusion of those who relapse ultimately makes other members more anxious: They know that if worst comes to worst, they will also be rejected. Choose a group that you feel is prepared to provide help no matter how you may fare.

Some support groups emphasize having the "right mental attitude" about illness, instructing members to visualize their white blood cells killing cancer cells or convincing them that illness can be cured only if they believe that it can. Having a positive outlook and trusting in one's medical treatment is helpful, but it is not a cure. Believing in mind over matter can leave patients feeling inappropriately guilty if the disease progresses despite their efforts to think themselves well. A good support group will not treat a physical condition as though it were a mental problem. A good support group will not blame patients for their illness, but help them face, understand, and cope with the illness. Remember: Social support does not provide a magical antidote. It should be used in conjunction with, rather than as a substitute for, traditional, aggressive medical care.

We die because we are mortal, not because we are lonely or have the wrong attitude. But we live more fully when we receive and take advantage of help from those around us. Although no one can fight our battles or do our living or dying for us, support groups can help do it *with* us. They can assist us in making the most of our physical resources to fight serious illness. They can help us acknowledge and bear the emotional costs of being ill while at the same time living our lives more richly.

THE BOTTOM LINE

A sense of social connectedness—joining together for safety and comfort—has had survival value for human beings since primitive times. From the day the helpless human infant is born, the support of others is crucial for survival. Now researchers are finding that a high level of social support may benefit our physical health, not only by influencing our behavior but by directly affecting our biological processes. Conversely, people who have negligible support systems—few or no family members or friends—tend to be less healthy and die younger.

Thanks to a growing body of research, evidence is mounting that social support in general and self-help groups in particular enhance our ability to cope better with physical illness. These groups provide a safe atmosphere in which to learn about the illness, ventilate feelings, and learn from the experiences and advice of fellow patients. Studies are just beginning to show that these groups provide a number of advantages. They not only seem to enhance their members' sense of control over their lives and ability to cope with the illness, but may also have biological effects, perhaps even helping the terminally ill to live longer.

The best way to find a group is through your physician, hospital, or other patients. To gauge whether a particular group is right for you, attend a session and see how you react. Support groups are no cure for disease, but they can help you live better—and perhaps longer.

HOW TO HELP A FRIEND OR LOVED ONE

You needn't feel completely helpless or irrelevant if someone close to you is diagnosed with a serious or life-threatening disease. The weight of scientific evidence says that family and friends can be enormously important in helping patients cope with disease.

But helpful social support doesn't mean merely having plenty of on-the-surface contact with other people—it means that the sick person must feel genuinely cared about. What matters is *how* people interact with the sick person—how much they show that they care about what happens to him or her, how often they make visits to the hospital, and how well they tend to the patient's needs after the return home. Concrete actions speak infinitely louder than hollow good wishes.

Here are some steps patients and their families can take to elicit the kind of social support they want from others:

1. *Banish secrets.* Families often want to protect each other from bad news, but hiding a person's serious illness from the rest of the family will backfire. Not only is keeping a secret quite stressful, but it cheats family members out of joining the common mission to help the sick person. The best strategy is to communicate directly and openly with close family members and friends about the illness. This will increase the degree of empathy and intimacy offered the sick person, who needs as much of both as possible.

2. *Include your children.* Although there may be limits to what young children can understand, if they sense they are being excluded, they will feel that they have done something wrong. Because young children tend to see themselves as the cause of whatever major events happen around them, they will view a parent's illness as punishment for some real or imagined wrongdoing of their own. You can reduce their anxiety and guilt a great deal if you explain the situation to them

clearly and come up with ways that they can help.

3. *Be selective.* Not everyone you know needs to be included in the patient's supportive network. Under the strain of serious illness, some relationships improve while others get worse. Both you and the patient should save your energy and use the illness as an excuse to disengage from unwanted social obligations. There are plenty of ingenious ways to keep in touch with people you don't have time for right now. To avoid the burden of information sharing, one husband jokingly suggested creating a telephone "voice mail" system to spare his wife the constant reporting of her condition: "Press 1 if you want to know how Martha slept; press 2 if you want to know the results of her bone scan. . . ."

4. *Tell family and friends clearly how they can help.* One cancer patient wrote a newsletter suggesting tasks friends could perform: bringing a meal once a month; calling other friends with information; driving the patient to medical appointments. Often patients are embarrassed or shy about asking for help, but friends and family usually *want* to help—you do them a favor if you tell them how.

Sometimes when a friend or relative becomes ill, you may back away because you don't know how to act around the sick person and her or his family. Here are three ways in which friends can be supportive of the patient in ways that will really count:

1. *Learn about the disease.* Ask the patient, friend, or family member whether she or he wants to discuss with you what is happening, and be prepared to listen.

2. *Help out.* Offer to do some of the less glamorous things that are terribly draining on someone who is ill or undergoing treatment: Walk the dog, do the laundry, drop the kids off at school. A group of friends who can help share the burdens of day-to-day life can be an enormous help to patients struggling to keep their family going.

3. *Give emotional support.* A hug and a few tears can go a long way toward helping someone who is ill to feel understood and cared about. If they start to cry when talking about their problems and fears, don't try to stop them. If you start to cry, let yourself. You will both feel closer.

21

HEALTHY ATTITUDES: OPTIMISM, HOPE, AND CONTROL

BY CHRISTOPHER PETERSON, PH.D., AND LISA M. BOSSIO

OPTIMISM HAS HAD A CHECKERED PAST. CONSIDER THE INSUFFERABLE Pollyanna, who preached that we should be glad for misfortunes because, after all, there's *always* a silver lining. Or the ridiculous Dr. Pangloss in Voltaire's *Candide*, who amid countless calamities still insisted we live in the best of all possible worlds. "Optimism," Voltaire wrote, "is a mania for maintaining that all is well when things are going badly."

But there is another brand of optimism that doesn't deserve this bad reputation. Optimists of this stripe view people as active participants in their own lives. They believe that expectations play a major role in determining what actually happens to them—not because they believe in mere wishful thinking, but because they know positive expectations lead them to take concrete steps that bring them closer to their goals.

Now there is good evidence that this sort of optimism can improve the quality of a person's life—and more. It can also play a key role in maintaining physical health.

The study of this connection is at the core of a growing body of research on the role of attitude in physical well-being. In the last few decades, a large number of studies have demonstrated a link between good health and positive psychological characteristics—not only optimism, but hope and a sense of

CHRISTOPHER PETERSON, PH.D., is a professor of psychology at the University of Michigan. LISA M. BOSSIO is a freelance writer and editor in the San Francisco Bay area.

control as well. The research leaves little doubt that when it comes to health, attitude does count.

HOW OPTIMISM IS MEASURED

One of the best research tools for measuring optimism is what psychologists call *explanatory style*: how people explain the bad events that befall them. For example, Mary Smith and Jane Doe both miss out on a big promotion. Smith is able to shrug off her disappointment: "It was just a bad break; maybe next time." Doe, however, keeps thinking, "I'm a poor excuse for a human being; I'll never succeed at anything important."

Obviously, Smith and Doe are miles apart on the optimism/pessimism scale. By analyzing how they explain to themselves what has happened, researchers can unravel three key components of their thoughts that identify them as optimistic or pessimistic.

First, the two women lay the blame for their misfortune at different doors. Doe, the pessimist, blames herself ("I'm a poor excuse for a human being")—what researchers call an *internal* explanation. It suggests some sort of fundamental personal flaw that will lead to similar failures in the future. Smith, however, believes that *external* factors like fate or chance—not some personal deficiency—were responsible for her disappointment.

The second component of explanatory style is whether a person believes the cause of the bad event is permanent or short-lived—to researchers, *stable* or *unstable*. If you see it as stable or long-lasting, that's pessimistic. Doe assumes that her own inadequacies won't change, so her future attempts to earn a promotion will end in failure as well. Smith, the optimist, assumes that her bad luck won't last forever.

Finally, optimists and pessimists differ in how pervasive they think their troubles are. Doe sees the problem as *global*—she thinks she will never succeed at anything. Smith sees her troubles as *specific* to her job, and doesn't expect them to affect other areas of her life.

Although these two women have had the same negative experience, they have interpreted it very differently. Optimistic Smith has an explanatory style that will probably further her chances of winning a promotion the next time out. Doe's pessimistic explanation is likely to result in a self-fulfilling prophecy, going hand in hand with low expectations for herself and leading to passivity and probable failure.

Usually, researchers measure explanatory style in one of two ways. The first is through a questionnaire that asks research subjects to think about hypothetical events that might happen to them and then asks them what they believe would be likely to cause those events. Subjects then rate these explanations along the three dimensions of explanatory style—internal versus external, stable versus unstable, and global versus specific—and average these ratings for an overall optimism/pessimism score. In the second approach, psychologists analyze written or spoken statements from their research subjects in the same way, by making the ratings themselves.

In real life, explanatory styles are rarely as clear-cut as Smith's and Doe's. The typical person falls somewhere in the middle of the optimism/pessimism spectrum. People may be relatively optimistic in one area of life and relatively pessimistic in another. Usually, though, there is some consistency in their style. (For a rough sense of where you may fall, see "Check Your Explanatory Style" on the next page.)

OPTIMISM AND HEALTH: THE EVIDENCE

Although folk wisdom has long held that optimism leads to good health, demonstrating this link in a rigorous, scientific manner has been quite difficult. Most people base their certainty that optimism is good for you on some personal encounter with an upbeat person who lived long and well. However inspirational these examples may be, striking cases are simply that: striking cases. They tell you only about one particular person's life and next to nothing about the underlying causes of his or her good fortune. But now, several well-designed studies have indeed suggested a strong link between optimism and good health.

In one of the first major studies in this area, one of us (Christopher Peterson) and his colleagues analyzed data previously collected during a 35-year research project, the Harvard Study of Adult Development. Begun in 1937, the study was designed to follow physically and emotionally healthy individuals through their lives. The 268 men in the study were drawn from the Harvard classes of 1942 through 1944. All were chosen for their academic success, good physical and psychological health, and high level of independence and accomplishment as determined by the college deans.

As undergraduates, the men went through numerous personality and intelligence tests. They were also rated by an examining psychiatrist who

CHECK YOUR EXPLANATORY STYLE

No one ever enjoyed being jilted, but the reasons people give themselves for having lost at love vary widely. Below are eight fairly typical reactions that fall at various points along the optimism/pessimism spectrum as measured by explanatory style. Imagine that a love interest has just walked out on you, or think back to a time when that did happen. How would you/did you react?

In general, optimists use external, unstable, and specific explanations for negative events, while pessimists tend toward internal, stable, and global explanations.

External
  Unstable
    Specific: "He/she was in a rejecting mood."
    Global: "People sometimes act that way."
  Stable
    Specific: "Intimacy is difficult for him/her."
    Global: "People have problems with commitment."
Internal
  Unstable
    Specific: "My conversation bored him/her."
    Global: "Sometimes I am boring."
  Stable
    Specific: "I'm unattractive to him/her."
    Global: "I'm unattractive."

attempted to predict each individual's likelihood of encountering future emotional difficulties. After graduation, the men completed annual questionnaires concerning their employment, family, and health. Finally, the results of their regular physical examinations, conducted by their own doctors, were sent to Harvard.

Among the many questionnaires completed by the subjects was a 1946 survey that proved well suited for examining their explanatory styles. The men had written essay-length answers to the following questions about their World War II experiences:

> What difficult personal situations did you encounter (we want details), were they in combat or not, or did they occur in relations with superiors or men under you? Were these battles you had to fight within yourself? How successful or unsuccessful in your own opinion were you in these situations? How were they related to your work or health? What physical or mental symptoms did you experience at such times?

For this study, we read through the responses of 99 of these men, picked at random, to find passages where they gave their explanations of bad events. An impartial panel of judges well versed in explanatory style theory then rated these statements according to the three dimensions: internal/external, stable/unstable, and global/specific. The ratings were averaged, and each subject was then given a score on a scale ranging from extremely optimistic to extremely pessimistic.

Finally, the Harvard men's optimism scores were compared with their health ratings as determined by their physicians from physical exams given at age 25 (about when the 1946 questionnaire was completed) and every five years thereafter. As expected, the men's health worsened on the whole as they became older. Even though all of the men started out in extremely good health, some nonetheless became quite sickly as they aged.

Significantly, the study found that men who scored optimistically in 1946 were healthier later in life than men who gave more pessimistic explanations. A relationship between optimism and good health became strongest at age 45, nearly two decades after optimism was assessed. This correlation held even when we took into account the slight differences among the men in their initial physical soundness and emotional health.

Next, we studied the relationship between explanatory style and physical health among 172 undergraduates enrolled at Virginia Polytechnic Institute. In the fall term of 1984, they completed three questionnaires: One measured optimism, another looked for depressive symptoms, and the third had the students describe all the illnesses they had experienced during the previous 30 days. For each illness, they reported the date that they first noticed symptoms and the last date that they felt them. The degree of illness was then calculated, based on the number of days that at least one symptom was present. One month later, the students were questioned about any illnesses they had experienced during the 30 days since they had completed the optimism questionnaire.

Finally, these men and women were contacted by letter one year later and asked the number of times they had visited a physician during the past year for diagnosis or treatment of any illness.

In the end, the study found that college students with an optimistic explanatory style had fewer days of illness in the subsequent month and made fewer doctor visits in the subsequent year than did their more pessimistic peers. These results held even when we factored in the subjects' initial health status and level of depression (since depressed people might complain more). During this time, the subjects in this group came down with infectious diseases only, usually colds or the flu. Because degrees of optimism and pessimism predicted these illnesses, the results hint that explanatory style may influence health by affecting the immune system.

Like the Harvard study, this experiment had some shortcomings. The students hardly comprised a cross-section of the population; on average, they were healthier, more intelligent, and more privileged than the population at large.

But while neither study alone was definitive, the converging results began to increase our confidence that a link really does exist between explanatory style and physical well-being. This confidence has since been strengthened further, as studies by other researchers have also linked optimism to aspects of good health.

For example, psychologist Leslie Kamen-Siegel and her colleagues at the University of Pennsylvania looked at the relationship between explanatory style and the competence of the immune system. They took 47 men and women between the ages of 62 and 87, interviewed them on a variety of topics, and determined their characteristic optimism or pessimism from their responses. A blood sample was also taken from each of the subjects at about the time of the interview and analyzed to yield a common measure of immunocompetence: the ratio between helper T-cells and suppressor T-cells (see Chapter 3). The more optimistic individuals had higher helper/suppressor ratios, suggesting that their bodies were better able to fight off disease.

Because Kamen-Siegel measured explanatory style and immunocompetence at the same time, the cause-and-effect relationship between these characteristics was not clear in her study. However, two additional studies of the link between optimism and good health suggest that explanatory style can affect the course of illness.

In the first of these studies, psychologist Sandra Levy and her colleagues at the University of Pittsburgh determined the explanatory style of 36 women with recurrent breast cancer. These women were followed for four years, during which time many of them died. Optimistic explanatory style was among the factors predicting a longer survival time.

In the second study, psychologists Gregory Buchanan and Martin Seligman at the University of Pennsylvania studied 160 men who had suffered heart attacks. Their explanatory style was measured from responses to an interview. The men were then followed for eight years, by which time 60 of them had died from cardiac causes, usually a second heart attack. Those men who still lived had had a more optimistic explanatory style at the beginning of the study than the men who died.

DISPOSITIONAL OPTIMISM: ANOTHER APPROACH

Several investigators have studied optimism by using different measures than explanatory style and have still found a connection with physical health—good evidence that the effect is real, not just an artifact of one particular kind of study design. Psychologists Charles Carver at the University of Miami and Michael Scheier at Carnegie-Mellon have studied an attitude they call *dispositional optimism*—defined as the degree to which someone expects the future to bring positive events rather than negative ones. Their straightforward questionnaire asks research subjects to indicate how closely they agree with such optimistic statements as "In uncertain times, I usually expect the best."

Using this measure, Carver and Scheier have shown in a series of studies that optimism is linked to good health and pessimism to poor health. Like our research with college students, one of their studies showed that pessimistic undergraduates developed more physical symptoms over time than their optimistic counterparts, even when they started out equally healthy.

In another study, Carver and Scheier found that dispositional optimism predicted how well men recovered six months after undergoing coronary artery bypass surgery. Compared to pessimistic patients, the optimists were more likely to have returned to work and to have resumed recreational, social, and sexual activities. They also were more likely to be exercising vigorously.

However it is measured, optimism does appear to play a role in good health. How large is that role compared with other factors? The answer is that our studies have found what statisticians call a "moderate correlation" between explanatory style and health. In fact, that's the most one could reasonably expect, considering the numerous elements that affect physical well-being, such as genetics, diet, exercise, income, social networks, and environmental hazards. But a moderate correlation can still have a major effect. In the study of the Virginia Tech college students, for example, a student with an optimism score in the top 25 percent went to the doctor only one-third as often, on average, as a classmate with a score in the bottom 25 percent.

THE ROLE OF HOPE AND CONTROL

Optimism and pessimism are not the only psychological attitudes that may affect physical health. Psychologist Charles R. Snyder and his colleagues at the University of Kansas have focused their research on hope—yet another way of understanding people's attitudes toward the future. According to these researchers, hope consists of two components: your determination to meet goals and your ability to create plans to meet them. Snyder has developed a questionnaire that measures hope by asking how much people agree with statements that reflect these two components—for example, "I energetically pursue my goals" (determination) and "I can think of many ways to get out of a jam" (creating plans).

In several studies, Snyder and his colleagues have shown that hope is linked to successful outcomes in various domains of life, such as work and school performance—and also health. In one study, for example, psychologist Timothy Elliott at Virginia Commonwealth University in Richmond found that patients paralyzed from a spinal cord injury who scored high on Snyder's measure of hope fared better emotionally and physically than those who scored low. Even if their levels of injury were comparable by objective measures, the more hopeful patients became more mobile than those who were relatively hopeless.

Another line of research has concerned itself with a person's sense of *control* over important life events—his or her ability to bring about good outcomes while avoiding bad ones. (This factor overlaps with optimism and hope.) Literally hundreds of studies have now shown that high-control individuals fare better in life than those who feel relatively powerless; they are more accomplished, happier, and indeed healthier.

A heightened sense of control can be beneficial even when it stems from a mere perception of one's circumstances, rather than the reality of the circumstances themselves. In one study, research subjects were exposed to loud bursts of noise and later tested to assess the effects of the noise on such mental tasks as proofreading. Some people in the study were told that they could stop the noise by pressing a button in front of them; others were not given this information. Those who were told about the button performed better on the later tasks, *even if they never pushed the button at all.*

The feeling of being in control matters whether you exercise it or not. And a sense of control is often more a matter of attitude—how you define your circumstances—than simply an objective reflection of your situation.

Evidence that a sense of control is good for health comes from a landmark study of nursing home residents by psychologists Judith Rodin of Yale and Ellen Langer of Harvard. The researchers gave half of the residents the right to make decisions concerning their day-to-day lives—such as whether they wanted to see a movie—to enhance their feelings of control. The other residents, in keeping with the home's usual procedures, were not given these options.

Over several weeks, the residents with enhanced control were more active, happier, and healthier than the others. And 18 months later, they were more likely to be alive. Only 15 percent of those with enhanced control had died, versus 30 percent of those without. This experiment showed that even increasing a person's control over apparently mundane things can have dramatic effects. Such research also suggests, however, that anything that depletes or diminishes control could undercut health.

Animal research has supported this conclusion. In the 1960s, psychologists Steven Maier and Martin Seligman at the University of Pennsylvania did a classic series of studies on dogs placed in painful situations they could not control. Their model has led to a whole series of studies on a concept, related to lack of control, that they termed *learned helplessness.*

In Maier's and Seligman's experiment, the animals were first given a series of brief electric shocks that they were unable to avoid. (The shocks were painful but not physically harmful.) One day later, the same dogs were placed in an enclosed box that had an electrified floor and a low barrier in the middle. When the shock was turned on, the dogs needed only to jump over the barrier in order to escape. They didn't; they just sat there and passively endured the shock. In contrast, when another group of dogs was first exposed to brief electric shocks that they *could* stop—say, by pushing a lever with their noses—they easily learned to jump over the barrier on the following day.

Why had the first group of dogs remained passive while the second group did not? Seligman and Maier proposed that the first group had learned initially that they could do nothing to control the electric shock and that this learning carried over into a situation where control was indeed possible. This phenomenon of learned helplessness has now been demonstrated in a variety of species, including human beings.

Learned helplessness has been linked to poor health in several lines of research. Further studies with animals have shown that exposure to uncontrollable shocks, but not controllable ones, can suppress immune functioning and increase susceptibility to tumor growth. (The relevance to human cancer is not entirely clear, however; see Chapter 5.) Human research shows, too, that a recent history of uncontrollable life events puts an individual at risk for a variety of illnesses, though various factors that affect a person's ability to cope, including one's overall sense of control over life, can largely determine how detrimental such stressful life events will be (see Chapter 2).

HOW ATTITUDE HELPS . . . OR HURTS

Several lines of research, using quite different procedures, now point to the same conclusion: "Positive" attitudes are linked to good health, and "negative" attitudes to poor health. Our next step is to uncover the mechanism that links positive attitudes and physical well-being. Clearly, the connection cannot be forged by magic. Our best guess is that there are several pathways, operating at different levels and each influencing the others. Research suggests that the following are the most likely routes, though we cannot yet say which are the most important.

THE IMMUNE SYSTEM
As described above, some studies with both animals and people have found that pessimism may adversely affect the immune system's functioning. These findings seem to support a plausible hypothesis: Pessimistic people may feel they are under greater stress, which in turn could interfere with their immune functioning, which could then lead them to fall ill. However, these results,

which come primarily from animal research, are difficult to interpret. It is important to remember that the immune system is just that—a system—and if one part is suppressed, another often takes over, in compensatory fashion. In other words, even if a negative attitude leads to low activity of a particular part of the immune system, it doesn't necessarily follow that pessimism weakens the immune system enough to make you ill.

BEHAVIOR

To date, the best-documented mechanism linking positive attitudes and physical well-being is that upbeat people are more likely than others to engage in health-promoting behaviors, such as exercising, eating well, and having regular medical checkups. They also respond to illness actively, seeing their doctors promptly and following whatever treatment plan is likely to help them get better quickly. Although these positive behaviors are undeniably beneficial, we don't know whether they are the most important factor linking optimism and health or just one of several.

FAMILY AND FRIENDS (OR LACK THEREOF)

Pessimistic people tend to be socially isolated, and isolation is a risk factor for poor health (see Chapter 20). In addition, their negative style may make it more difficult for pessimistic people to change their ways of thinking. Their pessimism fits within a certain social niche—a lonely one, filled with only a few other negative people—which leads them to maintain their pessimistic outlook. In some of our studies, we have found that family members tend to be similar in their degree of optimism or pessimism. If you find yourself surrounded by people who are gloomy, your attempts to be more upbeat are apt to be greeted with skepticism, if not downright hostility.

THE UNANSWERED QUESTIONS

Certainly, the evidence that attitudes influence health has important implications. But these findings do not boil down to simple messages or magical formulas for well-being. Questions remain, and it will take more study before we can offer definitive answers.

One unsolved puzzle is how specific the benefits of optimism may be. In other words, are positive attitudes a general boon to health, or do they confer protection against some illnesses more than others? We do not have a firm answer. Although the evidence suggests that the link is general, we have not systematically studied the range of human ailments in this regard, and there may well be some for which optimism proves irrelevant.

It is also not clear at what point in an illness your attitude is most likely to have an effect. Common sense suggests that attitude is probably least important at the very beginning and the very end of illness. In a recent study showing that stress can precipitate a cold among people exposed to the appropriate virus—described in Chapter 3—personality and attitudinal factors had no influence on whether a research participant fell ill. So optimism may not help keep you healthy if someone coughs in your face. Similarly, optimism is unlikely to rescue you from terminal illness. In a recent study of cancer patients whose disease was very far advanced, for example, personality and attitudinal differences showed no relationship to survival time. It is between these extremes that we believe psychological characteristics such as optimism, hope, and control play a role.

CAN OPTIMISM BE LEARNED?

There's an easy answer to that question: Of course! No one is born an optimist or a pessimist. Attitude is a product of our experiences and need not be fixed for life.

One way people can change is through a form of psychotherapy called *cognitive therapy*, developed by psychiatrist Aaron Beck at the University of Pennsylvania as a treatment for depression. Studies have now shown that cognitive therapy can be as effective as antidepressant medication, although some depressed people will still require drug therapy. A recent study has also shown that cognitive therapy techniques can help people learn to become more optimistic—not surprising, because pessimism and depression are closely linked. The psychological change seems to last. However, we don't yet have proof that cognitive therapy offers long-term benefits for physical health.

According to Beck, many people are depressed because they think in overly negative ways. Negativity has long been recognized as a sign of depression, but Beck believes it can be the actual cause. Further, Beck believes that people maintain their negative views because they think in irrational ways that keep them from changing their distorted perspective. Consider this typical exchange:

"What's wrong?"

"I'm such a loser. I'm so lonely. I have no friends."

"Well, have you considered going to the party that all of us at work were invited to?"

"No, I don't think so."

"Why not?"

"I won't have any fun. No one will talk to me."

"How do you know that?"

"I'm such a loser. I'm so lonely. I have no friends."

You get the idea, even if the depressed individual does not. Running through these negative statements is a clearly pessimistic theme. The negative outcome becomes "realistic" when it leads the person to create a world that indeed is gloomy and devoid of hope.

Cognitive therapy proceeds in several steps. First, patients are encouraged to see that their self-deprecating thoughts have an immediate effect on their mood, actually creating a state of depression. Second, they are helped to see that these thoughts are highly ingrained—in Beck's terms, they have become *automatic*—so that they can occur without people being fully aware of them; they only become aware of the depressed mood that follows the thoughts.

Patients are then taught how to identify such thoughts when they occur, to articulate them, and finally to ask themselves if these thoughts are warranted by the evidence. If not, they can replace them with more upbeat ways of thinking. And if these negative thoughts do seem consistent with their life circumstances, then the cognitive therapist can work with them to change those circumstances.

Cognitive therapy usually takes place in weekly sessions over several months. Whether it works by making a person more logical or by imparting a more pleasing view of an ambiguous reality, it does work, and in so doing, it makes people think more optimistically.

If you are depressed, we recommend that you consider cognitive therapy. (For some ways to do so, see Resources.) However, we have some hesitation about recommending cognitive therapy as a way of helping ordinary pessimistic people become more optimistic and improve their physical health. The health benefits of cognitive therapy have not been directly documented, although several researchers are now conducting the relevant studies. In addition, you may not be reimbursed for therapy by your health insurance policy, because "pessimism" is not officially recognized as a mental disorder.

TIPS ON RAISING OPTIMISTIC CHILDREN

Much of the research on optimism has looked into the *consequences* of this characteristic, rather than how it develops. However, we do have some inkling of the forces that shape our attitudes.

Optimism and pessimism apparently stretch back to two aspects of childhood. First, there are bad experiences: failures, losses, depressive episodes, harsh and inconsistent parents. The more of these you suffer during childhood, the more apt you are to be a pessimistic adult. Second are abstract lessons: what you hear parents or teachers say about the way the world works. Whatever their source, lessons in optimism or pessimism become internalized during childhood, influencing how we will view the world as adults.

Taken together, these ideas suggest the following strategies for raising an optimistic child:

1. Be consistent.
2. Be positive.
3. Be responsive.
4. To the extent you can, "program" the child's world to be consistent, positive, and responsive.
5. Give the child responsibility, and encourage independence.
6. Set realistic goals.
7. Involve the child in a variety of age-appropriate activities.
8. Teach the child not to generalize from specific failures.
9. Teach the child to have a general sense of confidence from his or her successes.
10. Encourage problem solving.
11. Help the child see failure as a challenge to do better next time.
12. Encourage humor as a way of coping.
13. Be a role model of realistic optimism.
14. If the child expresses pessimistic views, challenge them.
15. As best you can, screen the child's peers and teachers for pessimistic tendencies.

Can you become more optimistic on your own? It's possible. You'll find an excellent description of Beck's approach in *Feeling Good* by David Burns (see Resources). Perhaps the real title of the book should be *Thinking Good*, because that is what Burns urges his readers to do.

Here is some of our own basic advice for learning to be more optimistic:

1. Choose an area of your life in which you want to begin thinking and acting more optimistically.
2. Become mindful of your thoughts and beliefs in this area.
3. Ask yourself how realistic those beliefs are.
4. Set modest and immediate goals for changing your ways of thinking.
5. As you make those changes successfully, reward yourself.
6. Seek out the company of optimistic people.
7. Be playful about your venture into optimism.
8. Remember that optimism is healthy in part because it leads to action.
9. Ask your friends and family members to help you.
10. Make some positive changes in your life-style.
11. Be flexible. Use these suggestions in whatever way seems best to you. Expect some setbacks, and avoid blaming yourself if things go slowly.

We offer these tips with a warning: Merely reading this list will not make you more optimistic. Only action will.

Consider, too, that people are more likely to succeed in changing their attitude if another person helps. We follow this advice ourselves, because we are friends as well as colleagues. Not natural optimists, each of us helps the other to look on the brighter side. We agree to give each other some perspective when we get caught in negative thinking, and we remind each other of alternative interpretations, past triumphs, and future plans. We are hardly each other's therapists, but we have deliberately built this mutual encouragement into our friendship, and we can attest that it has helped each of us to be more optimistic.

If you want to become more optimistic, don't try to do it in a vacuum. Make changes that fit with your life. Cultivate new interests that will make you feel more competent and challenged by life. Do some volunteer work, seek out new friends, join your local health club, or find other activities you enjoy. Although we cannot guarantee that your health will improve if you take these steps, we can promise that your quality of life will.

THE BOTTOM LINE

When it comes to health, attitude does count. Numerous studies have linked such psychological characteristics as optimism, hope, and sense of control to increased physical well-being. Healthy optimism is not a Pollyannaish, unrealistic attitude, but one that embodies the belief that people can be active players in their own lives. Pessimism, on the other hand, breeds passiveness.

Although research on the link between optimism and health is technically difficult to undertake, several studies have now shown that optimism does help keep people healthy. Other psychological characteristics related to optimism—namely, hope and a sense of control—have been found to be important to physical health as well. Conversely, a lack of control can lead to a sense of passivity and defeat—what psychologists call learned helplessness—that is linked to poor health.

Attitudes probably influence health in a number of ways. Some studies suggest the immune system may be the mediating factor. Others point to interpersonal factors, such as social support, or to behavioral changes, such as eating well and exercising regularly. Most likely, all of these interrelated factors play a role.

Although questions remain about these links, clinicians are already exploring ways to change people's attitudes and thus enhance their physical well-being. One important tool may be cognitive therapy, originally designed to counteract depression, which seems to boost optimism as well. Although it is possible to change a negative attitude on your own, your chances of success are far better with outside help: a therapist or a friend who can help you look at the brighter side, interpret circumstances more realistically, and challenge dire expectations. Most of all, the key to success may be to change other aspects of your life at the same time that you work on becoming more upbeat.

22

PSYCHOTHERAPY AND MEDICAL CONDITIONS

BY JAMES J. STRAIN, M.D.

HARRIET PRIDED HERSELF ON HER INDEPENDENCE. A HEALTHY 84-YEAR-old widow with no children, she lived quite comfortably alone in her own New York City home. One evening, she tripped over the bedroom rug and was unable to stand up or crawl to the phone. The next morning—some 12 hours later—the woman who cleaned her home every week found her on the floor.

Harriet was rushed to Mount Sinai Hospital, where I am director of the Division of Behavioral Medicine and Consultation Psychiatry in the School of Medicine. She was diagnosed as having a broken hip, one of the most common medical problems among the elderly. (About four-fifths of the 270,000 Americans who break a hip each year are over age 65.) In the past, a broken hip often meant an elderly patient would be incapacitated for a prolonged period of time. But with current orthopedic treatments, a hip fracture patient should be able to walk with the assistance of a crutch or cane after six weeks, and by 12 weeks the patient can be essentially independent.

Harriet would not accept the fact that her prognosis was that good. She was convinced that she would never walk again, that she would have to give up her house and be forced into a nursing home. Like many elderly hip fracture patients, Harriet was thrown into a depression by her injury.

Often, this depression goes undetected or untreated and can lead to a self-fulfilling prophecy: Convinced their lives are over, depressed patients are un-

JAMES J. STRAIN, M.D., is a professor of psychiatry and director of the Division of Behavioral Medicine and Consultation Psychiatry at the Mount Sinai Medical Center in New York City.

able to work at rehabilitation. Because it is crucial that patients begin trying to stand and walk as soon as possible after surgery to rebuild muscle and prevent the development of dangerous blood clots, those who can't make the effort are more likely to end up incapacitated and dependent after all.

Fortunately for Harriet, her hospital stay coincided with a study we were conducting at Mount Sinai—in conjunction with the Northwestern University Medical School in Chicago—to determine the usefulness of psychiatric screening for patients with hip fractures. As part of the study, her depression was detected early. She received psychotherapy and antidepressant medication, which were critical in helping her make a full recovery.

When I first met with Harriet, I found it almost impossible to help her change her pervasive negative, despondent attitude. She was convinced she would never walk again. But eventually, Harriet revealed a striking and critical story from her childhood. After a long illness, her mother had died at an early age, leaving ten-year-old Harriet to manage on her own. After witnessing her mother's illness and decline, Harriet was convinced that her life was ending as her mother's had—being dependent on others and with no control over her life.

This childhood experience held the key to Harriet's despair: It had left her utterly convinced that the hospital care she was now receiving was futile. But through psychotherapy once a week for eight weeks, Harriet gained insight into the role that her childhood memory played in her current fears. I pointed out to her that medical science had made many advances since the days of her mother's illness, and I assured her that she had a different kind of illness, one from which she could regain her independence. She did not have to imagine herself fading away in some nursing home or having her life controlled by other people's wishes.

The medical team's confidence in her ability to improve relieved Harriet a great deal. She began to put more effort into rehabilitation. By the end of six weeks, she was able to return home from the intermediary care facility in which she had been placed after her hospitalization. At 12 weeks, she was indeed able to function on her own.

PSYCHIATRY IN A MEDICAL CONTEXT

Harriet is one of a growing number of medical patients who have benefitted from psychotherapeutic interventions. There is growing evidence of an enormous need for this type of psychological care, even though most people with medical illnesses are still unlikely to receive screening and necessary treatment for psychiatric symptoms.

The need has led to the development of a specialty called *liaison psychiatry*, practiced by psychiatrists like myself who concentrate on the psychological treatment of patients with serious medical conditions. The liaison psychiatrist, who generally works in a hospital, acts as a go-between, bringing knowledge of psychiatry into the general medical setting. The goal is to enable patients to be treated for mental or emotional problems that may result from their medical problems, and that may in themselves interfere with their treatment and recovery.

Liaison psychiatry is a close cousin of another type of practice called *consultation psychiatry*, in which a psychiatrist is called in by the primary-care physician to assess and perhaps treat a hospitalized patient who has been identified as having an emotional problem. Liaison psychiatry, however, offers a far more active approach, one in which the psychiatrist is considered part of the patient's medical team from the beginning of the hospital stay and works with the patient and his or her other physicians from the start, without waiting to be called. A related approach is taken by psychiatrists, psychologists, and others in the field of *behavioral medicine*, who use psychotherapeutic methods to alleviate medical problems—though not necessarily as part of a medical team. And recently, the Linda Pollin Foundation in Bethesda, Maryland, has been studying an approach called *medical crisis counseling*, a short-term counseling treatment for the medically ill.

Many physicians are unaware that their patients might benefit from psychotherapy or psychiatric treatment. Part of a liaison psychiatrist's effort is to educate other doctors to recognize and correctly treat mental disorders. Right now, about three-fifths of patients with psychological problems are seen only by primary-care physicians—internists, family physicians, obstetricians/gynecologists, pediatricians, and rehabilitation-medicine practitioners—and not by psychiatrists. In general, these physicians do not have the training, or the time under the current system of insurance reimbursement, to search for and identify mental or emotional problems in their patients. Yet research demonstrates that in any six-month period, one out of five Americans experiences a major psychological disorder—most commonly anxiety, depression, substance abuse, or acute confusion—and that the rate is even higher among patients with a chronic illness and among the elderly.

THE MAIN APPROACHES IN PSYCHOTHERAPY

Understanding the different kinds of psychotherapy can seem a forbidding task: There are more than 250 different, specific forms of therapy now practiced. Fortunately, they can be grouped under a handful of broad approaches.

In their book, *The Consumer's Guide to Psychotherapy*, psychologists Jack Engler and Daniel Goleman describe the five main approaches as follows:

Psychodynamic therapy derives from psychoanalysis and seeks to understand and resolve emotional conflicts that originate in your earliest relationships and repeat themselves in adult life. In psychodynamic therapy, sessions usually are devoted to exploring your current emotional reactions in terms of your past. This approach works best if your goal is to make some fundamental changes in your personality patterns (e.g., a history of self-destructive romantic relationships) rather than to change one specific behavior (such as a fear of flying).

Behavior therapy emphasizes changing specific behavior, like a phobia, by stopping what has been reinforcing it or by replacing it with a more desirable response. In behavior therapy, sessions are usually devoted to analyzing the behavior and devising ways to change it; you will carry out specific instructions between sessions. Behavior therapy is most effective with focused problems like a fear of public speaking.

Cognitive therapy is like behavior therapy in its focus on changing specific habits, but it emphasizes the habitual *thoughts* that underlie those habits. The general strategy is similar to behavior therapy, and the two approaches are often, but not always, combined. Cognitive therapy is best for problems where your habitual ways of thinking about yourself make things worse, like mild depression and low self-esteem.

Systems therapies focus on relationship patterns, either in couples, between parents and children, or within the whole family. This approach requires that everyone involved attend therapy sessions and often involves "homework" aimed at changing problem-causing patterns. Systems therapies are best for a troubled marriage or intense conflicts between parent and child, where the problem is in the relationship between them, not in just one or the other person involved.

Supportive therapy concentrates on helping people who are in an intense emotional crisis, such as a deep depression (which will generally also need to be treated with drug therapy). It focuses on the nuts and bolts of day-to-day problems and does not so much attempt to help you change as to help you handle overwhelming situations.

Research also indicates that primary-care physicians recognize cases of depression in only one-quarter to one-half of the patients who experience it, and they recognize other types of mental illness less than one-quarter of the time. But these same doctors write the majority of prescriptions for antidepressant and antianxiety drugs and may often prescribe them inappropriately: for the wrong illness, in the incorrect dosage, and for an inappropriate length of time. Clearly, there is a significant need for better recognition and management of the psychiatric conditions that so often accompany serious illness.

The most common psychological problems medical patients suffer from are "reactive" anxiety and depression—in other words, the emotional difficulty stems from a patient's reaction to his or her illness. Those with serious or terminal illnesses are particularly vulnerable. In other cases, psychiatric symptoms are directly caused by the patient's physical disease: The biochemical changes produced by cancer of the pancreas, for example, are often associated with depression. Still other patients experience a shift in their mental or emotional status due to medication; patients with collagen diseases or asthma, for instance, may react to the high levels of steroids that are sometimes required and that may induce a form of psychosis or depression. Finally, in the least common situation, the psychiatric and physical illnesses may be unrelated, as when a patient with long-standing depression suddenly suffers a coronary.

PSYCHOTHERAPY'S COST-EFFECTIVENESS

Whichever of these categories a patient falls into, if his or her emotional distress is identified and treated, the time spent in the hospital for the physical ailment is likely to decrease—a boon for the patient and an economic saving for the patient and health-care system alike. In other words, psychosocial treatment can be cost-effective.

One case in point is a 1987 study conducted jointly at Mount Sinai and Northwestern. Psychiatrist George Fulop of Mount Sinai and his colleagues (including myself) observed that patients hospitalized for medical or surgical reasons had significantly longer hospital stays if they also had concurrent psychiatric problems, especially if they were elderly. In other words, a patient who had a heart attack and who was also depressed tended to remain in the hospital for more days than a similar heart attack patient whose mood was normal. Fulop's study suggested that treating a medical patient's psychological disorders—through psychotherapy, counseling, or family therapy, or with medication if necessary—could not only improve psychological well-being, but have an effect on the patient's physical condition as well.

Several studies have now suggested that psychotherapy may reduce the use of medical services, enough to be cost-effective and to enhance the patient's quality of life. Effective therapy certainly lowers the medical bills run up by "somatizers"—individuals who develop physical symptoms for psychological reasons, even though they have no known underlying medical problem (see Chapter 13). But over the last several decades, researchers have also begun to assess whether psychotherapy can lower medical costs for patients with physical illnesses by reducing the number of doctor visits they make.

One well-known study—published in 1983 by psychologists Herbert J. Schlesinger and Emily Mumford and their colleagues at the University of Colorado School of Medicine—included patients with four common chronic diseases: airflow limitation disease (a group of illnesses including asthma and emphysema), diabetes, coronary heart disease, and high blood pressure. The researchers examined a group of Blue Cross/Blue Shield patients who underwent some form of psychotherapy after having been identified with one of these physical conditions, and compared them with a control group who did not receive psychological treatment after similar diagnoses had been made.

Three years after they received their medical diagnoses, patients who had undergone 7 to 20 mental health treatment visits had had lower medical charges than those who did not have psychological treatment. The total charges for the first group, including those incurred for psychotherapy and counseling, were $309 lower than for the other group. In other words, the savings on medical bills offered by psychotherapy more than compensated for its costs. After 21 sessions, the saving began to diminish as the cumulative cost of mental health care increased.

This study is often cited as "proof" of psychotherapy's financial advantages for the medically ill; it even led New York State to temporarily increase the psychotherapy benefits in its state employees' health insurance plan. However, the study was not without flaws. For example, it was a *retrospective* study, meaning that the researchers were looking back at the outcome for patients who had already been treated. More scientifically valid are *prospective* studies, which closely follow subjects selected at random from the beginning of treatment.

One specific limitation of this research approach was that the investigators could not clearly define the type of mental health problems the patients experienced or the specific treatment they received. The information used was from the Blue Cross/Blue Shield insurance claims submitted and could have encompassed a large variety of psychiatric interventions.

More rigorous research on specific forms of psychotherapy, including precise diagnoses, will be needed to reach firm conclusions about the economic benefits of psychological treatment for the medically ill. But there is already enough evidence to suggest that this cost/benefit research is important to pursue. For example, one review of 15 studies published between 1965 and 1980 demonstrated that patients who underwent psychotherapy used 13 percent fewer medical services than medical patients who were not in psychotherapy. And another assessment of 13 reports on the introduction of mental health services in different organizations described a 20 percent reduction in medical utilization for people who received psychotherapy.

MAXIMIZING THE BENEFITS

Our prospective research on elderly hip fracture patients is in some ways the culmination of many investigations into the relationship between the treatment of emotional disorders and recovery from a physical illness. Utilizing the findings from previous studies, this investigation included several factors likely to maximize the benefits to the patients we treated at Mount Sinai and Northwestern. The study clearly demonstrated that psychotherapy and psychiatric treatment for elderly hip fracture patients has physical as well as psychological benefits.

One crucial factor in the effectiveness of the psychiatric treatment was timing. Timing had proven essential in a previous study conducted by John Lyons, Jeffrey Hammer, and their colleagues at Northwestern University Medical School. Their study of 419 patients revealed that those who were seen by a psychiatrist early in their hospital stay (at least by the halfway point) were more likely to go home sooner. Those seen later had longer hospital stays.

Traditionally, hospitalized patients aren't evaluated by a psychiatrist unless the primary-care physician requests a consultation—and unfortunately, that request often comes late in the hospital stay (not uncommonly on the day of discharge). This leaves little or no time for appropriate psychiatric evaluation or for psychiatric treatment to have an impact. In the hip fracture study, therefore, we evaluated all patients within 72 hours of their admission to the hospital.

Another key to a successful psychotherapeutic intervention in a medical setting is ensuring that the psychiatrist is an ongoing part of the hospitalized patient's treatment team, rather than a one-time consultant. Previous research suggests that if a psychiatrist is not an integral part of the medical/nursing team caring for the patient, his or her recommendations are likely to be ignored by the primary-care physician and staff. Therefore, in the hip fracture study, the liaison psychiatrists were principal members of the patient's treatment team throughout the hospital stay.

Furthermore, it is essential to select patients appropriate for psychotherapy in the context of their illnesses. Not every patient with an emotional problem can necessarily benefit from short-term psychotherapy in a hospital setting. Substance abusers, for example, require long-term treatment and are unlikely to be sufficiently helped by psychotherapy and drug therapy for their emotional problems during a two-week hospitalization for infectious disease. Treatment can be started in the hospital, and appropriate referrals can be made for later care. But the period in the hospital may be too brief to demonstrate the medical and economic benefits of psychotherapy or treatment with psychiatric drugs.

The hip fracture study was designed with all these variables in mind. In addition, we knew that elderly hip fracture patients were prime candidates for psychiatric treatment; they tend to have psychiatric disorders that respond to treatment in a hospital context and can improve during the span of a typical hospital stay. For many of them, like Harriet, concerns about the injury's effects on their independence lead to depression. Their mood and mental alertness may also be affected by the blood loss that occurs during surgery, by the medications they are given, and by the foreign environment in which they find themselves.

In our study, 112 hip fracture patients were seen by a liaison psychiatrist as part of their ongoing medical care and were compared with a similar group of patients who received no psychiatric care. In addition to giving the treated patients psychotherapy and medications, the psychiatrist also participated in regular group meetings with the patient's medical team and worked with the patient's family, nursing home, nurses, social worker, doctor, and physical therapist.

When they left the hospital, those hip fracture patients who had been treated by a psychiatrist from the time of their admission were less depressed and confused than those who were not. Furthermore, they were discharged an average of two days earlier at Mount Sinai and also at Northwestern, as Jeffrey Hammer and John Lyons showed. And when they were followed up 6 to 12 weeks after leaving the hospital, the group screened and treated by a psychiatrist had fewer rehospitalizations and needed to spend fewer days in rehabilitation.

For these hip fracture patients, early psychiatric help not only improved their medical and psychiatric conditions, but reduced their medical costs as well. At the Mount Sinai Hospital, earlier discharge from the hospital saved $168,000 in costs for the group with psychiatric intervention, far outweighing the $20,000 cost of their psychiatric treatment. Their lesser need for rehabilitation or rehospitalization led to further cost savings as well.

WHO ELSE COULD BENEFIT?

Many medical institutions have begun to require early psychiatric screening for patients with hip fractures, reflecting the evidence that early identification and treatment of psychiatric disorders can have medical benefits and also be cost-effective. It is our hope that future research will offer information about other medical illnesses for which psychotherapeutic interventions can have an effect. (For example, David Spiegel has shown that ongoing group therapy increases survival in breast cancer patients; see Chapter 20.)

The Public Health Service and the Institute of Medicine are now promoting the use of guidelines for medical practice to improve the quality of care. With solid evidence of their benefits, psychiatric screening and treatment could become an accepted part of the treatment guidelines for several illnesses. (We would certainly hope that any future guidelines for the repair of hip fractures would take the need for psychiatric care into account.)

There is already some evidence that hospital patients in general—not just those with hip fractures—could benefit from psychiatric screening, and treatment when appropriate. Psychiatrist Stephen Saravay and his colleagues at the Long Island Jewish Medical Center followed patients for up to four years after they were discharged from the hospital. The patients had been screened for depression and other psychological problems at the time of admission.

The researchers found that those patients with psychological symptoms had longer hospital stays and higher rates of readmission after they were discharged. Those who suffered from depression or confusional states at their first admission also spent more days in the hospital for subsequent admissions up to four years after that first hospital stay. This important study shows that psychological factors continue to influence the course of medical illnesses after hospitalization and suggests that a timely intervention in the hospital may lessen the use of medical resources afterwards.

THE ROLE OF PSYCHOTHERAPY

Psychotherapy is a broad term that encompasses a number of methods used to help resolve a patient's emotional and psychological difficulties. It is only one of the types of treatment that liaison psychiatrists offer; they also use medication in treating patients with depression, dementia, anxiety, and psychotic states. But psychotherapy is a major vehicle for assisting patients with chronic illness.

In psychotherapy, medically ill patients are helped to verbalize their emotional conflicts. They begin to work through the anger and disappointment they may feel about being ill, in pain, unable to function mentally or physically, or concerned about continuing physical dysfunction and a potentially shorter life expectancy. Hospitalized patients with acute and chronic illnesses would often benefit from receiving psychotherapy because they are confronted with a unique set of stresses that compromise their ability to cope: the demands of a strange environment, anxiety at being separated from their loved ones, and fear that they will lose control of their mental and bodily functions, or even lose a part of the body itself.

Sometimes the therapist's major job is simply to undo a patient's misapprehensions about her or his illness. For example, approximately 20 percent of men refrain from working or having sexual relations after suffering a heart attack because of their fear (and often that of their wives) that these activities could kill them. Even if physiological tests demonstrate that they have sufficient heart function to work and to enjoy sex, they are reluctant to do so. In effect, they wind up as "cardiac cripples."

These men do not have a psychiatric illness, but have a misconception that is interfering with their full functioning. In this situation, the psychotherapist can help simply by pointing out to the patient that he is holding on to an erroneous belief—"sex or exercise will kill me"—that is not supported by current medical knowledge or his current medical status. The therapist helps the patient spell out his worries in detail and then attempts to work through them by pointing out the realities. For example, the therapist may examine the electrocardiogram with the patient and show him other evidence that his heart function is adequate. The therapist may also offer concrete examples of how little exertion certain activities actually demand; sexual intercourse, for example, requires no more energy than climbing one flight of stairs.

Therapy or counseling is also called for when patients are convinced they can do nothing to enhance their own recovery. Some elderly hip fracture patients, for instance, feel helpless and passive and insist they can't move or even attempt to stand up on their own. Doctors may be disinclined to push these elderly patients: after all, it's difficult to give orders to someone who is frail, pleads to be left alone, and reminds you of your grandmother. But in this situation, passivity on the part of the patient and the health-care team can be dangerous to the patient's health. Counseling can ensure that the patient is encouraged to take whatever steps are necessary for recovery.

Finally, for people who deny the fact that they are ill, psychotherapy can help them accept the reality of their medical condition. For example, a truck driver in his forties who had had a massive coronary refused to follow his doctor's orders to stay in bed. Rather, he spent his days running down the hospital hallway and doing pushups in front of the nurses' station in a frantic attempt to prove to them—and himself—that he was still in control, that he was a man, and that he was his old self. It was clear that he would not survive if he continued lifting the bed instead of lying in it.

Fortunately, we discovered he had a weak spot: He would never break a promise to his wife. So we explained the situation to her. She cried as she learned that he could die if he did not refrain from such vigorous endeavors. We had her ask him to promise to stay in bed for 48 hours. She told him that this mattered to her more than anything else in the world. "I always keep my promises to you," he told her. And sure enough, he stayed quietly in bed for two days and went on to recuperate from the heart attack.

For many patients, psychotherapy ends with their release from the hospital. But for others, the psychiatrist may recommend that treatment continue—at least until the patient has adjusted to being home again or the psychological problems seen in the hospital have been eased. In any case, psychotherapy for most patients with a medical illness can generally be short-term (although it may continue after they leave the hospital): It takes only a brief period of time for them to return to their accustomed pattern.

HELP OUTSIDE THE HOSPITAL

Of course, hospitalized patients are only a fraction of the people who can benefit medically from psychotherapy. There is growing evidence that it can be very useful for patients with a wide range of chronic medical problems, which can cause serious emotional problems that can, in turn, worsen the medical condition. Several studies have found that patients with medical illnesses who become severely depressed have a worse prognosis than those with similar medical conditions who are not depressed. One study of patients admitted to nursing homes found that those who suffered from serious depression were 59 percent more likely to die within a year of admission. Similarly, at the University of Minnesota, a study of 100 patients preparing to go through a high-risk procedure—bone marrow transplantion for leukemia—determined that 13 had major depression. All but one of these depressed patients died within a year of the transplant—but of the 87 patients who were not depressed, 34 were still alive two years later. And another recent study has demonstrated that men infected with HIV, the AIDS virus, develop AIDS more rapidly if they are depressed at the time that they test positive for HIV (see Chapter 23).

There is also evidence that treating depression can improve the physical well-being of people with chronic disease. Michael Von Korff, a psychiatrist at the Center for Health Studies of the Group Health Cooperative of Puget Sound, recently studied 250 people who were among the top 10 percent in their use of medical services—often because they suffered from severe chronic illnesses such as heart disease and diabetes. Two-thirds of those patients had severe depression or a history of it. But when the patients with severe depression were treated for it and their mood improved, the average number of days when they were incapacitated by physical problems dropped by 35 percent. For those with moderate depression who were treated, there was on average a 71 percent drop in the number of days of disability.

Many of the improvements in physical well-being may come simply from the patients' ability to take better care of themselves once their mental status is improved; for example, they become more willing to comply with treatment and increasingly interested in pushing themselves to recover. But there is also some preliminary evidence that a good therapeutic relationship itself may have direct physical benefits. Studies suggest that being able to confide your innermost thoughts and feelings (as you do in psychotherapy) can reduce physical signs of emotional stress, such as elevated blood pressure and heart rate.

THE KEYS TO SUCCESS

Although there is mounting evidence that psychotherapy and other psychiatric interventions are effective in assisting the medically ill, the mechanism is not at all clear. Because the psychiatrist engages in so many activities as part of the patient's medical team, it is difficult to pinpoint the major factors in the treatment's success. It may be that patients become more cooperative once their emotional needs are addressed. They may be less frightened about leaving the hospital because they have been helped through their anxiety or depression. They may also feel re-energized and therefore less resistant to rehabilitation. And, of course, patients who are less resistant to treatment, less hostile, and more grateful may naturally elicit more attention and care from their doctors and other caregivers.

Liaison psychiatrists interact with families and nursing home staff members as well, encouraging them to take the patient home as soon as he or she is ready. For example, the family and nursing home are often reluctant to cooperate with a patient's release if the patient is having delusions or hallucinations. But a psychiatrist who has followed the patient's case can offer reassurance that transient confusional states or strange ideas can be managed at home with psychiatric drugs. With such treatment and the support of an

WHO OFFERS THERAPY? AT WHAT COST?

If you have a serious medical illness, your physician may suggest that you consider psychotherapy to help deal with the emotional aspects of the disease. Because many physicians are not attuned to the medical usefulness of psychotherapy, however, don't hesitate to bring up the possibility yourself if you feel it would be useful to you. Either way, it's essential that you work with your physician to determine the best approach to psychotherapy for you, rather than simply go off to find a therapist on your own. Medical problems and psychological problems can be very closely intertwined, and your therapy should take your medical condition fully into account.

Many different kinds of professionals are trained in psychotherapy, including psychiatrists, clinical psychologists, clinical social workers, marriage and family therapists, and mental health counselors. Only psychiatrists are physicians permitted to prescribe medications. (Medication is especially helpful for obsessive-compulsive disorder, severe depression, manic depression, panic disorder, extreme anxiety, and psychotic states.) In general, psychologists and social workers can work effectively with a person with a medical illness as long as they consult with the physician in charge of the medical treatment and know that the physical aspects of the illness are being addressed.

If you want to use psychotherapy to help you cope with a serious illness, the most direct way to find a therapist is to ask your physician for a referral. Personal factors as well as professional credentials are important to the success of therapy: If you don't feel a basic level of comfort with a therapist, don't hesitate to ask for another referral.

The cost of therapy can vary widely, depending on several factors. In general, a private therapist will charge much more than a hospital, clinic, or agency charges for a therapist.

As Jack Engler and Daniel Goleman report in *The Consumer's Guide to Psychotherapy*, national surveys showed the following median fees per session for the main therapy professions in 1991. (Over the last several years, the cost of a therapy session has been climbing $5 to $10 every two years.) These are general guidelines; half of therapists in each profession charge more, half less.

Psychiatrists $100
Psychologists 85
Marriage and family counselors 75
Clinical social workers 70
Other counselors 65
Group therapy 40

Private therapists vary greatly in what they charge, from well under $50 per session to well over $100. Many therapists have a sliding-fee scale, however, and are open to negotiating their standard fee downward for those who cannot afford their standard fee. Insurance plans vary greatly in how much psychotherapy they will cover, if any.

accustomed environment, the patient may improve without spending additional time in the hospital or nursing home.

The basic message is clear: If a patient's emotional and psychological needs are being addressed, he or she is likely to cope more effectively with a chronic medical problem. Dealing with emotional issues can help medically ill people comply with their treatment, engage in rehabilitation therapy more vigorously, avoid unhealthy behaviors (such as smoking, drinking, and being sedentary), and be aware of any signs that their illness may be taking a turn for the worse that requires treatment.

PRIME CANDIDATES FOR PSYCHOLOGICAL CARE

Not every patient with a serious medical illness will need psychotherapy; many patients manage to cope with the stresses of illness and hospitalization very well on their own, with the support of family and friends. But psychotherapy and counseling efforts are crucial when a patient is in clear distress—and unfortunately, as mentioned earlier, many psychological problems are not immediately apparent or identified by the medical staff.

People with the most severe medical problems are especially likely to need psychological and emotional help. Severe liver disease, for example, is often accompanied by fear, anxiety, depression, and confusional states (such as delirium). When 40 candidates for liver transplant were evaluated at the Presbyterian University Hospital in Pittsburgh, three-quarters were found to be under moderate to severe stress, and half had psychiatric disorders ranging from delirium to major depression.

An assessment of the patient's mental status and ability to cope should be routine in medical care, as routine as checking the blood counts and examining the body for bleeding and strange swellings. Unfortunately, this is not yet standard medical practice. And even when physicians do attend to the psychological state of their patients, it takes considerable skill to find the true source of problems in people who are medically ill. Anxiety and depression, for example, may have a number of physical causes: They may result from a dysfunction in the heart or the kidney, from toxins produced by a faulty metabolism, or from a stroke or a blood clot. Drugs used to treat physical illness may also affect the mind and the function of the brain.

The unique role of the psychiatrist is to be able to tell whether anxiety, depression, or a confusional state is caused by emotional conflicts or is the product of a disordered body. This diagnostic step is critical before embarking on therapy. If it is omitted, a patient may be offered psychotherapy when the treatment should be for anemia, an infection, altered body chemistry, or a subdural hematoma (a pool of blood in the brain).

The need for a thorough, careful diagnosis of emotional difficulties is especially great for those medical illnesses and procedures that are most likely to involve psychological problems:

- AIDS
- bone marrow transplants
- severe burns
- heart or liver transplants
- end-stage kidney disease entailing dialysis
- hip fracture
- open-heart surgery
- plastic surgery

Patients with these medical problems—and probably others with certain severe illnesses—should have the opportunity to receive psychological care during hospitalization and convalescence as a matter of course. But a psychological consultation is appropriate for *any* patient who is having difficulty coping with hospitalization, who is not recovering at the expected rate, or who seems to be inappropriately burdened by mood disturbances, depression, anxiety, or confusional thinking. Undue concern about one's health even after the medical situation has stabilized, exaggerated fears of the future, profound isolation and withdrawal, feelings of shame about one's body, or failure to follow medical treatment—all are warning signs of the need for psychotherapeutic interventions.

THE BOTTOM LINE

Psychotherapy and psychiatric treatments can be very helpful for people with acute or chronic illness, even if the illness is completely physiological in origin (such as hip fracture in the elderly, end-stage renal disease, HIV infection, or cancer). These treatments are most effective when the source of the emotional problem is very carefully diagnosed, when treatment is started early, and when the psychiatrist or psychologist works closely with the patient's physicians.

For patients dealing with a chronic illness, psychotherapy can make it easier to cope with the day-to-day challenges and stresses the disease imposes. It affords the opportunity to view medical conditions more realistically, maximizes the benefit from medical treatment, and thereby contributes to physical and emotional well-being. Encouraged by a realistic understanding of the illness and the future, patients can make the most of their capacity to take care of themselves: exercising regularly, following dietary recommendations, taking medication as prescribed, and being appropriately in tune with bodily changes that should be reported to the doctor. Psychotherapy can help patients deal with the psychological ravages of a devastating illness, including feelings of rage and betrayal about having the disease.

Too often the despair over illness becomes more crippling than the physiological impairment itself. But psychotherapy and counseling can help people mobilize their energy to live more fully and productively. Psychotherapy and counseling are not a panacea, but they are a positive force for people with medical illnesses, helping them pursue health no matter how severe their physical problems may be.

23

STRESS MANAGEMENT: STRATEGIES THAT WORK

BY MICHAEL H. ANTONI, PH.D.

THERE WAS LITTLE UNIQUE ABOUT THE SETTING: A CONFERENCE ROOM at the University of Miami, dominated by a square wooden table. You could find men similar to those who sat around it in almost any corner of America these days. All of them were gay, and about one-third had just learned they were infected with HIV, the virus that causes AIDS. The men were meeting as part of our ten-week Cognitive Behavioral Stress Management program, which began at the university as part of a larger AIDS research project funded by the National Institute of Mental Health.

Our aim was to help these men face one of the most disturbing diagnoses in medicine—being HIV-positive—in as healthy and effective a way as possible. The type of stress management program we offered them is becoming a popular approach to helping people with chronic and deadly illnesses deal better with their distress. It includes instruction in a physical relaxation exercise to help calm both body and mind—but doesn't stop there. Fully half of the program is devoted to teaching specific strategies, such as assertiveness training, for coping with the stresses of daily life. The men in our program faced the turmoil of daily life compounded by all the uncertainties, anxieties, and distress that an HIV-positive diagnosis inevitably brings.

Throughout the program, the HIV-positive men were helped to find their way through the new, special circumstances they faced: dealing with the anxi-

MICHAEL H. ANTONI, PH.D., is an associate professor of psychology and psychiatry at the University of Miami, and an investigator at the Center for the Biopsychosocial Study of AIDS at the University of Miami School of Medicine.

ety triggered by every random ache or sneeze, telling family members of their infection, asserting themselves with recalcitrant health insurance companies or employers. Not surprisingly, many of the men finished the program saying they felt emotionally stronger, more confident, and better able to cope with their daily stress.

But emotional well-being was not our only interest. We were also investigating whether this psychological support delivered any physiological benefits, specifically by bolstering the men's immune systems. If a stress management program could offer medical improvement to people facing an illness as dire as AIDS, it might be promising for patients struggling with countless other difficulties as well.

Our results so far suggest this may indeed be the case. Men infected with HIV who underwent the program showed significant increases in their levels of helper T-cells—the immune system cells that are attacked by the AIDS virus—as well as in natural killer (NK) cells, which play a key role in suppressing tumor growth (see Chapter 3). In contrast, infected men who did not go through the program showed decreases in both immune system measures. Moreover, among HIV-positive men who went through our groups, those who attended more sessions were significantly healthier two years later than infected men who participated less frequently. By teaching these men how to cope better with the stress in their lives, we were apparently able to give their physical health a boost.

It's important to emphasize that we do not see our program as a treatment for AIDS itself, since the men had not yet developed signs of HIV infection or AIDS at the time they were in our group. Many of the men had normal helper T-cell counts at the start of our groups. There's no evidence that stress management will appreciably raise T-cell counts in patients in whom they have already declined substantially. However, our research suggests it may play a role in slowing the progression of HIV infection.

THE BASIC EVIDENCE

The stress management program that we designed was not unique. Such group training programs first became popular a decade or so ago. They were used initially to help people with psychological problems, such as depression or anxiety, and more recently to support patients with chronic diseases. Other researchers have used these methods with patients facing such disparate disorders as hypertension, herpes outbreaks, bulimia, breast cancer, and spinal cord injury. We chose to study men with the AIDS virus for two reasons: because they were a group clearly in need of help and because they served as good, if extreme, models of the stress a grave, chronic illness can create.

In general, HIV infection damages the body by attacking components of the immune system, most notably helper T-cells, that identify and attack viruses. Eventually, as these and other cells become ravaged, the immune system becomes so compromised that the body is left vulnerable to a host of life-threatening infections and rapidly progressing cancers, at which point the patient is considered to have AIDS. Because most studies suggest that virtually all people with HIV infection eventually develop AIDS, for which there is still no cure, people who learn that they are infected with the virus can be left shattered even if they do not yet have any physical signs of illness.

In 1985, when our research began, we were aware of previous studies that had linked certain psychological factors—a sense of lack of control over life, social isolation, and depression—to a decline in immune system cells, including helper T-cells. But no one had examined whether improving the psychological health of patients with HIV infection would help their physical health by strengthening the immune system or by stemming its decline. At the least, we reasoned, a stress management program would help infected people—especially those in the early stages—to grapple with the heavy psychological burden of the diagnosis.

We recruited 47 gay men from the Miami area, none of whom had been tested yet for HIV. Based on extensive physical exams, they all appeared healthy. In other words, there was no sign of physical deterioration that might lead them to suspect they were infected.

Half the men were randomly assigned to small groups for the ten-week stress management program, which entailed two weekly sessions, one devoted to coping techniques, the other to a relaxation exercise. The other men formed the control group and were not treated.

Five weeks into the program, both groups were tested for the AIDS virus. We discovered that about one-third of the men in each group tested positive for HIV. They were told of their infection in private interviews with a licensed social worker specially trained in counseling people after HIV testing. One week after we broke the news, the men returned for another blood test of immune function and for psychological testing, to assess the impact on their mood and their immune systems of learning they were HIV-positive.

We uncovered a significant difference between the two groups in both areas. HIV-positive men who had undergone the five weeks of stress management training showed little or no change in their levels of anxiety or depression in the week after being diagnosed. In the control group, however, we saw significant increases. For example, the depression scores for men in the pro-

KEEPING DEPRESSION IN CHECK

This graph shows changes in the level of depression from the week just before men were tested for the HIV virus to a point one week after testing. (The changes were measured by scores on a standard psychological test, the Profile of Mood States, or POMS.) Men who learned they were HIV-positive generally became more depressed, as would be expected. But the depression was much less severe in men who went into stress management groups. The level of depression went down slightly in men who tested negative, presumably because they were relieved to get a clean bill of health.

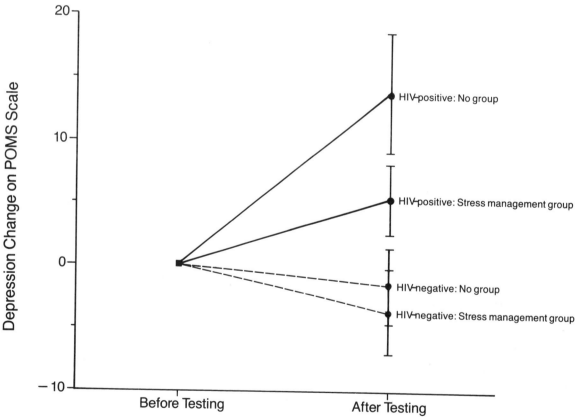

gram were just slightly higher than rates normally found in college students (see "Keeping Depression in Check"). But those in the control group were very upset: They scored within the range normally seen in psychiatric out-patients.

When we looked at the men's blood tests, we found a similar pattern. The control group showed slight drops in the levels and activity of helper T-cells and NK cells. But those in the stress management group actually showed a significant increase in the number and activity of these cells. Though the size of the groups was small, the differences between groups were large enough to be statistically significant in several cases.

In addition, we found that the increases in mood and immune measures were greatest in men who adhered strictly to what they were being taught. We assessed this by asking them whether they were practicing the relaxation exercise regularly at home.

Five weeks later, at the end of the stress management program, we tested all of the men again and found that the benefit of the program still held. It appears that stress management affects the immune system for the better both during an acute stressor—first learning of a deadly infection—and the early adjustment period afterward.

Our next step was to assess the *long-term* influence of this sort of program on the men's ability to cope and on their physical condition. Two years after the stress management training ended, we followed up 21 men who were HIV-positive—a group including men who had been through our stress management program, men who had completed an aerobic training program (another arm of our study), and men who had been assigned to the control group. We found that those who had been most distressed at diagnosis, used denial as a coping mechanism, and did not adhere to the stress management approach (if they were in the treatment group) were significantly more likely to have poorer immunologic status and more likely to have developed AIDS than the others. In fact, we were able to predict which men would progress to having full-blown AIDS over a two-year period based on the nature of their coping strategies. (We are now attempting to replicate this research with men who are symptomatic, though still without AIDS, when they enter the study, and we are beginning research focused on women and ethnic minorities.)

The way that people coped with their diagnosis also had long-term effects on mood. Men with poor coping strategies (such as denial) showed an increase in depression both five weeks and one year after diagnosis. But those who had mastered positive approaches—such as active coping and planning—had less depression as long as a year later.

Other researchers are now also finding that depression is linked to the progression of HIV infection. Researchers at the University of California, San Francisco, followed 330 HIV-positive men over six years. As they reported at the 1992 International Conference on AIDS, men who showed signs of depression at the start of the study had a more rapid drop in helper T-cells, developed AIDS sooner, and had twice the mortality rate of nondepressed men during the first three years of the study. By six years, the health of the two groups was similar; but since depression tends to wax and wane over time, the differences in mood between the groups could have evened out over those six years as well.

The UCSF study does not prove that depression speeds the progression of AIDS. It's possible, for example, that some unknown viral factor contributes both to depression and to immune system damage in people with HIV infection. But the study does add credence to the possibility that treating depression could slow down the decline of the immune system in HIV-positive people, as our own studies have shown.

Although our study focused on gay men facing HIV infection, our methods may be applicable to people confronting a wide range of medical difficulties. We are still running groups for HIV-infected men. But we are also exploring the effects of stress management on the health of people with certain types of cancer and chronic fatigue syndrome, maladies that are associated with impaired immunity.

TWO ROUTES TO RELIEF

We believe that one reason for the success of our program is its combination of relaxation exercises and techniques for coping with stress. To induce relaxation, men in our program spend one 45-minute session a week learning progressive muscle relaxation (see Chapter 14). In the first meeting, group members are taught to relax by tensing and releasing each of 16 muscle groups. Gradually, the muscle groups are combined into clusters; by the end of the ten weeks, members are able to relax their entire bodies through a simple countdown procedure. At eight weeks, we add an imagery exercise—envisioning themselves lying on a sunny, tranquil beach—to deepen the relaxation experience.

We call this relaxation training the "emotion-focused" component of the program because it is designed to help people cope with the feelings evoked by a stressful situation rather than the situation itself. This function can be equally well served by aerobic exercise, as our colleagues have found in a parallel study (see Chapter 19), and perhaps by other approaches as well.

The men also attend a second weekly meeting, which concentrates on teaching "problem-focused" methods for solving specific dilemmas they face. In contrast to relaxation, which helps people deal with unavoidable problems by changing their emotional reactions, problem-focused strategies help people master circumstances that *can* be changed. Part of the goal of treatment is to make group members more aware of the incidents that tend to alarm them and to teach direct strategies that will prevent or lessen their distress.

Both emotion-focused and problem-focused approaches are important in dealing with stress, because neither alone is the best approach to all situations. Circumstances, or at least a person's perception of them, may dictate which mode works best.

HOW NOT TO COPE

Left to shoulder the burden themselves, people with chronic disease may develop self-destructive ways of handling the challenges they face. One crucial goal of our stress management program is to make people aware of their automatic negative reactions, which simply exacerbate the stress. The program's problem-solving component focuses on becoming aware of any inadequate coping habits and learning to replace them with techniques that work.

We and others call inadequate methods of coping "indirect" because they are ways to avoid confronting one's problems squarely. They are common patterns, hardly unique to people with serious illness.

Some people use *behavioral avoidance*: rerouting their lives away from an uncomfortable person, place, or activity rather than handling the situation assertively. (An example would be a person who always skips staff meetings to avoid a hostile fellow worker.) In the extreme, this kind of avoidance can amount to a phobia.

Many people also make use of *cognitive avoidance,* in which they distance themselves from stress mentally by distracting themselves from the problem. A woman, for example, may keep thinking about the gift she plans to buy her daughter next week rather than focusing on the escalating fights she is having with her husband. Another tactic is outright denial: keeping pain out of consciousness by pretending it doesn't exist. An HIV-positive man who convinces himself that there is no threat to his health, even after he has been diagnosed, would be using this strategy.

Although these avoidance strategies are common, they do little to ease the burden. And our studies show that they can lead both to negative emotional consequences, such as depression, and to greater impairment in immune function, at least in HIV-positive men.

The other major indirect approach to handling stress focuses on avoiding the emotions triggered by stressful circumstances. Common strategies include increased smoking, eating, and use of alcohol and recreational drugs. Some people use even more extreme measures: They give up emotionally, feel completely helpless, even faint rather than face their feelings. Like behavioral and cognitive avoidance, these approaches to coping with emotions can be psychologically and perhaps physically problematic.

When people continually avoid dealing with stressful situations and the emotions they cause, they tend to get more and more stuck in their ways and unable to make effective changes. At that point, it does little good just to tell them to break their bad habits, stand up to their fears, and clean up their act. Often this approach simply reinforces how helpless they feel to change things. Even realizing that their ways of coping are ineffective may increase their sense of incompetence, helplessness, and hopelessness, which in turn contributes to self-destructive thoughts and behaviors.

People who have trouble coping with one problem often begin to consider themselves incapable of success in other areas of life as well. The result is a set of erroneous thinking patterns, or *cognitive distortions*. People begin to tell themselves they're just no good ("I'll always be second-rate"), give up their attempts to improve things ("I have no right to expect more"), and isolate themselves socially ("I don't need any help from anyone").

By helping people become more aware of the degree to which they use poor coping strategies and the damage they can cause, stress management programs can make them willing to learn more constructive approaches to handling stress. Specifically, the stress management program we offer teaches people four major approaches: cognitive restructuring, assertiveness training, using information, and enhancing social support. Although our initial work has been with gay men facing HIV infection, the strategies described below can be useful for managing burdens in your own life, whatever your situation.

COGNITIVE RESTRUCTURING

One of the goals of a stress management program is to clear up distorted ways of perceiving distressing situations. This approach is based on cognitive therapy, developed by psychiatrist Aaron Beck and his colleagues at the University of Pennsylvania (see Chapter 21).

Cognitive distortions are harmful in part because they can lead to and reinforce upsetting emotions. So our sessions encourage people to focus on the link between the way they *think* and the way they end up *feeling*. Before you can experience an event as upsetting, you must first process it in your mind and assign it some personal meaning. If your perceptions of an event are distorted in some way, your emotional response may be extreme—for example, depression or pervasive anxiety. But making a minor adjustment in your perceptions can enable you to understand things more clearly, just as you would fix the tuning on your radio if it were blasting static instead of playing music.

Although this may seem simple, it takes a lot of practice to do it effectively. Our first step is to introduce group members to ten of the most common cognitive distortions, such as "jumping to conclusions." We provide group members with a "book definition" of each distortion along with a tangible example of how this sort of thinking might take form in real-life situations. Next, we encourage group members to discuss ways in which they see these distortions in their own thought patterns. Once all members grasp how these distortions work, they are given a weekly assignment to record at least one stressful or emotionally uncomfortable event each day and note the way they respond to it.

After members have become adept at identifying these distortions, we teach them ways to turn around the thoughts—a process called *rational thought replacement*. One key way is by listening carefully to the words they use to describe their experiences. Words like *never* ("I'll never get it right"), *always* ("I always screw up"), and *should* or *ought* ("I should call my sister") are giveaways that the person is not thinking rationally. Group members are taught to be alert to their speech and thoughts and to replace these words with more neutral ones—for example, "*Sometimes* I make mistakes" or "My sister *wants* me to call her."

An important tool for replacing cognitive distortions is role playing, a common psychological technique used in groups. Each member presents to the group a stressful situation he or she experienced and is encouraged to reenact the situation with one other group member while the "audience" provides feedback.

ASSERTIVENESS TRAINING

This segment of the program teaches specific skills for managing difficult interactions with others. After all, if you cannot communicate your thoughts and feelings to fellow workers, family members, friends, and romantic partners, you are probably headed for conflict and stress. By responding assertively in such situations, you can often minimize the stress involved or eliminate it altogether.

In our first session, we alert members to the three styles of communicating: nonassertive (or passive), aggressive, and assertive.

In the passive approach, you don't directly alert other people to your needs or wishes. In effect, you let them guess and choose for you. When they don't choose wisely, you're left feeling hurt, anxious, and resentful.

At the other extreme is aggressive communication, which people often confuse with being assertive. Delineating the subtle differences between these two approaches is an important part of training. It is the difference between yelling at a waiter because your steak arrives charred (aggressive) and simply pointing out the problem and requesting a replacement (assertive).

Obviously, aggressive behavior is hostile and invasive. It leaves people feeling put down and turned off. Hence, they are likely to react aggressively toward you or walk away from you. In the end, you are left feeling tense and isolated—an unpleasant and unhealthy combination.

Assertiveness, on the other hand, means exercising your personal rights to state your opinion or feelings while simultaneously respecting the rights of others and hearing them out. In assertive exchanges, the communication channels are left open and messages are less likely to be blocked or distorted, so both people remain fairly relaxed, even while discussing difficult topics. Assertiveness allows you to deal with stressful topics efficiently, resolve conflicts quickly, and put less of a strain on yourself and your relationships.

In our work with gay men, we taught them assertive techniques for dealing with several life situations they were actually facing, such as talking with their physicians about their diagnosis (if they were HIV-positive), claiming their legal rights in the workplace, and negotiating "safer sex" with prospective partners. As with training in cognitive restructuring, role playing is an important part of learning assertive behavior in the groups.

INFORMATION

The educational component of stress management programs includes information on the nature of stress, the problems it can cause if not handled properly, and the various physical sensations that are signs of it. The goal is to help people become "stressperts" who can recognize when they are feeling burdened and act immediately to improve the situation. In our groups for gay men, the information portion of the sessions also touched on such topics as immune system functioning, HIV testing, viral transmission, safer sex, and the nature of the human stress response.

SOCIAL SUPPORT

It's critical to know there are people or institutions that you can count on for different levels of help. Because social support is so important to emotional and physical health, the program includes training in understanding its value, recognizing the numerous forms it may take, and assessing one's own support network. Although most people don't realize it, there are at least five major categories of social support:

- *Emotional support*: An expression of caring that lets another person feel liked, loved, or esteemed.
- *Positive regard*: Expressing agreement with a person's beliefs and feelings, or at least acknowledging that they are appropriate.
- *Information*: Providing knowledge that may be helpful to someone.
- *Physical support*: Providing physical aid or an opportunity to work.
- *Financial support*: Providing money.

These kinds of support can come from different sources and have different benefits.

People's social support networks may be stronger in some areas than others. We have group members answer a questionnaire that assesses how they are doing in the five major domains; for example, it asks how many times in the past month they have asked a friend for a loan, called someone for help with their car, or sought out a shoulder to cry on. The questionnaires are scored and translated into bar graphs that show the status of each person's social support in the five key areas. All members share these "maps" with the group.

Usually, the members have different strengths and weaknesses; one person may have plenty of people he feels he can comfortably ask for money, but none he can turn to for emotional support. The group members offer each other suggestions on shoring up the weak spots in their networks. For example, many members are reluctant to ask friends for emotional support for fear of being rejected, because their friendships have been based primarily on having a good time. When other group members recount how much deeper their friendships became when they opened up to such friends, it becomes easier to take the risk. We also provide group members with information on the whereabouts of several formal support organizations in the community.

An important aspect of our social support instruction is teaching members how to differentiate positive from negative support. Although social support can have many benefits, there is a risk in "negative support," which leaves you feeling down and insecure rather than recharged and upbeat. A prime example of negative support: A friend who wants to be your drinking companion, joining you in drowning your sorrows—and subverting your efforts to cope with stress more effectively.

One of the best examples of positive social support is the group itself. In fact, the support it offers is one reason why a group setting is the most potent and long-lasting way to learn stress management skills. In the initial session, group members are paired in a buddy system that remains intact throughout the program. Beyond that, all members are encouraged to interact with one another and the group leaders.

In these groups, there is a sense of warmth and security that can come only from caring human beings who know your situation firsthand, people who have been there themselves. We believe that groups in which everyone has the same chronic condition—whether HIV infection, diabetes, breast cancer, or something else—offer the most effective emotional support. The supportive and open group environment in our program encourages the honest expression of feelings. Members are offered nurturance, unconditional positive regard, reassurance of their worth, and a general sense that they can turn to the others at any time. But because we know the groups are limited to ten weeks, we also work with their members to help them use the resources of people in their communities, jobs, and homes to the fullest.

If nothing else, the success of our program shows that a multitude of strategies can help people manage stress. If relaxation exercises don't work well for you—or aren't enough—there is an arsenal of techniques that you can deploy, whatever the medical circumstances or other challenges of your life.

THE BOTTOM LINE

Group stress management programs for people with chronic illness are becoming a common mind/body treatment. Research has long shown that such groups are an extremely effective way of teaching people more successful ways to shoulder the psychological burden their illness causes. And recent research on gay men infected with the AIDS virus adds evidence that these groups can offer physiological benefits as well.

Stress management groups teach relaxation techniques that calm the body and mind in the face of distress, but this is only one component of their approach. The groups also teach four specific coping strategies that can help group members face particularly stressful circumstances in everyday life:

Cognitive restructuring helps them recognize irrational thinking patterns that can cause or exacerbate negative emotions and helps them replace those thoughts with rational ones.

Assertiveness training teaches ways to express their wishes concretely while still respecting the needs and desires of others. Learning this productive way of communicating can short-circuit stressful encounters, putting less wear and tear on the body, mind, and relationships.

Information on the causes and signs of stress—and on the specific illness or problem group members share—is another key part of stress management.

Social support is a major focus of these groups. Members learn to recognize the many types of support and their benefits in coping with stress. They learn how to augment weak areas of their current support networks. And the group itself serves as a model of good social support, offering members a safe place to learn and share.

V

BECOMING AN
ACTIVE PATIENT

24

PREPARING FOR SURGERY AND MEDICAL PROCEDURES

BY HENRY L. BENNETT, PH.D., AND ELIZABETH A. DISBROW, M.A.

WHEN WE WALK DOWN THE HALLS AT THE MEDICAL CENTER OF THE UNIversity of California, Davis, we hear staff members refer to patients by their illness or surgery rather than by their names: "the bowel resection," "the endo chole," "that hot ectopic." When we first started working as psychologists in the Department of Anesthesiology, we felt that this habit seemed to strip patients of their humanity, reducing them to a pathology to be treated or fixed. In time, we have come to understand the reason for this shorthand: It immediately conveys useful, specific information to the operating room team in a way that saying, "George Jones is here for his first surgical experience," obviously doesn't.

Still, the clinical, technical approach of a medical team can be tough on a patient. Undergoing a difficult medical procedure—surgery, in particular—means confronting your vulnerability and mortality. Alone, stripped of everything including your clothes, you are likely to feel defenseless and fearful.

In a surgical situation, there are two opposite camps: a well-trained team ready to perform a medical procedure and an unprepared patient feeling anxious, uncertain, and helpless. Patients sometimes turn to the surgeon, anesthesiologist, or nurses to help them manage psychologically, but this strategy

HENRY L. BENNETT, PH.D., a psychologist, is an associate clinical professor in the Department of Anesthesiology at the University of California, Davis, Medical Center, where ELIZABETH A. DISBROW, M.A., is a staff research associate.

often backfires. These medical professionals are trained mostly in the technical aspects of medicine, not in hand-holding.

However, health-care professionals are beginning to understand the benefits of helping patients cope with the psychological stress of surgery. Research shows that if your anxiety over an operation is eased and you feel some degree of control, you are likely to experience less physical discomfort after surgery and recover more quickly. Someday, most hospitals may have surgery preparation programs to help patients harness their psychological abilities to help themselves through surgical procedures. Meanwhile, it's largely up to patients to prepare themselves for surgery by following specific steps to make the experience less taxing physically and more tolerable emotionally.

THE POWER OF CONTROL

There's an old saying among doctors: "The way the patient goes into anesthesia is the way the patient will come out of it." In other words, people who approach surgery with a truly cheerful demeanor and a sense of being in control do much better both during and after surgery than highly anxious patients who feel overwhelmed by the situation.

Contrary to popular belief, anesthesia does not "shut off" your brain entirely for the duration of surgery. Anesthesia is designed to provide three things: lack of movement; analgesia, or freedom from pain; and amnesia, or lack of memory for the surgery. When it is properly administered, anesthesia does provide unconsciousness, but your brain still works and seems to maintain some unconscious awareness of its surroundings. In fact, a number of well-designed studies suggest that under certain conditions, surgical patients can actually hear operating room conversation (see "Can Patients Hear During Surgery?").

For the past four years, our team at the University of California, Davis, has been developing a "comfort monitor" that assesses the unconscious effects of surgery on patients through microscopic analysis of their facial muscles. Although invisible to the human eye, electrical pulses of extremely small voltage are emitted by the facial muscles, even when drugs that paralyze muscles are used for anesthesia (as is common).

By measuring which facial muscles are most active, we can detect a patient's expression. For example, if the machine registers a relatively high degree of frowning/wincing and jaw clamping, these are signs that the patient is

CAN PATIENTS HEAR DURING SURGERY?

One of us (Henry Bennett) first became interested in the psychology of surgery by pursuing an academic question: Are patients aware of the speech and other sounds around them when they're under general anesthesia, even though they don't remember anything when they awaken? While the evidence is mixed, there have now been three international conferences on the topic, resulting in two books.

A number of well-designed studies now suggest that under certain conditions, which are not well understood, surgical patients can subconsciously pick up operating room conversation and be affected by it postsurgically. About 20 research centers (most of them in Europe) are trying to determine how, where, when, and why this can occur. This research has two basic implications.

For physicians who perform surgery, the message is simple: Watch your language. An offhand comment—for example, a surgeon saying, "Look how her cancer has spread!"—may be perceived by the patient, making the experience of surgery more stressful and hindering physical and emotional recovery after surgery.

For patients, the message is: Protect yourself during surgery by using earplugs or, preferably, a cassette player. These devices can do more than block out disturbing sounds in the operating room; they can also provide you with sounds that have a positive effect. Soothing music or other sounds can help you relax as you are entering anesthesia and may help you subconsciously once you are under.

In addition, there's some evidence that verbal suggestions can be heard subconsciously during surgery and can help promote recovery afterward. A well-controlled study by anesthesiologist T. McLintock and colleagues at the Royal Infirmary in Glasgow showed that women who listened to a tape of "positive therapeutic suggestions" while undergoing a total abdominal hysterectomy required 24 percent less pain medication the day after surgery than patients who were given a blank tape instead. The benefit of the suggestions was totally unconscious: After surgery, all of the patients said they didn't remember anything.

uncomfortable. Higher brow and cheek muscle activity indicates a smile—a comfortable patient. If there is no difference in voltage across facial muscles, we assume the patient is at ease.

One of our goals is to find a way of detecting an unusual but serious surgical problem: In rare circumstances, patients may regain conscious awareness during surgery under general anesthesia (though they don't necessarily feel pain). This can occur if the inhalation agents that keep them unconscious must be turned down or even turned off in an emergency situation. Although this problem appears to be rare, a five-year survey at UC–Davis has found about 50 patients so far out of 30,000 undergoing anesthesia who say they remember having this experience; many of them were traumatized by it.

If a patient does become conscious during surgery, he or she generally has no way to signal the surgical team because modern anesthesia utilizes powerful relaxants that paralyze the muscles. At present, hospitals do not monitor whether you are aware during anesthesia; it is simply assumed that the anesthesia is working. Our work could give surgical teams a way to detect a change in the patient's consciousness and adjust the dose of anesthesia accordingly.

Beyond providing a tool for dealing with a rare problem, our "comfort monitor" is starting to shed some light on the experience that patients generally have under anesthesia. The great majority register significant discomfort. Of 70 patients we have closely monitored over two years, only one essentially remained "at ease" throughout a major intra-abdominal operation.

This patient's story, however, may symbolize the benefits of being emotionally prepared for surgery. She happened to be the only patient in this group who took the prospect of major surgery quite seriously. She employed a psychological counselor and spent several sessions planning her strategy. She then brought a cassette player to the operating room and listened to soothing music through headphones both before and during surgery.

This woman awakened after surgery feeling calm and comfortable and was discharged from the intensive care unit to a regular ward room on the second day. She was relaxed and pleasantly in control, she needed minimum medication, and her bowels were working fully. In contrast, other patients undergoing similar surgery were highly anxious, needed far more medication, had much longer stays in intensive care, and did not have functioning bowels for approximately one week.

Although one patient alone proves nothing, this woman's experience echoes the findings of numerous studies on the benefits of psychological preparation for surgery. She intuitively understood that the way she went into anesthesia would be the way she came out.

A FASTER RECOVERY

It has long been suspected that intense preoperative anxiety can have a negative effect on recovery. And conversely, there is good evidence that psychological preparation for surgery can improve the physiological response to the procedure.

Over the last three decades, researchers have performed many experiments to determine what sorts of psychological preparation would most help surgical patients. Over the last 30 years, a variety of techniques have been shown to be useful in different situations. For example:

- Hypnosis prior to surgery can reduce the length of a hospital stay and analgesic use after surgery.
- Relaxation instructions given to patients undergoing abdominal surgery can reduce their pain when they become mobile again after surgery and reduce their need for analgesics.
- Giving patients educational information before chest and abdominal surgery can improve their breathing capacity afterward.
- An informational preoperative session can reduce circulatory complications after surgery.
- Small group therapy sessions before surgery can reduce postoperative blood pressure.
- A group of people who went through several educational sessions before surgery returned to work earlier than similar patients who did not attend such sessions.

Research has now clearly established that psychological and behavioral preparation for surgery can affect the body's recovery. When psychiatrists Malcolm Rogers and Peter Reich at Harvard Medical School did a thorough review of the literature, they found the most consistent benefits were in reducing postoperative pain and shortening the length of hospitalization, although other physiological improvements (as well as psychological ones) were also shown in some studies. Another review of 13 studies, done by

CHOICES TO CONSIDER

In our experience, the following questions are often sources of anxiety and uncertainty for patients planning to undergo surgery. Dealing with these issues actively can do a lot to reduce the anxiety.

How do I know I really need surgery? Before having an operation, get at least one other medical opinion from a physician in the same specialty, outside your local community. You may also want to get an opinion from a specialist in a different field of medicine, because this can alert you to alternative treatments. A classic example is therapy for lower-back pain: A surgeon will usually recommend an operation, while an internist is more likely to suggest medication to stop muscle spasms. A surgical quick fix may sound appealing, but it's often not the cure-all it appears to be. To confirm that surgery is the right option, you may need to undergo some specific diagnostic tests.

Which type of facility is better: a small, intimate hospital close to home or a large medical center or specialty hospital? The answer depends on the type of surgery you are having. If the procedure is commonplace—such as a hernia repair, gallbladder operation, or hysterectomy—chances are that your local hospital will offer good pre- and postoperative care, provided the general surgeon you use is board certified and has performed the surgery often. But if you are facing a complicated or very invasive operation, it is generally best to go to a specialty hospital or regional medical center, where you're more likely to find a surgeon highly experienced in that particular procedure.

What should I do if I may need a blood transfusion during surgery? Ask the surgeon ahead of time if you're likely to lose enough blood to require replacement. If so, consider autologous blood donation, in which you donate your own blood several weeks before the surgery, in case you need it.

Another alternative is the recently developed "cell saver." As blood is lost during surgery, it is transferred to a sterilized canister and the healthy red blood cells are then recycled back into your veins through the IV. This system can salvage about half of the blood lost in an operation. If the hospital you're considering doesn't offer it, and you may lose a lot of blood, consider going to a different hospital.

Some people make use of directed blood donations from friends and relatives. But the complication rates are high. You are more likely to receive tainted blood from an untested friend than from your local blood bank, which has ongoing donors whose health and blood are checked regularly.

researcher Emily Mumford and her colleagues at the University of Colorado, showed that psychological preparation reduced hospital stays by 2.4 days on average.

Although many different psychological approaches can be helpful, research is demonstrating that the greatest physiological benefits come from the patient's taking an *active* approach to surgery, not simply trying to relax. When you undergo an invasive medical procedure, the health-care team often says, "Just relax, we'll take good care of you. We'll be putting you to sleep." But while the "sleep" metaphor may sound comforting, it is far from accurate. Brain activity during anesthesia is unrelated to that of normal sleep.

Moreover, undergoing surgery takes a great deal of energy—much like running a marathon. The opening of the body and repair of tissues and organs puts tremendous demands on the body. Throughout the operation, stress hormones surge as the body mobilizes to meet the test. For hours or even days afterward, a surgical patient may feel tired, relieved, relaxed, or exhausted.

As with an athletic event, successful surgery requires that you train, know the course to follow, and have the right equipment. Imagine setting out on a marathon or steeplechase course, being told you *must* complete it, but having no idea about the rules, successful strategies, or the results of those who went before you. No wonder so many surgical patients feel helpless—a feeling that can inhibit their physical recovery.

The key to coping with surgery effectively is to rethink your role, from that of a passive body being worked on by professionals to that of an athlete in the midst of an especially challenging event. One especially powerful approach for doing that—one that seems to be more effective than either relaxation alone or simply gathering information about the procedure—is an approach called *instructional intervention*.

In this method, a health-care professional works with you before surgery, starting by helping you focus your attention (though formal hypnosis isn't necessarily used). He or she then gives you very specific instructions or suggestions for influencing functions controlled by the autonomic nervous system—such as pain perception, bowel contractions, blood flow, and perhaps even immune functioning—that will influence recovery from the surgery you are about to undergo. Doctors used to think these autonomic activities were wholly outside of our voluntary control, but the growing field of mind/body research indicates that both animals and humans can learn to alter them somewhat. Even if your doctor is unfamiliar with these techniques, you may want to make a tape yourself, using some of the suggestions given below, and listen to it as part of your preparation. If nothing else, going through this kind of preparation can enhance your feeling of control over the situation.

Here are the most common functions that people can learn to control, and thus speed their recovery.

PAIN CONTROL

Although relaxation and psychological preparation are generally helpful in reducing postoperative pain, some approaches are more helpful than others. Some studies have shown that postoperative pain can be reduced by teaching patients simple coping techniques or by giving them educational information before surgery. However, other studies have shown no benefit in pain prevention from offering presurgical patients group therapy, information about the surgical process, reassurance, or advice in redirecting their attention away from the pain. Also ineffective was a presurgical program that included self-hypnosis with *nonspecific* suggestions for relaxation and distraction from pain.

Specific physiological instructions seem to be particularly useful in controlling postsurgical pain. In a classic study in the early 1960s—performed by a group of researchers led by anesthesiologist Larry Egbert at Massachusetts General Hospital—46 patients were told by their anesthesiologist that they could relieve pain around the site of incision by relaxing the surrounding muscles; the patients were then instructed on how to do this. These patients requested lower doses of morphine for pain relief and returned home sooner than a group of similar patients who did not receive these instructions.

More recent studies confirm that specific training in relaxing the muscles around the site of the incision helps to reduce discomfort after surgery. In one study, people who used biofeedback specifically to relax their abdominal muscles reported less pain and used lower doses of analgesics after surgery. Simple, specific verbal instructions to relax the appropriate muscles can also be valuable. As part of our patient preparation program, developed on the basis of published studies, we often give our patients suggestions like the following:

> All of your muscles in your [site of surgery] will be completely relaxed as you come out of the operation. It is very important that all of these muscles remain completely relaxed, even limp, like a rag doll, limp and relaxed, so that blood will flow into that area so much better to heal you, so that the pain medicine will work so much better. With relaxed muscles, you know what to do. With relaxed muscles, you will recover more quickly and more comfortably. Therefore all of the muscles in your [site of surgery] will be completely relaxed after surgery and will remain relaxed.

STOMACH AND BOWEL ACTIVITY

Surgery to the gastrointestinal tract can lead to several unique postoperative side effects. Among the most important is ileus: the cessation of contractions in various digestive organs, such as the stomach and large and small intestines. Without this movement, the patient cannot begin eating normally again.

In a study we conducted in 1990, we were able to speed patients' recovery by giving them specific instructions. First, a nurse randomly assigned 40 patients about to undergo abdominal surgery to one of two counseling groups. In a 15-minute interview, the first group was simply given information and instructions about how to clear their lungs after surgery. The second group was also given information and then direct, physiologically precise suggestions that their gastrointestinal systems would begin functioning soon after surgery.

The two interviews differed only in the use of the physiological instructions. For example, the patients who got those instructions were told: "Your stomach will churn and growl, your intestines will pump and gurgle, and you will be hungry soon after your surgery." The patients were also asked what foods they were looking forward to eating after surgery. They were then told that thoughts of favorite foods often lead to stomach growling, and the suggestion was given: "So you can get back to eating [the favorite food] just as soon as possible, your stomach and intestines will start moving and churning and gurgling very soon after surgery. . . ."

Patients in this instructional group showed a significant reduction in the amount of time their stomach and intestines remained inactive after their operations. Their bowels began to move in an average of 2.6 days, compared to 4.2 days in the first group. (The patients' susceptibility to hypnosis, as determined by a psychological scale, did not influence how affected they were by the instructions.) Finally, patients who were in this second group left the hospital an average 1.5 days sooner than those in the other group—a saving of about $1,200 per patient.

In contrast, simply reassuring patients before abdominal surgery or telling them what to expect without giving them specific instructions have been shown to be only marginally effective when tested as ways to prevent other side effects of this surgery. Several researchers have tried to use such approaches to reduce postoperative vomiting, a common complication of surgery. One research team had a nurse sit with and reassure patients immediately before surgery, but the benefits were not significant. Another conducted small, hour-long group sessions in which patients received information about what to expect and discussed their anxiety; but this approach, too, did not lessen postoperative nausea or vomiting. A specific instructional approach remained the most effective.

BLOOD LOSS

Two patients undergoing similar surgery can lose very different amounts of blood; the loss is not easy to predict or control. A large amount of blood loss is dangerous for the patient and hinders the surgeon's view of the surgical site, making the operation more difficult. However, research has shown that giving people appropriate verbal instructions can actually lead them to redirect their blood flow around specific parts of the body. In the mid-1980s, one of us (Henry Bennett) and colleagues decided to see whether that principle could be applied to patients undergoing a certain type of spinal surgery that generally leads to profuse blood loss (enough to require a transfusion).

In our study, 94 patients scheduled for spinal surgery were randomly divided into three groups before the operation for a 15-minute intervention, delivered by a psychologist. The first group received only information about neural monitoring of spinal cord function, a procedure that patients in each of the groups would go through. The second group was also taught how to relax their muscles while entering and emerging from anesthesia.

The third group, which we called the *blood-shunting* group, was given all of the instructions the first two groups received and was then told how important it was that they conserve blood during the surgery. To help these patients believe that they could control their blood flow through words alone, they were reminded of the phenomenon of blushing, a change in blood flow that reddens the face, which can be triggered just by being embarrassed by someone else's words. Then they were given these specific instructions:

Blood vessels are made of smooth muscle, and like any muscle, they contract or relax in localized areas to alter blood volume to the area. To make sure you will have very little blood loss in your surgery, it is very important that the blood move away from [the site of surgery] and out to other parts of your body during the operation. Therefore, [spoken slowly] the blood will move away from [site of surgery] during the operation. Then, after the operation, it will return to that area to bring the nutrients to heal your body quickly and completely.

This instruction was given without hypnosis or practice sessions. And yet, patients assigned to the blood-shunting group lost significantly less blood (a median of 500 cc) than those assigned to either the control group or the relaxation group, where the median blood loss was nearly a full liter (900 cc). The amount of blood lost by patients in all three groups was within the normal range, but the blood shunters were at the low end of the spectrum. Even when other circumstances related to blood loss were factored in, such as the length of the incision and time under anesthesia, the presurgical instructions that patients had been given remained a significant variable.

INFLUENCING THE IMMUNE SYSTEM

Several studies have shown that the functioning of the immune system is altered, often depressed, after surgery. Levels of the stress hormone cortisol are often high, a state associated with low levels of antibodies and white blood cells, particularly the natural killer cells (see Chapter 3). At the Veterans Administration Hospital in Miami, physicians Bernard Linn and Nancy Klimas and psychologist Margaret Linn found that poor immune function was linked to a more complicated recovery—and that people who have a more pronounced response to everyday life stress had more difficult recoveries as well.

Conversely, if cortisol levels can be kept relatively low, immune system functioning improves and the patient has a more robust recovery from surgery. And there is preliminary evidence that direct instructions, usually given during hypnosis or a relaxation exercise, can positively influence immune functioning. In one study, Karen Olness and her colleagues at Minneapolis Children's Medical Center found that children who received specific instructions to increase their immune function did indeed show the suggested changes in salivary levels of immunoglobulins (the building blocks of antibodies), whereas just relaxing produced no effect (see Chapter 16).

Some researchers are just beginning to apply similar techniques to improve immune functioning after surgery. For her doctoral dissertation in nursing, Carole Holden-Lund at the University of Texas gave patients instruction in relaxation and imagery based on specific physiological processes of wound healing and found that cortisol levels were lower and the wounds of surgery healed more quickly after surgery.

WORKING WITH YOUR HOSPITAL

When patients feel a sense of control over surgery and know what to do, especially physiologically, their recovery is more robust and speedier, they and their surgeons are happier, costs go down, and insurance companies save money. And yet it's the rare hospital that offers a patient preparation program. Those programs that do exist, usually run by the nursing department, do not generally offer specific physiological instructions. Instead, they offer mainly reassurance and information, which have only a limited physiological benefit.

One of us (Henry Bennett) has given presentations on active participation by patients to surgical departments at several hospitals, encouraging them to implement a trial program, but so far none has. The hospital administrators and nurses claim such a program would not be effective enough to warrant disrupting the hospital's way of doing business. Hospitals tend to be organized to accommodate the staff more than the patients, and active-participation programs are typically seen as burdensome, time-consuming, and inefficient. In fact, it takes little time to provide a structured session that can motivate a patient to help repair his or her body "from the inside."

In the future, perhaps hospitals will become less resistant to these approaches. Twenty years ago, hospitals treated childbirth as if it were a disease; now it is seen as a natural, family-bonding experience. This change came only when pregnant women and their husbands pressured hospitals to offer natural childbirth as an option and voted with their pocketbooks by choosing to give birth in those facilities that did.

Unfortunately, patient activism may be harder to generate in the case of surgery. It is a private experience, often tinged, unnecessarily, with shame or guilt that "there's something wrong with me." Unlike pregnant women, most surgical patients do not feel the need to have "the right experience." Yet the psychological quality of the surgical experience can have great consequences for both physical and emotional health.

DESIGN YOUR OWN PRESURGICAL PROGRAM

Until hospitals begin offering patient preparation plans, it's up to you to design your own presurgical program. But there are results from 30 years of research to guide you.

The basic rule for undergoing surgery is this: Bring with you to the operating room the thoughts and attitudes that will put you at ease and help you feel in control. Enter surgery already prepared with specific plans for what you are going to do during and following the event.

Here are some suggestions for coaching yourself through an operation:

TAKE THE SURGERY SERIOUSLY
If you had to run a marathon, you would naturally be anxious, but you would prepare in order to make the experience as tolerable as possible. Channel your anxiety into your own program for undergoing the operation. Know what premedication, anesthesia technique, and postoperative pain regimen will be used, and discuss your options with your physicians. Decide what props you want: If you are going to be hospitalized for any length of time, you may want your own bathrobe, slippers, cassette player and headphones, family pictures, serene posters, and other comforting objects.

HAVE YOUR COGNITIVE STRATEGY READY
Know where you will be going in your mind when you begin drifting into anesthesia. If you want to use music and headphones as part of this strategy, preset the volume, and coordinate your plans with your anesthesia provider.

As to the content of your cognitive strategy, you might practice a script like this: "I am going to a comfortable place in my mind, one I already know, a place that is safe for me, comfortable and warm, where I can spend a few hours." Visualize a place you have been that is warm and soothing, such as a beach or your sunny backyard—not a physically cold place. Repeat this exercise to yourself in the days before surgery so that the thoughts become second nature. This will make things easier on the day of your operation.

INSTRUCT YOUR BODY BEFOREHAND

As we have described, the most direct mind/body approach for encouraging physical recovery from surgery is a specific instruction that helps you wield some control over the responses of your autonomic nervous system, such as muscle tension, blood flow, and the movement of food through your digestive tract. If you have a supportive surgeon, you can get an idea from her or him as to which autonomic responses will factor most significantly into your surgery and recovery, then create instructions for yourself accordingly. If appropriate, you can also use the instructions given above for relaxing your muscles at the site of surgery, controlling blood flow, or speeding gastrointestinal recovery.

You can simply give yourself the instructions mentally over the days before the surgery, much as an athlete does when "psyching" for a big event. Another option is to record the instructions on an audiocassette and play them back to yourself before the operation—and during the surgery as well, if you wish.

PROTECT YOURSELF DURING SURGERY

Because studies show that patients may be able to hear in some circumstances even under general anesthesia, you can use foam earplugs (available at any pharmacy) to block out noise or potentially disturbing conversation in the operating room. Better yet, bring an autoreverse, battery-operated cassette player with earphones. The tape can run your selection of comforting music or sounds (the ocean, for example) throughout the operation. The important thing is to choose tapes that you find familiar and soothing. (Tell your surgeon beforehand about your plans to use a tape player so that there are no surprises in the operating room.)

You can also intersperse or substitute the music with positive therapeutic suggestions like those mentioned above. A set of tapes specifically for use during surgery is available from Linda Rodgers, a counselor at P.I.P. Surgical Associates in Katonah, New York. Her series includes tapes to be used before, during, and after surgery; they include music intermixed with soothing instructions and suggestions for local, regional, or general anesthesia (see Resources).

If you bring a cassette player, be sure to use fresh alkaline batteries. With the earphones on, set the volume so you can hear at a low level. Set auto-reverse to "on." Then place tape over the controls so that the player doesn't switch over to the radio if it gets jostled (which will result in loud static blasting your ears).

RESPECT YOUR COPING STYLE

You will cope with surgery best if you are aware of your preferred way of handling stressful situations. Research shows that people generally use one of two major coping styles.

Some people are *avoidant copers*, who don't want to be overwhelmed with information or asked to make too many decisions. If you are this type, absorbing a great deal of information about the surgery itself can raise your anxiety. Don't ask questions simply because you think you "should."

People who fall into the second category, called *vigilant copers*, do best under the opposite strategy: They want to feel a sense of control over the situation and hence seek out a great deal of information before surgery. If you are a vigilant coper, be sure to ask the hospital staff for all of the information you need to feel as comfortable as possible.

Both approaches are valid ways of confronting the life crisis of surgery. And both allow you to take steps to make your surgery more comfortable. An "avoidant" person may not want to know any of the physical details of surgery, but may still want to use strategies for relaxing before surgery, listen to soothing music during the operation, and so on. A good hospital support program should ideally be flexible enough to accommodate the needs of both types of patients.

BE ASSERTIVE WITH HOSPITAL STAFF

Once you determine what kind of support you need from the hospital staff, don't wait for them to give it to you. *Ask* for it. As part of your strategy for coping with surgery, you may even decide you'd like to have your hand held, your brow rubbed, or your arm stroked right before the procedure, especially as you go into anesthesia. Sometimes a simple request gets a big result.

You need to respect the framework established by the surgical team to enable them to do their jobs safely and effectively. Rather than fighting them, you'll want to work *with* them, on their terms. Even so, you can insist on personal choices in some matters.

For example, you should certainly consider asking to sign the informed consent form for anesthesia a few days before you are wheeled into surgery. To save time, the anesthesia team may prefer not to meet with you until immediately before surgery or even when you are in the operating room ("Just read this and sign here so that we can get going, please"). But reading of all the possible (albeit rare) complications at that time can add enormous stress to surgery.

DISCUSS YOUR MEDICATION PLAN

It can feel like a real violation of your rights if, before you're even in the operating room, you begin to feel funny and the anesthesiologist announces, "I've just given you something." To avoid this, be sure to speak with the anesthesiologist ahead of time about what medications will be used before, during, and after surgery. Practitioners differ, often remarkably, in the ratio of safety to comfort they use in determining their plan for your anesthesia. As the consumer, you may need to lobby for the comfort part of the formula, although it is unrealistic to expect that you will be utterly without discomfort.

Before receiving anesthesia, it is common to be given preparatory medication. However, this is not necessary for all patients. A patient given far more medication than she or he needs can feel out of control and stressed—the opposite of the desired result. The right amount of medication for you may be none, a little, or a great deal. You should not be overmedicated simply for the convenience of the staff.

In general, it is best to have medication that is short-acting, if possible; if necessary, you can always be given added doses or infused with it continuously. Avoid such medications as droperidol and scopolamine, which have effects that can last for several days (a "locked-in" syndrome). To maintain control, you may need to inform the anesthesiologist that you would like "titration to effect," that is, just enough medication to make you feel comfortable without oversedating you.

Some people want to be "knocked out" before they go to the operating

room, but this is not possible. Only general anesthesia provides true unconsciousness, and this cannot be started until you are in the operating room.
However, some potent sedatives, such as midazolam (*Versed*) can erase all
later memory of coming to the operating room, yet still leave you conscious at
the time so that nurses and anesthesiologists can ask you questions, such as
whether you are allergic to certain substances, in order to ensure your safety.

During surgery itself, a number of different substances may be used for anesthesia. To learn more about the options, see "Anesthesia Today: Just Enough."

TAKE CHARGE OF YOUR PAIN CONTROL

As part of your presurgical program, you should obtain information about
postoperative pain management as well. Make arrangements with your surgeon for the type of medication you'll want and need; then make sure the
anesthesiologist concurs. You'll also want to ask the anesthesiologist practical
questions about maintaining pain control, such as what happens if the epidural catheter in your back fails at 3:00 A.M.

In the last few years, there have been two major advances in postsurgical
pain control. The first is a system called *patient-controlled analgesia* (PCA), in
which a pump provides a small dose of medication, usually morphine, into
your IV when you push a button. This system puts the patient in charge of
pain control and does away with the sometimes agonizing wait for a nurse to
supply a new dosage of painkiller every time the drug runs out. By allowing a
nearly constant level of morphine in the blood and reducing patient anxiety,
this device has revolutionized postoperative pain management. Unfortunately,
many hospitals still do not offer PCA.

The other major advance in pain relief is the recognition that patients can
safely be given large doses of narcotics in a hospital setting without becoming
addicted. For years, doctors were afraid that patients would not be able to
give up these drugs once the physical need for them had diminished. But
recent studies have clearly refuted this notion.

In 1992, the U.S. Department of Health and Human Services recommended that doctors aggressively treat pain in postsurgical patients. Rather
than waiting for the patient to complain about pain before intervening, the
report said, doctors should try to prevent the discomfort from building. Both
the American Medical Association and the American Nurses Association have
endorsed these federal guidelines. (Significantly, these guidelines include presurgical relaxation training as an important part of a pain control program.)

ANESTHESIA TODAY: JUST ENOUGH

Some people refuse anesthesia during surgery or request only a minimum amount because they fear the medication is dangerous. But the anesthetics used today are very safe, and it is foolish to reject them out of fear. It is important to have enough anesthesia to maintain your comfort. On the other hand, it's wise not to have more anesthesia than is necessary.

As a rule of thumb, you should seek the least invasive procedure that will give you the desired result. Discuss the options with your anesthesiologist well in advance of surgery. From least to most intrusive, here are the various types of anesthesia available.

LOCAL ANESTHESIA

An injection of a local anesthetic is enough for many procedures. This will numb the area around the incision but leave the rest of the body unaffected. Some people are afraid a local anesthetic will not be enough and ask to be "knocked out" even for minor surgery. But there are drawbacks to such overkill. For example, after a wisdom tooth extraction, it is important that the tooth sockets stay clean. If you have systemic drugs that make you unconscious, you may vomit later, which can loosen the blood clots in the sockets, leading to increased pain and perhaps complications.

REGIONAL ANESTHESIA

This approach, useful for surgery below the chest, numbs the site of the surgery and the surrounding area. The main types of regional pain blocks are spinal—in which medication that lasts about two hours is injected—and epidural, in which a catheter (a tiny, threadlike device) delivers anesthesia to the area right next to the spinal cord and remains in place so that additional drugs can be readily infused. Either approach allows you to maintain consciousness (you may want to use a cassette player to keep the troublesome sounds of surgery at bay). An advantage of regional anesthetics is that if you feel uncomfortable, you can tell the surgical team so. With an epidural, the catheter can also be left in and used to provide pain medicine after surgery.

GENERAL ANESTHESIA PLUS REGIONAL ANESTHESIA

A combination strategy may be the best option for long operations performed below the chest, such as a total hip replacement. A regional anesthetic numbs the area of surgery, while a light general anesthetic is used to maintain unconsciousness, primarily because lying still for several hours is nearly impossible while conscious. The advantage to this technique is that the general anesthesia needn't be heavy enough to block pain, but simply enough to keep you unconscious: The epidural anesthesia does the job of preventing pain signals from reaching the brain. Once again, the epidural catheter can remain in place to deliver pain medication after surgery as well. From the standpoint of your comfort, this is an excellent method for major surgery.

GENERAL ANESTHESIA

This continues to be the mainstay of anesthesia practice. It entails administering multiple medications in order to create unconsciousness, elimination of pain, and amnesia for the surgical experience.

Unconsciousness can be induced in two main ways in adults, both of which use an IV. The standard is sodium thiopental (*Pentothal*). It causes rapid loss of consciousness, which can be unpleasant if you're not expecting it or if you feel out of control in the few moments when it is taking effect. It can also leave you with something of a hangover effect. A newer drug for induction of anesthesia is propofol (*Diprivan*). Though it can be irritating when injected, it seems to produce a smoother transition into unconsciousness—more a "slipping away" than a "slam in the head"—and that could aid in a smoother emergence from anesthesia.

Once unconsciousness is induced, most practitioners use inhaled gases to maintain anesthesia in their patients. The potent agent in these cases is now almost always isoflurane (*Forane*). It is remarkably safe and stands in great contrast to ether, which was used previously and could be horribly unpleasant. Almost all anesthesiologists mix *Forane* in the gas with far larger dosages of nitrous oxide, inexpensive and considered safe. However, nitrous oxide has a hangover effect and has been implicated in postanesthetic nausea and vomiting.

FACE YOUR FEARS

There is good reason to be apprehensive—even terrified—about the prospect of your body being operated upon. However, if you allow these feelings to control you, undesirable consequences could ensue, including a much more difficult and exhausting recovery, wound complications, and further invasive medical treatments.

Often, patients who experience the greatest anxiety over a looming operation are those who have had surgery and anesthesia before. If you had surgery as a very young child, you may remember it more strongly than you realize. It is very common for parts of the brain and nervous system to retain unconscious memories of previous trauma and respond with anticipatory fear to the prospect of another operation.

You may be comforted to know, however, that anesthesia has changed dramatically in the last decade. It is now safer and less toxic and ensures a better state of unconsciousness.

If you are fearful, your best strategy is not to deny the anxiety but to honor it and even "talk" to it. Acknowledge your fear, but remind yourself that you have made the decision to enter surgery for good reasons and that there is every chance the surgery will benefit you. Rehearse such positive thoughts repeatedly as you approach surgery, and plan a strategy that will maximize your comfort and sense of control.

THINK POSITIVELY

You may be best able to handle surgery if you keep the reason for it in focus: It is to improve your functioning in your life. Remember, this is *your* operation. You can, and should, take some responsibility for planning the experience.

Remember, too, that you are renting the operating room and paying the nurses, the surgeon, and the anesthesia provider. You are entitled to ask for anything you feel will enhance your ability to deal with this stressful situation. Do your best to work *with* the surgical team, not against them; these people are highly trained professionals, and you must respect their knowledge and skill. If you are appropriately assertive, however, you may find that they are quite willing to try to meet your needs.

Once you have set up your presurgical program, relax. You have done what you can to make the operation as stress-free as possible; leave the rest to your surgical team.

Finally, after surgery, give yourself the time you need to heal. Remember that the presurgical program you followed has given your body a boost on the road to recovery.

PREPARING FOR INVASIVE MEDICAL PROCEDURES

Just as with surgery, the most common types of anxiety associated with undergoing an invasive medical procedure stem from fear of the unknown and the anticipation of unpleasantness or pain. In some cases, as with magnetic resonance imaging (MRI), the body's reaction to severe distress and anxiety may lead to both unsatisfactory scan images and great discomfort.

While several approaches, including relaxation techniques, can help reduce your anxiety, increasing your knowledge about what to expect is one of the best things that you can do. Psychologist D. Thorp and his colleagues found that patients with prior knowledge of the MRI or CT scans and experience with invasive tests had a better subjective experience of the MRI scan. Because many other studies indicate that familiarity with the procedure (together with relaxation) can significantly reduce anxiety, here is a brief summary of what to expect with several of the most common procedures.

MAGNETIC RESONANCE IMAGING (MRI)

MRI is painless and noninvasive, but the scan takes place within a confined space that many people find uncomfortable. It usually lasts from 30 to 90 minutes, during which time you must remain still. You may be strapped down, but you experience no physical sensations other than the occasional sound of thumping produced by the machine. Based on the reports of 40 men and women, the two most unpleasant features of undergoing MRI are the confined space of the machine and the requirement that patients hold still for an extended period of time.

Fortunately, entrepreneurs have developed music systems specifically designed for MRI applications, and these have been shown to reduce dramatically the subjective discomfort of confinement in the machines. Because there is a strong magnetic field within the MRI, ordinary cassette players won't work in this environment. Instead, MRI music systems use earphones similar to the long tubes used on airplanes for the same purpose. Check to see if the MRI facility has these, and lobby for them if it does not. A supplier is listed in the Resources section.

COMPUTED TOMOGRAPHY (CT) SCANS

People who receive CT scans have experiences similar to those of people who undergo MRI, but to a less intense degree. They are also required to hold still for an extended period of time, but the CT scanner is not as confining. The other main difference is that CT requires the use of a radioactive dye, which is either taken orally or injected. In a study by psychiatrist John Peteet, a few patients reported several sources of moderate discomfort associated with this injection, including flushes, tingling, or dizziness (which lasts only a few seconds), nausea, and minor reactions to the dye. Very few people had complaints about the procedure itself. Again, prior knowledge of the procedure and experience with it reduced a patient's overall anxiety and improved the patient's comfort level.

UPPER ENDOSCOPY

Gastrointestinal endoscopy is a more invasive procedure than MRI or CT scanning. You will probably be sedated (with *Valium*, for example), but you will remain fully conscious throughout the procedure. An IV is started so that medications can be easily administered. The larynx is usually sprayed with a topical anesthetic, and a bite block is inserted to protect your teeth. You will lie on your side as a flexible, lubricated tube is passed down the throat and into the stomach. The scope will be passed into the back of the throat; and as it is passed into the esophagus, you will be asked to swallow. Through the tube, the physician can inspect, photograph, and biopsy the inner lining of the stomach. The procedure usually lasts 20 to 30 minutes.

Psychologist Suzanne Gattuso and her colleagues found that patients who were instructed in both relaxation and coping methods and who were confident about their ability to cope with the procedure reported significantly less distress and a lower incidence of gagging than people who received either relaxation training or procedural information alone. (In fact, the information alone was especially distressing to people who tended to cope with difficulties by avoiding thinking about them.) In another study, 48 people undergoing gastrointestinal endoscopy were studied before and after the procedure. Patients who were well informed in advance about the procedure, including those who watched a videotape of it, tended to be less uncomfortable than the less informed patients.

LOWER ENDOSCOPY

A lower endoscopy, or colonoscopy, allows the physician to examine your colon and rectum for pathological changes. About 24 to 48 hours before the

CARDIAC SURGERY: SPECIAL CONSIDERATIONS

Cardiac surgery, more than other types of surgery, is especially likely to be followed by psychological disturbances. The heart-lung machine, used to provide circulation and oxygenate the blood during surgery, is one cause. Despite excellent filtration systems, tiny blood clots formed in the machine can enter the body and lodge in the brain, creating confusion and cognitive problems after surgery. These problems are difficult to prevent, but fortunately, they are usually temporary.

Other kinds of psychological problems are caused by the anesthesia itself. Because your heart is not working well, the anesthesiologist will use medication before surgery to lower the stress of coming to the operating room and undergoing the induction of anesthesia. Often anesthesiologists will use scopolamine or droperidol, medications that "lock you in" just before, during, and after surgery. The sense of unreality they create can be disturbing, and your memory for it may be clouded, except for the feeling that "something is not—or was not—quite right." Ask about alternatives to these medications, which could help you avoid these problems.

Finally, during the operation itself, the anesthesiologist may use only narcotics and paralyzing muscle relaxants—drugs that do nothing to block the processing of sound in the brain. If these medications are used during your surgery, playing a tape of music or positive suggestions may be especially valuable. Several recent studies have shown physiological benefits from playing therapeutic suggestions during cardiac surgery. You would do well to use a cassette player during the operation and ask that your wish to use a sound system be respected.

procedure, you will be asked to begin a clear-liquid diet and to drink a bowel preparation fluid.

You will be awake but sedated, with medications given through an IV. The procedure is usually done with the patient on her or his side. Some discomfort may occur when air is introduced through the scope to aid in visualization, which can cause flatus and a bloated feeling in the abdomen.

The entire process takes from 30 to 120 minutes, depending on the procedures that are necessary.

CARDIAC CATHETERIZATION

In this procedure, also known as an arteriogram or angiogram, an IV will be started, and electrodes will be placed on the side of your chest to monitor your heartbeat. A tube (catheter) will then be placed in an artery or vein in your arm or leg and moved forward until it reaches the heart. (The skin around the incision will be numbed first.)

Once the catheter reaches the heart, dye is injected so that the state of the coronary arteries and heart valves can be seen on an X-ray. When the dye is injected, patients often report a warm or hot feeling; it usually lasts about 30 seconds and does not recur. Some patients also have feelings of nausea or experience extra heartbeats. If you aren't informed that these feelings are normal, they can be unnecessarily alarming.

The procedure usually takes one or two hours, and often involves an overnight stay in the hospital. If a leg artery is used, your movement will be restricted for several hours after the procedure. If an arm artery or vein is used, you will probably need several stitches after the catheter is removed.

ANGIOPLASTY

Angioplasty is a nonsurgical treatment designed to open clogged arteries—the coronary arteries that supply heart muscle with blood, the arteries supplying the kidney, or blood vessels elsewhere in the body. In this treatment, a catheter with a small balloon on the end is inserted into a groin artery and threaded up until it reaches a clogged artery. The balloon is then inflated and deflated several times to try to flatten the deposits against the artery wall and improve blood flow.

When you arrive in the X-ray suite, an IV will be started. You will be awake during the procedure, but you can receive medications through the IV to help you relax. As with cardiac catheterization, the tissue around the point of incision will be numbed, electrodes will be attached to monitor your heartbeat, and dye will be injected so that an X-ray can be taken of the blocked artery. You may also be asked to help with placement of the catheter by coughing or taking deep breaths.

When the catheter is in place, the balloon is slowly inflated. Be warned: Your original symptoms may recur at this point, because the balloon will temporarily block blood flow. This is common, but it is important to tell your doctor right away so that she or he can deflate the balloon.

Angioplasty does not work for everyone, and there is no way to predict success ahead of time. In rare cases, the procedure may actually block the artery further. Five percent of all angioplasty patients experience total blockage, and three percent require emergency surgery to correct it. Life-threatening complications occur in less than one percent of all cases. The frequency of complications diminishes as physicians refine their skills, so make sure that your doctor has had plenty of experience performing this procedure.

THE BOTTOM LINE

Any invasive medical procedure can be anxiety-provoking, and undergoing surgery can be extraordinarily stressful. But research indicates that the more you know what to do and expect before, during, and after surgery, the more likely that it will go smoothly and you will recover rapidly. Few hospitals offer patient preparation programs to get you ready to withstand surgery's physical and emotional onslaught, but there are steps you can take yourself. The best approach is to think of yourself as an athlete training for a major event, rather than as a passive body being handed over to the surgical team.

Enter surgery already prepared with specific plans for what you'll do before, during, and after the event. In addition to learning about the surgery beforehand, consider giving yourself specific instructions or suggestions for controlling autonomic processes that play major roles in your physical recovery—most notably, muscle relaxation and blood flow. (You can ask your surgeon well ahead of time what physiological functions would optimize your recovery.) Plan to use earplugs or, better yet, a cassette player during surgery, to block out any disturbing sounds that you may perceive unconsciously, and to provide comforting sounds, music, or verbal suggestions.

At every step, work closely with your surgical team. Communicate your needs assertively, but respect their professional judgment as well. Don't be afraid to discuss all aspects of your treatment, from premedication to anesthesia to postsurgical pain control.

As with an athletic event, preparation, rehearsal, and coaching can all help you deal with a surgical event. By devising an active plan, you will limit the emotional trauma of undergoing surgery and put yourself on a more rapid road to recovery.

FOR CHILDREN: SURGERY WITHOUT TRAUMA

It is an all too common scenario: At first, your child seems content to be taken out of your arms by the surgical team. But as stranger and stranger things begin to happen, your child becomes increasingly distressed. By the time the operation must begin, a nurse is holding your struggling child down on the operating table while the anesthesiologist is forcing the mask over the little one's face. The child feels betrayed, which has negative implications for how smoothly he or she will emerge from anesthesia and recover from surgery. Longer term, this episode can make the child distrustful of authority—including the parent, whose last words were probably something like, "Don't worry, they'll take good care of you."

There are steps you can take to avoid this outcome, as one of us (Henry Bennett) did recently. When my two-year-old son needed surgery under general anesthesia to implant "ear tubes," I insisted that I be allowed to stay with him through the induction of anesthesia. I "suited up" for the operating room along with my son and accompanied him, presenting it as a new and interesting place. At the anesthesia station, he sat on my lap, feeling safe and secure while he looked around.

He was given the breathing mask to play with and soon began inhaling halothane, which is routinely used to induce general anesthesia in children. After a few moments, he began to feel different and gave me a "What's going on, Dad?" look. I smiled and remained calm. A few moments later the boy's eyes closed and he became "floppy" as he comfortably lost consciousness. Then I left the operating room before surgery began.

Of the six toddlers in the recovery room later that morning, my son was the only one who emerged without screaming, crying, or being agitated. He simply opened his eyes, saw me, smiled, and reached for me within a few moments. About 30 minutes later, we left the hospital. When anesthesia is handled this successfully, it could be called the "Zen of medicine": Lots of effort is expended so that it seems as if nothing has happened.

Many specialists in pediatric anesthesia recognize the value of having a parent present while anesthesia is induced, but hospitals can be resistant. Operating-room health-care workers often think the parent will panic and go berserk; faint, hit the floor, and introduce a new medical emergency to the situation; disrupt the normal social atmosphere of the operating room; or prolong the induction process, throwing them off schedule.

The best strategy for a parent who wants to be present during anesthesia is to make the arrangements well ahead of time. Gently but relentlessly insist—and, if necessary, threaten to go to an alternate hospital that is more cooperative. The more that parents lobby to accompany their children to the operating room, the more obliging hospitals will become.

Another change for the better in children's surgery is the improvement in sedatives for premedication. These drugs for children are delivered rectally, nasally, or through the skin. It is not unreasonable to give children a sedative if it helps them feel more comfortable. After all, that is part of your goal in protecting your child during this vulnerable time.

25

WORKING WITH YOUR DOCTOR

BY TOM FERGUSON, M.D.

IN 1975, WHILE I WAS A STUDENT AT THE YALE UNIVERSITY SCHOOL OF Medicine, I made a decision that changed my life. Rather than pursue a conventional clinical practice, I decided to focus my interest on the patient's role in the health-care system. I wanted to understand all the things people do, or could do, to take better care of their health—not only the ways they keep themselves healthy, but the ways they manage and adapt to illness.

My medical school professors were brilliant and totally committed to their profession. But much as I admired them, I was shocked that they failed to take into account the way people's life circumstances contribute to illness and the extent to which people are able to affect the course of disease. The ability of people to care for themselves can be a tremendous resource that my professors seemed to ignore or discount.

Most of our patients' illnesses were due to factors beyond any doctor's control, yet they were still often within the control of the patient. The majority of their illnesses were caused or worsened by lack of information, lack of social support, unhealthy patterns of eating, lack of exercise, other poor health habits, or psychological problems. Yet we medical students were taught that regardless of the complexity of a patient's life and all the factors contributing to the illness we were treating, we should be able to give the patient a diagnosis, and prescribe an appropriate drug or surgical procedure (or, all too

TOM FERGUSON, M.D., a graduate of the Yale University School of Medicine, is a nationally known expert on self-help and self-care. He was the founding editor of *Medical Self-Care* and currently edits *Tom Ferguson's Health in the Information Age Letter* in Austin, Texas.

rarely, psychotherapy)—and we should perform this minor miracle within a limited number of brief clinical visits.

I found it painful to see patients—even highly educated, professional people—who were treated by their doctors as powerless and who had come to have no confidence in their own ability to prevent or manage their health problems. Both the patients and doctors were playing by the rules that governed medical care at the time. Physicians were supposed to be expert technicians, and medical information was a professional secret, limited to doctors. It was not considered important or even appropriate for patients to seek information or to question a doctor's orders. Patients who did attempt to shape their own medical care risked being labeled as "uppity," "difficult," or "uncooperative." The roles that physicians had to assume were burdensome to them as well as to patients; we doctors were supposed to be miracle workers, to fit an almost magical image that nobody could live up to.

After I completed medical school, I became the founding editor of *Medical Self-Care*, a medical journal for lay people designed to help them take charge of their health. That journal and my work since then have been driven by the simple idea that lay people can and should take a great deal more responsibility for their health—and that health-care professionals should help them do it.

In retrospect, I was in the right place at the right time. Beginning in the mid-1970s, a number of forces began to change our health-care system profoundly. That system is now in the midst of an extraordinary transformation, of which mind/body medicine is a part. Together, physicians and lay people are developing a more open and cooperative vision of what it means—and what it takes—to live in good health.

The older, more mechanistic view of medicine was based on a model that fit the Industrial Age. The hospital was, in effect, a medical factory. Physicians were the expert technicians who ran the factory. And patients, with little say in their medical fate, were controlled by their doctors.

The new approach to health care—often called "patient-centered" health care—is much more in tune with the themes and metaphors of the Information Age. It begins with a sharing of information and of responsibility for the choice of treatments between physicians and their patients. This type of health care makes for diversity, individuality, and self-responsibility, both in wellness and in illness. It treats health as a complex network of interacting mental, emotional, and physical processes, all closely linked with the physical environment and connected to far-reaching social and information networks.

The patient-centered approach recognizes that only a tiny fraction of our health-care needs is actually provided by professionals. It encourages lay people not to be passive recipients of professional services, but rather to become key providers of health care for themselves, their family, and their friends.

The development of this new approach has been closely intertwined with the development of mind/body medicine, for three reasons. All mind/body techniques, from meditation to the use of support groups, obviously require the individual's active participation. Significant, also, is the fact that the patient-centered approach has focused attention on the psychological issues involved in doctor-patient communication. And mind/body research now suggests that the very act of taking greater control of your medical treatment can itself contribute to physical health.

SHARING MEDICINE'S PROFESSIONAL SECRETS

Information, more than anything else, is the key to patient-centered health care. For centuries, doctors followed the lead of Hippocrates, who advised physicians not to discuss with patients the nature of their illness or its treatment. But uninformed consumers can't make reasonable decisions about their own care, nor are they likely to notice professional mistakes.

Although passive patients may console themselves by believing that their doctor has a magical cure for every illness, in reality they are missing an important opportunity to contribute to their own care and they are setting themselves up for a major disappointment if the treatment fails. "Public expectations of health care in this country are substantially removed from reality," says Dennis O'Leary, president of the Joint Commission on Accreditation of Hospitals. "Blind trust in medical treatment is not in anyone's best interests. Consumers can make better decisions if they have better information about all their available choices."

Fortunately, the past two decades have seen an explosion in the amount of medical information directly available to ordinary people. According to Jonathan Fielding of the UCLA School of Public Health, health information on the major television networks increased 29-fold between 1975 and 1987.

Coverage of health matters in newspapers and magazines has also greatly increased.

Hospital and medical librarians around the country now routinely help consumers find the medical information they need. Specialized consumer health information libraries can help consumers obtain the same medical information that has long been available to their physicians. And anyone with access to a fax machine can now receive a state-of-the-art review of current treatments and prognoses for nearly any type of cancer by calling the National Cancer Institute's telephone database, known as CancerFax (see Resources for Chapter 5).

Such new developments are welcome: They not only give patients more choices but serve as an antidote to the old style of medical care that kept them ignorant and powerless. In addition to making patients confused and uncomfortable, the old approach may well have worsened the course of their disease. As Ivan Illich observed in his book *Medical Nemesis*, "Medical procedures turn into black magic when, instead of mobilizing his self-healing powers, they transform the sick man into a limp and mystified voyeur of his own treatment."

THE COMMUNICATION GAP

Major hospitals, medical specialty organizations, and research institutes are now taking steps to help patients become better informed. But many individual physicians still have poor communication skills that often severely hinder their ability to help their patients.

The "bedside manner" of many physicians is, in a word, abysmal. The typical general practitioner spends only seven minutes with the average patient, down from 11 minutes per patient in 1975. And physicians spend much of this time talking, not listening. A study by internist Howard Beckman and sociolinguist Richard Frankel at the Wayne State University School of Medicine found that most doctors interrupt their patients within the first 18 seconds of their efforts to explain their problems.

While surveys still show that most Americans say they are satisfied with their personal physicians, the polls are beginning to turn up a significant communication gap. In a 1991 American Medical Association survey, many consumers agreed with statements that were critical of America's physicians. Only 42 percent felt that doctors usually explain things well to their patients, and only 31 percent said that most doctors spend enough time with their patients. On top of that, 69 percent agreed with the statement, "People are beginning to lose faith in their doctors."

Several years earlier, in 1984, a Harris Poll interviewed people who had changed physicians and asked them why they had made the switch. Their answers focused on communication issues. They complained that:

- The doctor didn't spend enough time with them (51 percent).
- The doctor wasn't friendly (42 percent).
- The doctor didn't answer questions honestly and completely (40 percent).
- The doctor didn't explain problems understandably (30 percent).
- The doctor didn't treat them with respect (27 percent).
- The doctor wasn't always available when needed (27 percent).

Small wonder that a study of more than a thousand letters of complaint to a large Michigan health maintenance organization, undertaken by Richard Frankel (who is now at the University of Rochester), found that more than 90 percent of the complaints concerned the manner in which medical staff communicated with patients.

You can usually tell if your physician is willing to take a patient-centered approach within the first few minutes of an office visit. Doctors who are poor communicators commonly behave in a way that would be considered downright rude in anyone else. They keep tight control of the medical interview, interrupt, ignore your questions, and frequently change the subject before the previous topic has been dealt with to your satisfaction. They are impatient and abrupt. They may ignore or downplay your feelings of pain or distress and may dismiss heartfelt questions with such patronizing phrases as "Just let me worry about that" or "You needn't concern yourself with that." And they may use medical jargon that leaves you confused, frightened, or upset.

The harm done by this poor style of communication can be more than psychological. Studies show that such physicians frequently overlook or ignore concerns that are important to treating the patient. One recent study found that 80 percent of physicians didn't even listen to all the details of a patient's chief complaint and thus may have missed some vital information.

The way in which doctors talk to patients about their condition may also cause psychological and even physical harm. The late Norman Cousins, working at UCLA's Brain Research Institute, interviewed 600 people with malignancies. He found that in many cases their diseases took a sharp turn for the worse shortly after they received their diagnosis. Cousins believed that the way some doctors presented the diagnosis might actually intensify the disease. He set out to observe various physicians as they informed patients of a serious diagnosis and found many who delivered the news in a devastating way.

One doctor Cousins observed put the patient through an extensive battery of tests, then kept the patient and his family waiting in apprehension. "After some time," Cousins recalled, "the doctor arrived. He didn't sit down. He spread his hands, shook his head, and looked grim. 'Well, Charlie,' he began. 'What can I say? Your kidneys are crapped out. Your liver is crapped out. Everything's crapped out. There's not a hell of a lot we can do. I'm really sorry.'"

Another example occurred when a San Francisco woman went in for a breast biopsy. In Cousins's words, "She was quite naturally concerned and telephoned the oncologist the next day to ask what he'd found. She was told that no diagnoses were given over the phone and that she would be receiving the results in a letter.

"Several anxious days later, a certified letter arrived. It said: 'I regret to say that your biopsy was positive.' Can you imagine how devastated and abandoned she must have felt?"

Fortunately, an increasing number of physicians and other health professionals are now practicing in a more patient-centered way. These health professionals treat their clients with respect and will invite them to discuss their situation in an atmosphere of privacy and comfort, without distracting interruptions, and will display empathy and use good communication skills. Above all, these physicians are good listeners, always seeking to shift the balance of conversational initiative back to the patient.

In marked contrast to the physicians above, Cousins found these skills in a Houston cancer specialist:

"When he gets a patient with a new diagnosis of cancer, he sits down with them and tells them he's convinced they are going to make it. He tells them it's nonsense to equate the word 'cancer' with death. He tells them he has an excellent treatment for their condition, and that they have an excellent treatment of their own—their body's own natural healing processes.

"'And you can activate that healing process,' he tells them, 'by building up your confidence in yourself and your confidence in me. By building up your joy, your appreciation of life, your urge to do everything you've always wanted to do.' He tells them they're in possession of the most magical system the world has ever known for the treatment of disease.

"'Now,' he says. 'Here's the partnership I propose. I'll work with you on the things you'll be doing to build up your confidence, your joy, your hope, your faith. Beginning tomorrow, I'm going to introduce you to five other patients who had exactly the same kind of cancer you have and came through it successfully. I'm going to make sure you receive the best treatment medical science has to offer. We're going to have a lot going for us, and I'm convinced that we can whip this thing and that you can make it.' Then he holds out his hand and says, 'Now how about a partnership?' They always take his hand."

To their credit, leading medical organizations are now taking steps to encourage more doctors to become like that Houston oncologist. The American College of Physicians and some medical specialty organizations have begun major studies to evaluate the quality of doctor-patient communication in hospitals and in office visits. And under a pilot program now being run by the National Board of Medical Examiners, physicians-in-training are put through a test of their communication skills—using mock office visits with actors playing the parts of patients—that could soon be a required part of the examination needed to obtain a medical license.

PUTTING THE PATIENT IN CHARGE

Physicians and physician organizations are taking communication seriously because research has shown it can have a real impact on the course of medical care. Recent studies suggest that the patient benefits physically from taking an active role in the medical interview. For example, a study reported in the journal *Diabetes Care* found that diabetics who were trained to be more assertive during visits to their doctors showed a significant drop in blood sugar and had fewer physical limitations than a control group after four months.

In other studies of people with ulcers, hypertension, or diabetes, Tufts University researchers actually taught patients a set of skills that enabled them to be more assertive with their doctors—with good results. Internist Sheldon Greenfield and social psychologist Sherrie Kaplan developed a 20-minute "assertiveness coaching session" for patients waiting to see their physicians. Trained aides reviewed the patients' medical records with them, helped them think of questions they wanted to ask, and urged them to take an active role. The aides also offered techniques for overcoming embarrassment and anxiety.

The result: The coached patients established a much higher level of control when they saw the doctor. They directed the conversation, interrupted their doctors when necessary, and obtained a good deal more medical information. Four months later, the coached patients had missed less work, reported fewer symptoms, and rated their overall health as significantly better than patients who had simply followed doctor's orders.

Being assertive, as these patients were trained to be, means coming into a doctor's office knowing what you want to accomplish. It means telling your doctor about your observations, feelings, fears, and preferences without being hindered by anxiety or guilt.

Assertiveness should not be mistaken for aggressiveness: It's important to express your feelings and your views while also respecting your clinician. Assertiveness without aggression leads to the best medical care.

At first, you may find it difficult to be open and assertive with your physician. Many physicians, too, can become defensive in the presence of what they perceive as a suddenly demanding patient. Keep in mind, however, that few physicians have been trained in the communication skills that would make it easier for them to meet your needs for information.

While many physicians may find it hard to shift their communication style, they may benefit from the change as much as their patients do. Studies show that doctors with good communication skills find their work more rewarding and take pleasure in the knowledge that their patients are more satisfied with their care. And as a bonus, physicians with good communication skills are much less likely to be sued than the average doctor.

You can help your doctor communicate more effectively by being aware of—and responding to—the person behind the professional manner. Let your doctor know you appreciate his or her efforts and attention. You can also help the process by sharing your real feelings. If you feel frightened or embarrassed, simply saying so can go a long way toward changing the emotional tone of the interaction.

You may find it hard to be so direct. But the more you are able to express your feelings, the better you'll feel. It's the feelings you *don't* express that make you most uncomfortable. And the more you communicate your needs, the better your doctor will be able to understand and respond to them. The following guidelines can help you communicate more effectively.

HOW TO TALK TO YOUR DOCTOR

Many factors can affect your communication with your doctor, beginning with your choice of a physician. Different doctors have very different kinds of practices and appeal to different kinds of patients. You have the right to choose a doctor who shares your personal style and philosophy. If you feel there isn't a good match between your doctor's style and your own, start shopping for a new doctor.

If you have found a physician you're comfortable with, however, there are still many steps you can take to improve communication.

- *Plan the interview in advance.* Decide what you want to get out of this visit to a doctor. Make a list of your most important questions and concerns. Have this list in mind—or on a piece of paper—when you walk into your doctor's office. If you have a question that you are embarrassed or uneasy about, write it out, practice it, and ask that question first.
- *Take charge of the interview.* You have to set goals and control the interview to a large extent. You also need to make sure you really understand everything that your doctor says.
- *Be assertive.* Being assertive doesn't mean you need to be challenging or confrontational. It *does* mean you have to state your questions, concerns, and preferences clearly.
- *Consider getting a second opinion.* If you are uncomfortable with your physician's recommendations, ask for a consultation with an appropriate specialist. Such consultations are commonplace, and your physician should welcome such a request. If he or she is unwilling to arrange a consultation, find another physician.
- *Be a good observer.* Keep a record of each symptom you experience. When did it start? How did you treat it? What other symptoms have you had? Have you experienced dizziness, nausea, coughing, diarrhea, unusual bleeding? Be as specific as possible. If your observations are lengthy or complex, write them down.

- *Make sure you understand what you and your doctor have concluded.* Don't leave your doctor's office uncertain about the diagnosis, the treatment, or the self-care measures you should take. If something is unclear, review your understanding of key points with your doctor to make sure that you are both on the same wavelength.
- *Become an expert in your own condition.* If you develop a health problem, look it up in the medical literature. Use a bookstore, public library, or hospital or medical school library to find the information you want. On-line computer searches can provide you with in-depth information on virtually any medical topic.
- *Know what to ask if your doctor suggests a medical test.* For a simple blood test, you may want to ask only a few brief questions. However, if the test is complex, expensive, painful, or potentially harmful, you should ask about the test in some detail. Here are some questions to begin with:

Why do I need this test?
How should I prepare for the test?
How is the test performed?
How will the test feel?
How much time will it take?
What are the risks?
How will the results affect what we do next?
How much will the test cost?
Will the test be covered by my health insurance?

If all else fails and you decide to look for a new doctor, get advice from family, coworkers, and friends, particularly those in health-care professions. Nurses, pharmacists, and other health professionals usually know who are the best local doctors. You may wish to check out any recommended physicians by going in for an interview, a physical, or a consultation for a minor illness. When you find the right doctor, you will come out of the office feeling secure and reassured.

Once you have chosen a new physician, write or call your former doctor's office and ask to have copies of your medical records sent to the new doctor. Be businesslike about it. You need not offer any explanation; changing doctors is a common practice.

BRINGING A FRIEND ALONG

One strategy you may find useful is to ask a friend to accompany you when you go to see your doctor. Although this may not be necessary for routine medical care, it can be especially helpful when you are facing an important medical decision or are confronted by a serious diagnosis. Taking a friend along under such circumstances can help in several ways:

- Your friend's presence helps you stay relaxed and focused, which can help you get what you want out of the visit.
- With a friend on hand, you'll be less likely to feel intimidated. Having an observer there, too, may encourage your doctor to take more time and communicate more clearly.
- Your companion can help bring up questions or concerns the two of you had discussed earlier. And after the visit, your friend can help you recall the details of what was said and what you agreed to do.
- Your friend can remind you of the practical aspects of your plans and decisions: Who drives you to the hospital to have a test? Who takes care of the kids if you have to go in for surgery?

Lowell Levin, a leading self-care expert and professor at the Yale School of Public Health, is a strong advocate of taking a friend along on a clinical visit. "If you encounter resistance to the idea of bringing a friend, write your doctor a follow-up letter explaining your feelings about the matter," he suggests. "Send a copy to the medical chief of staff and another to the chief hospital or clinic administrator. Such feedback can be an important part of letting our doctors know that bringing a friend along is our perfect right."

The key is to pick a doctor you like *before* there is an emergency. Otherwise, you may end up being treated by people you don't really know or like.

FROM PASSIVE PATIENT
TO HEALTH-ACTIVE CONSUMER

Taking responsibility for your health is not always easy. Despite the changes of recent years, many people still tend to approach their health care passively. John Fiorillo of New York's Health Strategy Group, a market research firm, has described three categories of health consumers.

Passive patients, in Fiorillo's typology, regard the vicissitudes of health and illness with grim resignation; they take little or no responsibility for their health because they feel there is little they can do to prevent disease or manage illness.

Concerned consumers often ask questions of their physicans and may even seek out a second opinion, but ultimately they almost always go along with whatever the doctor recommends.

Health-active/health-responsible consumers are determined to play an active role in their own health: They are tireless seekers of health information and refuse to relinquish control of the key decisions having to do with their own care. They ask lots of questions, do not hesitate to disagree with their physicians, and often choose to explore alternative therapies. Even so, they are not necessarily antidoctor: They question the doctor because they want to understand their condition and make the key choices about their treatment.

Based on market research, Fiorillo believes that Americans are beginning to shift from being passive patients to being concerned consumers when it comes to health. The health-active group is still small, but it's growing rapidly.

The trend away from passivity is certainly a positive development. But it would be a mistake to think that everyone should try to take maximum control of all medical decisions at all times. The real goal of taking an active role in your health care should not be to match yourself against some idealized image of a perfect patient, but rather to choose a style of interacting with your doctor that suits both your personal preferences and your medical and psychological condition.

There are times when it pays to take charge—for example, if you need to make an important medical decision, or if you think your physician or nurse may have made a mistake or overlooked important information. But there are also times when making a conscious decision not to think about your poor medical condition, and simply hoping for the best, may be the wisest course—for both your psychological and your physical health.

In general, the healthiest approach is to take an active role in deciding the course of your care, but to be ready to leave your care in professional hands once you have done everything you reasonably can. And whatever your medical situation, you need to take your personal predispositions into account and adopt an approach to your health care that feels comfortable for you and your family.

SELF-CARE: THE FOUNDATION OF ALL HEALTH CARE

Taking charge of your health doesn't just mean communicating well with your physician: It also means dealing effectively with the many health problems that don't require a physician's care. The best health care combines self-care with professional advice.

The concept of self-care may seem a bit less radical when you consider how frequently most people practice it already. When family physician Raymond Demers and his colleagues at the University of Washington Medical Center asked a group of Seattle residents to keep a diary of all health problems that arose over a three-week period, they found that only 5.4 percent of the problems recorded were ever brought to a physician's attention. The rest were treated with self-medication, home remedies, or a wait-and-see approach. And among the problems that were seen by professionals, self-care still tended to play the most important role in treatment.

When asked why they had not sought medical care, the people in Demers's study said:

- The problem could be treated effectively by self-care measures.
- The problem would heal by itself without treatment.
- They had decided to wait and see if it progressed.
- The problem was not something a doctor could do much about.

The researchers concluded that "medical care, as provided by physicians, is neither central to nor a necessary part of the health-care seeking process."

In a particularly interesting study of self-care, Christopher Elliott-Binns, an English researcher, sat in a general practitioner's office and interviewed a thousand patients who came in with new problems. He asked the patients if they had sought information and advice or used self-care before coming to see the doctor.

Ninety-six percent answered yes to one or both questions: Fully 88 percent had received advice or information from friends or family members and 52 percent had used at least one form of self-treatment. In addition, 16 percent had sought information in books, magazines, or other media. The patients in the study frequently conducted a wide search: One patient, a boy with acne, had received information or advice from 11 different sources.

Moreover, in the opinion of a panel of physicians, the advice the study participants had received from friends, family members, and nonphysician health-care professionals was surprisingly sound. The best advice came from pharmacists, nurses, and family members—particularly wives. Given these findings, Elliott-Binns asked rhetorically, "Is it justifiable to call the family doctor the source of primary care?"

Indeed, it would be difficult for physicians to handle the extra load that might come should there be a movement away from self-care. Economist Simon Rottenberg of the University of Massachusetts has calculated that if a mere 2 percent of over-the-counter drug consumers in the United States chose to visit a primary-care practitioner rather than using self-medication, there would be a 62 percent annual increase in patients' office visits.

WHAT IS SELF-CARE?

The term *self-care* does not refer to any single, pat response to a health-care problem. It simply refers to the extensive, and often untapped, ability of lay people to provide a wide range of health services for themselves. By its nature, self-care is flexible, responding as needed to the situation at hand.

Traditionally, health care has been divided into three levels: primary, secondary, and tertiary. Primary care includes visits to a general practitioner, family physician, internist, pediatrician, or other general clinician. Secondary care involves a visit to a specialist or a stay at a community hospital. Tertiary care refers to care by a subspecialist or admission to an academic medical center. All these categories refer to levels of professional care, with no consideration of self-care approaches.

The patient-centered approach recognizes six levels of health care, spanning the spectrum from complete independence on the part of the consumer to a full but informed delegation of responsibility to a health-care provider. People with health problems typically begin with the first two levels, moving on only if these approaches do not solve the problem. By thinking about this structure, you may become more aware of your own options in managing different aspects of your health.

1. INDIVIDUAL SELF-CARE

When people become aware of a relatively minor health concern—such as athlete's foot, menstrual cramps, or a sprained back—they typically try to solve it on their own, often with the help of over-the-counter medications. Individual self-care is also used to manage flare-ups of chronic problems, such as arthritis, for which the person has already consulted a professional. This level of care is commonly used to manage psychological, social, or stress-related problems, too, through meditation, relaxation, or physical exercise.

2. INFORMAL SELF-HELP NETWORKS

This approach involves asking others for help, support, and advice. People typically begin by turning to those to whom they feel closest, then moving further out through a network of social contacts until they find someone with the required information or expertise. Surveys indicate that, except for wives who ask their husbands, the people sought out for this type of information and support are usually women. Informal self-help networks also include health professionals people know socially.

3. FORMAL SELF-HELP GROUPS

If advice from friends and loved ones doesn't solve the problem, the next step may be to seek the support of a formal or semiformal self-help group or community program. People may call a self-help hotline, sit in on a meeting of a local Alcoholics Anonymous group, or join one of the specialized self-help groups that have sprung up in recent years. A great deal of self-help networking now takes place over electronic "bulletin boards"—especially valuable for people with disabilities or chronic illness, who have the greatest need for support groups yet who find it most difficult to attend them.

4. HEALTH PROFESSIONALS AS FACILITATORS

At this level of health care, the client or consumer remains in charge and the health professional plays the role of adviser and support person. Nurse practitioners, physicians' assistants, home health-care workers, and other nonphysicians have taken the lead in promoting this approach, which has been widely used in the mental health field for many years. But a growing number of

SURVIVAL TIPS FOR A HOSPITAL STAY

If a hospital stay is necessary, you needn't approach it with panic or dread. Some basic strategies can do a lot to enhance your comfort and sense of control, factors that could aid your recovery.

- *Talk with friends and family members who have had the same procedure you are planning to have.* You may learn more about the upcoming experience from them than from a dozen doctors.
- *Get a tour of your hospital floor before you check in.* If possible, do this a few days before you are admitted.
- *Be nice to the hospital staff.* Get to know your nurses and other hospital staff members. Try to understand their problems and concerns. Be a friend. Share your resources with them. Give them small gifts if it's appropriate—candy or fruit are always welcome—with a thank-you card. If a hospital staffer goes beyond the call of duty on your behalf, send a note to the person's supervisor.
- *Be assertive.* If you want something, don't be afraid to ask. Most nurses and other hospital staffers want to do a good job of meeting your needs. But they can't do this if you don't let them know what your needs are. Don't be concerned about asking for a lot of care—that's what hospitals are for.
- *Insist on being an individual.* Customize your room. Bring your own music and reading matter. Wear your own robe and pajamas.
- *Take charge of your visitors.* Some people feel that when they are in the hospital, they must be at the mercy of any and all visitors. In fact, you are in charge of setting your own visiting hours. Ask visitors to come at the times most convenient to you. And if you don't feel like seeing anyone, say so.
- *Ask questions.* Hospitals can be mysterious places. You can demystify things by asking lots of questions. You have the right to ask questions about every drug, every test, every person, and every piece of medical apparatus that is a part of your care. If you don't know what something is for, by all means ask. If you ask a question and the person doesn't respond, don't give up. Simply say: "I under-

stand that you may be busy right now, but I really want to know what this piece of equipment is for." Continue asking until your questions are answered.

- *Resolve complaints quickly.* If you have a problem or a complaint while in the hospital, first speak to the person involved. Be assertive, not aggressive, and be willing to compromise. If that doesn't resolve the problem, talk to the person's supervisor, the nursing supervisor, or the head of the department. You may also wish to use an advocate—either a patient advocate provided by the hospital or a friend or family member. If that still doesn't help, talk to the hospital administrator. And if all else fails, complain to your doctor.
- *Know when to let your doctor take over.* There's nothing to be gained by obsessing about situations you can't control. When things are out of your hands, the best advice is to stay relaxed and hope for the best. In many cases, when you are going in for surgery or a high-tech medical test, it makes sense to tune out anxiety and let your doctor do the worrying.

physicians are also coming to realize that their patients can often manage their own health problems if they are provided with the appropriate tools, skills, information, and support.

5. HEALTH PROFESSIONALS AS PARTNERS

Certain conditions are best managed by a physician-patient team. For example, doctors may need to order tests or medicines, recommend a course of treatment or a program of rehabilitation, or do other things patients cannot do for themselves. But even so, both parties realize at this level of self-care that the contribution the patient can make to managing the overall problem is at least as important as anything the professional can do.

6. HEALTH PROFESSIONALS AS AUTHORITIES

This has been the traditional mode of practice, and it can still sometimes be the most appropriate one. In some situations, the patient may well want to delegate to the physician the responsibility for making all necessary medical decisions for a certain period of time. This is inevitable if someone is going to be unconscious or incapacitated, for example, or has chosen to undergo surgery or some other complex test or treatment that will make it temporarily impossible to make key choices. But health professionals and their patients alike should remember that this level of care is appropriate for only a small minority of all health problems.

HEALTH EMPOWERMENT

Everything you do to become a more active participant in your own health care adds up to a stronger sense of control over your medical destiny, a process I call *health empowerment*. This is more than just a way of feeling good about yourself; it can be a key to real changes in your physical health.

In a classic study (described in Chapter 21), psychologists Ellen Langer and Judith Rodin gave a group of nursing home residents the power to make some choices about their environment. In this experiment, the people who took control and made their own choices were not only more active and happy than those who were not given this opportunity, they also lived substantially longer.

A more recent study of the Arthritis Self-Help Course, described in Chapter 10, also showed the benefits of taking control. People with arthritis were offered a course on arthritis self-management designed to help them manage their disease and its treatment. Those who completed the course reported a dramatic decrease in pain, experienced less disability than others with the disease, and required fewer visits to their physicians.

When the researchers analyzed the results to see which elements of the course fostered these positive effects, they found that the greatest benefit did not come from the exercises or the medical information taught in the course, but from an increase in what they called *self-efficacy*. People who experienced the greatest increase in well-being had developed a positive, take-charge attitude and the confidence that they could deal with their disease more effectively. This subtle but profound shift in personal perspective had made all the difference.

Health empowerment means becoming aware of—and coming to believe in—the many ways that you can exert influence over your own health and thus influence the direction of your own life. This is not just a matter of wishful thinking; it is the systematic exploration of the ways in which you can take responsibility for your situation.

Although you cannot always determine your circumstances, you *can* determine your response to those circumstances. The arthritis patients who benefited from the class were able to shift their perspective: to see that they held the power to affect their condition in their own hands and that they were not powerless victims of their disease.

THE BOTTOM LINE

Although a physician's advice and treatments can be lifesaving and modern drugs and medical devices are extremely useful tools, many people have given up a great deal of their power to heal themselves by trusting only in their doctors. The growth of patient-centered medicine puts power and control back into the hands of the individual.

Better doctor-patient communication is critical to making medical care more equitable and effective, and medical organizations are beginning to work with their members on this issue. But patients, too, can learn techniques for talking to their doctors more effectively. Studies have shown that active, assertive patients fare better medically than more passive ones. Even so, there are certain situations in which patients can have only limited control and where the wisest course may be to decide to leave everything to the doctor.

Approaching health actively means knowing how and when to use self-care, as well as knowing how to work well with a physician. The vast majority of medical problems are handled by the people who experience them, without their ever being brought to a doctor's attention. Written resources, social networks, and self-help groups can all play a role in making self-care effective.

As ordinary people take more responsibility for their health, many physicians are learning to listen to their patients more carefully and treat them with new respect. They are beginning to speak to their patients as equals, in their patients' own language, and with full appreciation of their patients' deepest concerns. This new conversation has the potential to be a healthy one indeed.

THREE PILOT PROGRAMS IN PATIENT-CENTERED CARE

As people become more interested in taking an active part in their health care, some new institutions are developing to help them do it. Here are three of the best.

1. PLANETREE'S PATIENT-CENTERED HOSPITAL

You are on the second floor of a modern medical center, but you would never know it. The Planetree Model Hospital Unit does not feel, look, or sound like a hospital. Classical music plays softly in the background. Patients wear their own robes and pajamas, sleep on flowered sheets, and are encouraged to sleep in as long as they like.

There is no nurse's station: It has been replaced by a convenient study area where patients are encouraged to read their own charts and write in them as well. There are no visiting hours: Friends and family are welcome at all times convenient for the patient. Family members cook for their ailing loved ones in a special patients' kitchen. Interested family members are trained to serve as active care partners, changing dressings, flushing out permanent IV lines, and performing other vital nursing services. Family members who learn these techniques in the hospital can continue them at home after the patient is discharged.

At Planetree, it's clear from the very beginning that things are arranged for the convenience of the patient, not the medical staff. This patient-centered model has already begun to spread to a number of other hospitals across the country, and is now being formally tested at major medical centers in California, Oregon, and New York. As a nurse on the unit explains, "Once patients get a taste of the Planetree model, they simply won't permit themselves to be admitted anywhere else."

For further information:
Planetree Model Hospital Unit
2300 California Street, Suite 201
San Francisco, CA 94115
(415) 923-3696

Planetree also operates one of the most sophisticated consumer health information libraries in the country. Planetree librarians help visitors and callers locate the health and medical information they want, drawing on an impressive collection of sources. They can also put together a customized information packet on virtually any medical topic and can perform customized computer searches of the medical literature for a modest fee.

For further information:
Planetree Health Resource Center
2040 Webster St.
San Francisco, CA 94115
(415) 923-3681

2. THE COMMONWEAL CANCER HELP PROGRAM

This program, located in Bolinas, California, is for people with cancer who are receiving the best available medical care but want to do something more. Founder and director Michael Lerner, a recipient of a MacArthur Foundation "genius" grant, used the fellowship to visit 30 of the world's best-known alternative cancer treatment centers. He returned from his research convinced that a common characteristic of many of the best centers was a high concentration of active, health-responsible patients seeking to integrate the best of conventional and alternative cancer therapies.

Lerner, medical director Rachel Naomi Remen, and their colleagues at the Commonweal Cancer Help Program now offer week-long seminars eight times a year at Commonweal's rural coastal retreat an hour north of San Francisco. Participants are invited to use imagery, meditation, gentle yoga stretching, a vegetarian diet, massage, art therapy, guided support groups, and classes on informed choice in cancer therapy. They are encouraged to develop their own highly personalized approaches to recovery, which often include elements of a psychological or spiritual quest. Goals for healing that emerge from the program may include changes in diet, lifestyle, relationships, living arrangements, or work.

Participants often report that as a result of the seminar they are able to develop a less frightened and more hopeful relationship with their illness. As one recent participant commented, "The retreat experience was one of the richest experiences of my life. I learned to see healing in a whole new way: as an effort to discover who we really are."

For further information:
Commonweal Cancer Help Program
P.O. Box 316
Bolinas, CA 94924
(415) 868-0970

3. THE AMERICAN SELF-HELP CLEARINGHOUSE

This center was originally set up as a telephone switchboard to help New Jersey residents find local self-help groups addressing their specific concerns. Over the past several years, it has become something more: Edward J. Madara, the center's director, has become a leader in the movement to help interested people start their own self-help groups.

Callers on the center's helpline are given information about the specific groups of interest to them. If no suitable group exists, the center can refer callers to local organizations that can help them establish their own mutual support group. The staff and volunteers at the New Jersey center have been responsible for the formation of an estimated 850 new groups over the past 12 years.

The center also publishes *The Self-Help Sourcebook*, the best national directory of self-help groups. Call or write for ordering information. A free brochure, "Ideas and Considerations for Starting a Self-Help Group," is available on request; send a stamped, self-addressed, business-size envelope.

For further information:
The American Self-Help Clearinghouse
St. Clares–Riverside Medical Center
25 Pocono Road
Denville, NJ 07834
(201) 625-7101

RESOURCES

This listing is keyed to the 25 chapters of this book. Each chapter list (with a few exceptions) is divided into the following sections:

Groups and Organizations. In general, these are support groups for people with specific illnesses; organizations that can help you find skilled practitioners of a particular mind/body technique; or organizations that disseminate information on a particular topic. Where appropriate, clinics that specialize in mind/body approaches are listed. These organizations and clinics are listed on the recommendation of the authors of individual chapters and have not been evaluated by the editors or endorsed by Consumers Union.

General References. This section includes publications at a level appropriate to the general reader, with annotations to help readers find the resources that will be most useful to them. In the chapters on specific illnesses, we have concentrated on resources that focus on mind/body aspects of those diseases, but have also included a few sources that give general information on coping with those diseases. Instructional audiotapes are listed where appropriate.

Professional References. This section is primarily for researchers, educators, and health-care professionals who require more detailed scientific information. However, many of these references will also be accessible to the lay reader with some knowledge of psychology or medicine. (We have included a few references that are out of print, as noted, because they are good basic references and should still be available in academic libraries.)

1. WHAT IS MIND/BODY MEDICINE?

The following are good general resources for information on the field of mind/body medicine as a whole.

Borysenko, Joan. *Minding the Body, Mending the Mind.* New York: Bantam, 1988. Draws on findings in mind/body research and on the author's experiences with over 2,000 patients at New England Deaconess Hospital.

Cousins, Norman. *Head First: The Biology of Hope and the Healing Power of the Human Spirit.* New York: Viking Penguin, 1990. Describes research on the possible physiological benefit of positive attitudes.

Dienstfrey, Harris. *Where the Mind Meets the Body.* New York: HarperCollins, 1991. Profiles seven researchers who have investigated key areas of mind/body medicine: Type A behavior, the relaxation response, psychoneuroimmunology, biofeedback, neuropeptides, hypnosis, and imagery.

Goleman, Daniel. *The Meditative Mind: The Varieties of Meditative Experience.* Los Angeles: J.P. Tarcher, 1990. Compares the major approaches to meditation, reviews data on their benefits for physical health and emotional well-being, and offers basic instruction for meditation.

Gordon, James S.; Jaffe, Dennis; and Bresler, David. (eds.) *Mind, Body and Health: Toward an Integral Medicine.* New York: Human Sciences Press, 1984. A pioneering collection of essays on the applications of the mind/body approach in health-care practice.

Gordon, James S. *Stress Management.* New York: Chelsea House, 1990. Traces the ways stress affects the body and describes some of the programs that can help manage stress before it becomes destructive.

Locke, Steven E., and Colligan, Douglas. *The Healer Within: The New Medicine of Mind and Body.* New York: NAL–Dutton, 1987. An overview of psychoneuroimmunology and other research on the ways in which emotions and attitudes can affect physical health.

Ornstein, Robert, and Sobel, David. *The Healing Brain.* New York: Simon & Schuster, 1988. Presents an account of key findings in mind/body medicine and explores their implications for health.

Ornstein, Robert, and Sobel, David. *Healthy Pleasures.* Reading, Mass.: Addison-Wesley, 1990. Presents evidence that positive experiences are especially important in health maintenance.

Advances: The Journal of Mind-Body Health, a quarterly journal, reports on developments in mind/body medicine and explores their implications for health care, medical training, and further research. It provides a forum for health-care professionals and general readers concerned with these issues. For subscription information, contact:

The Fetzer Institute
9292 West KL Ave.
Kalamazoo, MI 49009
(616) 375–2000

2. BETWEEN MIND AND BODY: STRESS, EMOTIONS, AND HEALTH

General References

Farquhar, John W., *The American Way of Life Need Not Be Hazardous to Your Health.* Reading, Mass.: Addison-Wesley, 1987. With a focus on preventing heart disease, this book demystifies medicine with a practical, proven approach to preventing chronic disease and disabilities.

Pelletier, Kenneth R. *Holistic Medicine: From Stress to Optimum Health.* Magnolia, Mass.: Peter Smith, 1984. Builds upon the clinical research in stress to include nutrition, physical activity, psychosocial, and environmental influences for attaining optimal health.

Pelletier, Kenneth R. *Mind as Healer, Mind as Slayer.* (Revised ed.) New York: Delacorte, 1992. Considered a classic in the mind/body medicine field, it details the development of stress-related chronic diseases as well as practical, clinical interventions for prevention.

Selye, Hans. *The Stress of Life.* (2nd ed.) New York: McGraw-Hill, 1978. Describes the research and clinical basis for Selye's pioneering insights into the stress adaptation response.

Professional References

Chrousos, G.P., and Gold, P.W. "The Concepts of Stress and Stress System Disorders." *Journal of the American Medical Association*, 267(1992):1244–1252.

Friedman, H.S., and Booth-Kewley, S. "The 'Disease-Prone Personality.'" *American Psychologist*, 42 (1987):539–555.

Gorman, J.M., and Kertzner, R.M. *Psychoimmunology Update.* Progress in Psychiatry Series, No. 35. Washington, D.C.: American Psychiatric Press, 1991.

Johnson, R.T. *Behavioral Influences on the Endocrine and Immune System: A Research Briefing.* (Report of the Panel on Behavioral Influences on the Endocrine and Immune Systems.) Washington, D.C.: Institute of Medicine, 1989. (Limited distribution.)

Miller, A.H. (ed.) *Depressive Disorders and Immunity.* Washington, D.C.: American Psychiatric Press, 1989.

Pelletier, K.R. "Mind-Body Health: Research, Clinical, and Policy Implications." *American Journal of Health Promotion.* 6(1992):345–358.

Rahe, R.H. "Epidemiological Studies of Life Change and Illness." *International Journal of Psychiatry in Medicine*, 6(1/2)(1975):133–146.

Stein, M.; Miller, A.H.; and Trestman, R.L. "Depression, the Immune System, and Health and Illness: Findings in Search of Meaning." *Archives of General Psychiatry*, 48(1991):171–177.

3. MIND AND IMMUNITY

General References

Schindler, Lydia W. *Understanding the Immune System.* (Revised.) Bethesda, Md.: National Institutes of Health, 1991. (NIH Publication No. 92–529.) A concise review of current research in immunology for the general reader.

Professional References

Professionals interested in this field may want to follow the journal *Brain, Behavior, and Immunity*, edited by Robert Ader with Nicholas Cohen and David Felten. Published by Academic Press, the journal covers research on psychoneuroimmunology on a regular basis.

The following reference works are also recommended:

Ader, R.; Felten, D.; and Cohen, N. (eds.) *Psychoneuroimmunology* (2nd ed.) San Diego: Academic Press, 1990.

Borysenko, M. "The Immune System: An Overview." *Annals of Behavioral Medicine*, 9(1987):3–10.

Cohen, S.; Tyrrell, D.A.J.; and Smith, A.P. "Psychological Stress and Susceptibility to the Common Cold." *New England Journal of Medicine*, 325(1991):606–12.

Cohen, S., and Williamson, G.M. "Stress and Infectious Disease in Humans." *Psychological Bulletin*, 109 (1991):5–24.

Kiecolt-Glaser, J.K., and Glaser, R. "Psychoneuroimmunology: Can Psychological Interventions Modulate Immunity?" *Journal of Consulting and Clinical Psychology*, 60(1992):569–75.

Kiecolt-Glaser, J.K., and Glaser, R. "Stress and the Immune System: Human Studies." In Tasman, A., and Riba, M.B. (eds.) *Annual Review of Psychiatry*, 11 (1991):169–180. (Washington, D.C.: American Psychiatric Press)

Kiecolt-Glaser, J.K.; Dura, J.R.; Speicher, C.E.; Trask, O.J.; and Glaser, R. "Spousal Caregivers of Dementia Victims: Longitudinal Changes in Immunity and Health." *Psychosomatic Medicine*, 53(1991):345–362.

4. HOSTILITY AND THE HEART

Groups and Organizations

Support groups can play an important role in helping heart-disease patients cope better with their illness. Nearly every hospital of any size has a cardiac rehabilitation program that includes a support group in addition to the standard components of supervised exercise and guidance in reducing risk factors. Those whose local hospital may not have such a program can obtain information about sources of help for heart patients by contacting the Mended Hearts program at the following address:

Mended Hearts
7272 Greenville Ave.
Dallas, TX 75231
(214) 706-1442

General References

Friedman, Meyer, and Ulmer, Diane. *Treating Type A Behavior and Your Heart.* New York: Fawcett, 1985. Describes the program that Friedman and his colleagues employed to help men who had suffered heart attacks reduce their Type A behavior.

Karasek, Robert, and Theorell, Töres. *Healthy Work: Stress, Productivity, and the Reconstruction of Working Life.* New York: Basic Books, 1990. Good review of job stress by the leading researchers on this important source of stress.

Lerner, Harriet G. *The Dance of Anger: A Woman's Guide to Changing the Patterns of Intimate Relationships.* New York: HarperCollins, 1985. The title says it all.

Ornish, Dean. *Dr. Dean Ornish's Program for Reversing Heart Disease.* New York: Ballantine, 1992. Covers managing stress, exercise, even cooking gourmet, heart-healthy meals (recipes included).

Tavris, Carol. *Anger: The Misunderstood Emotion.* (Revised ed.) New York: Simon & Schuster, 1989. This widely read book dispels many of the myths about anger.

Williams, Redford. *The Trusting Heart: Great News About Type A Behavior.* New York: Times Books/Random House, 1989. A detailed review of the research showing that hostility is the only toxic component of Type A behavior.

Williams, Redford, and Williams, Virginia. *Anger Kills: Seventeen Strategies for Reducing the Hostility that Can Harm Your Health.* New York: Times Books/Random House, in press. How to tell if you have a hostile personality and what to do about it if you do.

Professional References

Dembroski, T.M.; MacDougall, J.M.; Costa, P.T.; and Grandits, G.A. "Components of Hostility as Predictors of Sudden Death and Myocardial Infarction in the Multiple Risk Factor Intervention Trial." *Psychosomatic Medicine,* 51(1989):514-522.

Frasure-Smith, N., and Prince, R. "The Ischemic Heart Disease Life Stress Monitoring Program: Impact on Mortality." *Psychosomatic Medicine,* 47(1985):431-445.

Friedman, H.S. (ed.) *Hostility, Coping, and Health.* Washington, D.C.: American Psychological Association, 1991.

Shekelle, R.B.; Gale, M.; Ostfeld, A.M.; and Paul, O. "Hostility, Risk of Coronary Heart Disease, and Mortality." *Psychosomatic Medicine,* 45(1983): 109-114.

Smith, T.W. "Hostility and Health: Current Status of a Psychosomatic Hypothesis." *Health Psychology,* 11(1992): 139-150.

Suarez, E.C., and Williams, R.B. "Situational Determinants of Cardiovascular and Emotional Reactivity in High and Low Hostile Men." *Psychosomatic Medicine,* 51(1989): 404-418.

Williams, R.B.; Barefoot, J.C.; Califf, R.M.; et al. "Prognostic Importance of Social and Economic Resources Among Medically Treated Patients with Angiographically Documented Coronary Artery Disease." *Journal of the American Medical Association,* 267(1992): 520-524.

Williams, R.B.; Haney, T.L.; Lee, K.L.; et al. "Type A Behavior, Hostility, and Coronary Atherosclerosis." *Psychosomatic Medicine,* 42(1980):539-549.

5. EMOTIONS AND CANCER: WHAT DO WE REALLY KNOW?

Groups and Organizations

The National Cancer Institute provides general information on the various aspects of cancer and cancer treatment. It may also be able to give you information on community resources for people with cancer in your area.

National Cancer Institute
Office of Cancer Communications
Building 31, Room 10A16
Bethesda, MD 20892
Cancer Information Services:
(800) 4-CANCER. Evenings: (800) 638-6694

The Institute has also recently launched CancerFax, which provides current recommended treatment guidelines for virtually any type of cancer by fax at no charge. CancerFax operates 24 hours a day, 7 days a week. To receive a listing of topics available from the service, dial (301) 402-5874 from the telephone receiver on your fax machine. A recorded message provides directions; after requesting a listing of topics, you choose the information you want by punching in the 6-digit number for each selected topic. If you have any trouble using CancerFax, call (301) 496-8880 for technical assistance.

The following organizations provide various kinds of support for people with cancer and their families:

American Cancer Society
1599 Clifton Rd. NE
Atlanta, GA 30329-4251
(404) 320-3333

Consult local listings to find the nearest office and for information on support groups such as CanSurmount, an educational and support program for patients and their families; I Can Cope, a psychological support system for cancer patients; and Reach for Recovery, which offers physical and psychological rehabilitation for women who have had mastectomies. The American Cancer Society will also know about local support groups for patients with certain types of cancer or those undergoing treatment, and can direct you to therapists experienced in working with cancer patients.

American Association of Sex Educators, Counselors
and Therapists
435 N. Michigan Ave., Suite 1717
Chicago, IL 60611
(312) 644-0828

Offers referrals to sex counselors experienced in problems resulting from physical illness.

Candlelighters Childhood Cancer Foundation
7910 Woodmont Ave., Suite 460
Bethesda, MD 20814
(301) 657-8401, or
(800) 366-2223

Provides information for children with cancer and their families.

Commonweal
P.O. Box 316
Bolinas, CA 94924
(415) 868-0970

Holds regular retreats for individuals with cancer. (For a full description, see Chapter 25.)

The National Coalition for Cancer Survivorship
1010 Wayne Ave., Fifth floor
Silver Spring, MD 20910
(301) 585-2616

Serves as an advocacy group for cancer survivors. Encourages research and influences health policy.

National Hospice Organization
1901 N. Fort Myer Dr., Suite 901
Arlington, VA 22209
(703) 243-5900
Helpline: (800) 658-8898

Offers referrals to nearly two thousand local hospice groups, and provides information on how to begin a group if none is available in your area.

Ontario Cancer Institute
500 Sherbourne St.
Toronto, Ontario, M4X 1K9
Canada
(416) 924-0671

Provides support groups for individuals with cancer.

Post-Treatment Resource Program
Memorial Sloan-Kettering Cancer Center
410 East 62 St., Room 740
New York, NY 10021
(212) 639-3292

Provides support and information for individuals who have undergone treatment for cancer.

The Wellness Community
2200 Colorado Ave.
Santa Monica, CA 90404
(310) 453-2200

Provides support groups and information for persons with cancer. Has branches in other cities.

General References

Dreifuss-Kattan, Esther. *Cancer Stories: Creativity and Self-Repair.* Hillsdale, N.J.: Analytic Press, Inc., 1990. A vivid depiction of the inner life of the cancer patient, drawing on works by writers, poets, and artists who struggled with the disease.

Fiore, Neil A. *The Road Back to Health: Coping with the Emotional Aspects of Cancer.* (Rev. ed.) Berkeley, Calif.: Celestial Arts, 1991. A compassionate guide to dealing with the trauma of cancer, written by a physician who is a cancer survivor himself.

Laszlo, John. *Understanding Cancer.* New York: HarperCollins, 1988. A clear, comprehensive guide to understanding the disease, written by a vice president for research of the American Cancer Society.

Morra, Marion, and Potts, Eve. *Triumph: Getting Back to Normal When You Have Cancer.* New York: Avon Books, 1990. Advice on coping with the illness.

Mullan, Fitzhugh, and Hoffman, Barbara. (eds.) *Charting the Journey: An Almanac of Practical Resources for Cancer Survivors.* Yonkers, N.Y.: Consumer Reports Books, 1990. Covers a wide range of issues relating to cancer, including insurance, job discrimination, effects of cancer treatment, and emotional aspects.

Schover, Leslie. *Sexuality and Cancer.* (Revised ed.)

New York: American Cancer Society, 1991. This booklet comes in two versions: one for men, one for women.

Sontag, Susan. *Illness as Metaphor and AIDS and its Metaphors.* New York: Doubleday, 1990. A classic critique of psychological theories of cancer causation, from a humanistic and literary standpoint.

On Videotape

A teaching videotape, *No Fears, No Tears,* is a resource for parents and professionals working with children with cancer. Produced by Leora Kuttner, it demonstrates how to use various interventions, ranging from simple distraction to hypnotic induction, to reduce discomfort associated with medical treatment. For information, contact The Canadian Cancer Society, British Columbia Yukon Division, 565 W. 10th Ave., Vancouver, BC V5Z4J4, Canada; (604) 872-4400.

Professional References

The American Cancer Society's Second Workshop on Methodology in Behavioral and Psychosocial Cancer Research. (Santa Monica, Calif., Dec. 5-8, 1989.) Proceedings. *Cancer,* 67(3 Suppl.)(1991):765–868.

Bovbjerg, D.H.; Redd, W.H.; Maier, L.A.; et al. "Anticipatory Immune Suppression and Nausea in Women Receiving Cyclic Chemotherapy for Ovarian Cancer." *Journal of Consulting and Clinical Psychology,* 58(1990):153–157.

Derogatis, L.R.; Morrow, G.R.; and Fetting, J. "The Prevalence of Psychiatric Disorders Among Cancer Patients." *Journal of the American Medical Association.* 249(1983):751–757.

Fawzy, F.I.; Cousins, N.; Fawzy, N.W.; et al. "A Structured Psychiatric Intervention for Cancer Patients: I. Changes Over Time in Methods of Coping and Affective Disturbance." *Archives of General Psychiatry.* 47(1990):720–725.

Fawzy, F.I.; Kemeny, M.E.; Fawzy, N.W.; et al. "A Structured Psychiatric Intervention for Cancer Patients: II. Changes Over Time In Immunological Measures." *Archives of General Psychiatry.* 47(1990): 729–735.

Holland, J.C. and Rowland, J.H. (eds.) *Handbook of Psycho-Oncology: Psychological Care of the Patient with Cancer.* New York: Oxford University Press, 1990.

Lederberg, M.F., and Holland, J.C. "Psych-Oncology." In Kaplan, H.I., and Sadock, B.J. (eds.) *Comprehensive Textbook of Psychiatry/V.* (5th ed.) Baltimore: Williams & Wilkins, 1989; Vol. 2, pp. 1249–1263.

Moorey, S., and Greer, S. *Psychological Therapy for Patients with Cancer: A New Approach.* Oxford: Heinemann, 1989.

Redd, W.H. "Behavioral Approaches to Treatment Related Distress." *Ca: A Cancer Journal for Clinicians.* 38(1988):138–145.

Telch, C.F., and Telch, M.J. "Group Coping Skills Instruction and Supportive Group Therapy for Cancer Patients: A Comparison of Strategies." *Journal of Consulting and Clinical Psychology.* 54(1986):802–808.

6. CHRONIC PAIN: NEW WAYS TO COPE

Groups, Organizations, and Clinics

The following groups provide useful information and other services to chronic pain sufferers and their families:

American Chronic Pain Association
P.O. Box 850
Rocklin, CA 95677
(916) 632-0922
Self-help organization with over 500 groups internationally. Publishes workbooks and a newsletter.

National Chronic Pain Outreach Association
7979 Old Georgetown Rd., Suite 100
Bethesda, MD 20814-2429
(301) 652-4948
An information clearinghouse. Publishes a newsletter and makes referrals.

American Council for Headache Education
875 Kings Highway, Suite 200
West Deptford, NJ 08096
(800) 255-2243
Organization dedicated to education, research, and helping people understand the problems of headache.

The following two professional organizations jointly offer a directory that can help you scout a quality pain clinic. For each facility, the directory lists staff and programs offered, and indicates whether the facility is accredited by the Commission for the Accreditation of Rehabilitative Facilities (CARF), the Joint Commission on the Accreditation of Health-Care Organizations (JCAHO), or both.

American Pain Society
5700 Old Orchard Rd., 1st Floor
Skokie, IL 60077-1024
(708) 966-5595

The American Academy of Pain Medicine
(Same address as American Pain Society)
(708) 965-2776

General References

Corey, David, with Solomon, Stan. *Pain: Free Yourself for Life*. New York: NAL–Dutton, 1989. Provides a comprehensive description of the gate control theory and describes many of the self-help techniques discussed in this chapter.

Headley, Barbara J. *Chronic Pain: Life Out of Balance*. (2nd ed. by Monsein, Matt, and Carish, Sharon.) St. Paul, Minn.: Pain Resources Ltd., 1988. A booklet that clearly summarizes current knowledge of pain.

Mohr-Catalano, Ellen M. (ed.) *Chronic Pain Control Work Book*. Oakland, Calif.: New Harbinger, 1987. Includes information to assist people in understanding various types of pain and discusses home strategies to reduce pain and to cope with discomfort.

Solomon, Seymour, and Fraccaro, Steven. *The Headache Book*. Yonkers, N.Y.: Consumer Reports Books, 1991. A comprehensive volume that reviews current theories of the causes of headaches and describes both drug and nondrug treatments.

Stacy, Charles B.; Kaplan, Andrew S.; and Williams, Gray. *The Fight Against Pain*. Yonkers, N.Y.: Consumer Reports Books, 1992. Reviews the range of pain syndromes, the gate control theory, and many psychological techniques discussed in this chapter.

Sternbach, Richard A. *Mastering Pain: A Twelve-Step Program for Coping with Chronic Pain*. New York: Putnam, 1987. Describes a sequential strategy for coping with pain.

Professional References

Blanchard, E.B.; Appelbaum, K.A.; Radnitz, C.L.; et al. "A Controlled Evaluation of Thermal Biofeedback and Thermal Biofeedback Combined with Cognitive Therapy in the Treatment of Vascular Headache." *Journal of Consulting and Clinical Psychology*, 58(1990): 216–224.

Flor, H.; Fydrich, T.; and Turk, D.C. "Efficacy of Multidisciplinary Pain Treatment Centers: A Meta-Analytic Review." *Pain*, 49(1992):221–230.

Funch, D.P., and Gale, E.N. "Biofeedback and Relaxation Therapy for Chronic Temporomandibular Joint Pain: Predicting Successful Outcome." *Journal of Consulting and Clinical Psychology*, 52(1984):928–935.

Holroyd, K.A.; Nash, J.M.; Pingel, J.D.; Cordingley, G.E.; and Jerome, A. "A Comparison of Pharmacological (Amitriptyline HCl) and Nonpharmacological (Cognitive-Behavioral) Therapies for Chronic Tension Headaches." *Journal of Consulting and Clinical Psychology*, 59(1991):387–393.

Holroyd, K.A., and Penzien, D.B. "Pharmacological Versus Nonpharmacological Prophylaxis of Recurrent Migraine Headache: A Meta-Analytic Review of Clinical Trials." *Pain*, 42(1990):1–13.

Meichenbaum, D. *Cognitive-Behavior Modification: An Integrative Approach*. New York: Plenum, 1977. (Out of print.)

Melzack, R., and Wall, P.D. "Pain Mechanisms: A New Theory." *Science*, 150(1965):971–979.

Pennebaker, J.W. *The Psychology of Physical Symptoms*. New York: Springer-Verlag, 1982.

Turk, D.C.; Meichenbaum, D.; and Genest, M. *Pain and Behavioral Medicine: A Cognitive-Behavioral Perspective*. New York: Guilford Press, 1983.

7. DIABETES: MIND OVER METABOLISM

Groups and Organizations

The American Diabetes Association provides general information for people with both Type I and Type II diabetes. The organization publishes a monthly magazine for patients, *Forecast*, and has an 800 number for patient information. The Juvenile Diabetes Foundation serves people with Type I diabetes.

The American Diabetes Association
149 Madison Ave.
New York, NY 10016
(212) 947-9707
For patient information: (800) 232-3472

The Juvenile Diabetes Foundation
432 Park Ave. South
New York, NY 10016
(212) 889-7575

General References

Brackenridge, Betty; ed. by Hoel, Donna. *Diabetes 101*. Minnetonka, Minn.: Chronimed, 1989. A general guide to diabetes and its treatment, written for patients.

Surwit, Richard S., and Feinglos, Mark. *Behavior and Diabetes Mellitus*. Kalamazoo, Mich.: Upjohn W.E. Institute for Employment Research, 1988. An introduction to the role of behavior and psychology in diabetes, for students and professionals.

Professional References

Cox, D.J., and Gonder-Frederick, L. "Major Developments in Behavioral Diabetes Research." *Journal of Consulting and Clinical Psychology*, 60(1992):628–638.

Surwit, R.S.; Feinglos, M.N.; and Scovern, A.W. "Diabetes and Behavior: A Paradigm for Health Psychology." *American Psychologist*, 38(1983):255–262.

Surwit, R.S.; Schneider, M.S.; and Feinglos, M.N. "Stress and Diabetes Mellitus." *Diabetes Care*, 15 (1992):1413–1422.

8. THE SKIN: MATTERS OF THE FLESH

Groups and Organizations
The following organizations offer information and support for people with a range of skin disorders. (For allergic problems, consult the Asthma and Allergy Foundation, listed with resources for Chapter 11.)

National Alopecia Areata Foundation
710 C St., Suite 11
San Rafael, CA 94901
(415) 456-4644

Eczema Association for Science and Education
1221 Southwest Yamhill, Suite 303
Portland, OR 97205
(503) 228-4430

Herpes Resource Center
P.O. Box 13827
Research Triangle Park, NC 27709
(919) 361-2120

National Psoriasis Foundation
6443 Southwest Beaverton Highway, Suite 210
Portland, OR 97221
(503) 297-1545

United Scleroderma Foundation
P.O. Box 399
Watsonville, CA 95077-0399
(408) 728-2202

National VD Hotline
(800) 227-8922

Human Papillomavirus (HPV) Support Program
American Social Health Association
P.O. Box 13827
Research Triangle Park, NC 27709
(919) 361-8400

General References
Grossbart, Ted, and Sherman, Carl. *Skin Deep: A Mind/Body Program for Healthy Skin.* (2nd ed.) Santa Fe: Health Press, 1992. A clear guide to how emotions trigger and heighten skin problems. Provides a practical, research-based workbook of techniques to help alleviate skin symptoms and their emotional impact.

Professional References
Koblenzer, C.S. *Psychocutaneous Disease.* Philadelphia: W.B. Saunders Co., 1987.

Panconesi, E. (ed.) *Stress and Skin Diseases: Psychosomatic Dermatology. Clinics in Dermatology,* Vol. 2, No. 4. Philadelphia: J.B. Lippincott, 1984.

Whitlock, F.A. *Psychophysiological Aspects of Skin Disease.* Philadelphia: W.B. Saunders, 1976. (Out of print.)

9. GUT FEELINGS: STRESS AND THE GI TRACT

Groups and Organizations
The Crohn's and Colitis Foundation of America
444 Park Ave. South, 11th Floor
New York, NY 10016-7374
(212) 685-3440
Maintains a list of support groups for inflammatory bowel disease, which exist in most states.

International Foundation for Bowel Dysfunction
P.O. Box 17864
Milwaukee, WI 53217
(414) 964-1799
Provides information on support groups and a newsletter addressing the concerns of people with irritable bowel syndrome.

General References
Janowitz, Henry D. *Your Gut Feelings: A Complete Guide to Living Better with Intestinal Problems.* New York: Oxford University Press, 1989. Written by a gastroenterologist, this book describes the most common diseases of the large intestine and diagnostic tests doctors may perform for bowel symptoms. Especially useful for preparing for a visit to the physician.

Shimberg, Elaine F. *Relief from IBS (Irritable Bowel Syndrome).* New York: Ballantine, 1991. A self-help guide concerning IBS, written by someone with the disorder, including a detailed discussion of the role of stress and suggestions on controlling it.

Professional References
Camilleri, M., and Prather, C.M. "The Irritable Bowel Syndrome: Mechanisms and a Practical Approach to Treatment." *Annals of Internal Medicine,* 116(1992):1001–1008.

Drossman, D.A., and Thompson, W.G. "The Irritable Bowel Syndrome: Review and a Graduated, Multi-Component Treatment Approach." *Annals of Internal Medicine,* 116(1992):1009–1016.

Whitehead, W.E., and Schuster, M.M. *Gastrointestinal Disorders: Behavioral and Physiological Basis for Treatment.* San Diego, Calif.: Harcourt Brace Jovanovich, 1985.

10. ARTHRITIS: WHAT DOCTORS CAN LEARN FROM THEIR PATIENTS

Groups and Organizations

The Arthritis Foundation provides free brochures, low-cost handbooks and guidebooks, and lists of support groups and arthritis specialists. It also conducts the Arthritis Self-Help Course throughout the country. For information, call your local Arthritis Foundation branch or the national office:

The Arthritis Foundation
P.O. Box 19000
Atlanta, GA 30326
(800) 283-7800

General References

Lorig, Kate, and Fries, James. *Arthritis Helpbook.* (3rd ed.) Reading, Mass.: Addison-Wesley, 1990. A valuable resource with many practical suggestions for self-management, used in the Arthritis Self-Help Course.

Sagan, Leonard A. *The Health of Nations: True Causes of Sickness and Well-Being.* New York: Basic Books, 1989. An epidemiologic view of underlying psychosocial and economic causes of disease in individuals and societies.

Trien, Susan F., and Pisetsky, David. *The Duke University Medical Center Book of Arthritis.* New York: Fawcett, 1992. Offers a medical perspective with clear descriptions of disease mechanisms and treatments for all types of rheumatic disease.

Professional References

Antonovsky, A. *Unraveling the Mystery of Health: How People Manage Stress and Stay Well.* San Francisco: Jossey-Bass, 1987.

Bandura, A.; Adams, N.E.; and Beyer, J. "Cognitive Processes Mediating Behavioral Change." *Journal of Personality and Social Psychology,* 35(1977):125–139.

Callahan, L.F.; Brooks, R.H.; and Pincus, T. "Further Analysis of Learned Helplessness in Rheumatoid Arthritis Using a 'Rheumatology Attitudes Index'". *Journal of Rheumatology,* 15(1988):418–426.

Callahan, L.F.; Kaplan, M.R.; and Pincus, T. "The Beck Depression Inventory, Center for Epidemiological Studies Depression Scale (CES-D), and General Well-Being Schedule Depression Subscale in Rheumatoid Arthritis: Criterion Contamination of Responses." *Arthritis Care and Research,* 4(1991):3–11.

Lorig, K.; Seleznick, M.; Lubeck, D.; Ung, E.; Chastain, R.L.; and Holman, H.R. "The Beneficial Outcomes of the Arthritis Self-Management Course Are Not Adequately Explained by Behavior Change." *Arthritis and Rheumatism,* 32 (1989):91–95.

Pincus, T. "Formal Educational Level—A Marker for the Importance of Behavioral Variables in the Pathogenesis, Morbidity, and Mortality of Most Diseases?" *Journal of Rheumatology,* 15(1988):1457–1460 (editorial).

Spergel, P.; Ehrlich, G.E.; and Glass, D. "The Rheumatoid Arthritic Personality: A Psychodiagnostic Myth." *Psychosomatics,* 19(1978):79–86.

11. ASTHMA: STRESS, ALLERGIES, AND THE GENES

Groups and Organizations

Information concerning asthma and allergies is available from:

The Asthma and Allergy Foundation of America
1125 Fifteenth St. NW, Suite 502
Washington, DC 20005
(202) 466-7643

The National Jewish Center for Immunology and Respiratory Medicine in Denver runs a free phone service for information on asthma and other lung disorders; call (800) 222-5864.

General References

Altman, Nathaniel. *What You Can Do About Asthma.* New York: Dell, 1991. A guide to understanding the nature of asthma, with a focus on specific forms of treatment.

Shayevitz, Myra, and Shayevitz, Berton. *Living Well with Chronic Asthma, Bronchitis, and Emphysema.* Yonkers, N.Y.: Consumer Reports Books, 1991. A practical guide to dealing with the symptoms of respiratory illness, with a primary focus on these problems in adulthood.

Professional References

Knapp, P.H., and Nemetz, S.J. "Acute Bronchial Asthma. I: Concomitant Depression and Excitement, and Varied Antecedent Patterns in 406 Attacks." *Psychosomatic Medicine,* 22(1960): 42–56.

Lehrer, P.M.; Hochron, S.M.; McCann, B.; Swartzman, L.; and Reba, P. "Relaxation Decreases Large-Airway but Not Small-Airway Asthma." *Journal of Psychosomatic Research,* 30(1986):13–25.

McNichol, K.N.; Williams, H.E.; Allan, J., et al. "Spectrum of Asthma in Children—III: Psychological and Social Components." *British Medical Journal,* 4(1973):16–20.

Morrison, J.B. "Chronic Asthma and Improvement with Relaxation Induced by Hypnotherapy." *Journal of the Royal Society of Medicine*, 81(1988): 701–704.

Mrazek, D.A. "Asthma: Psychiatric Considerations, Evaluation, and Management." In Middleton, E.; Reed, C.E.; and Ellis, E.F. *Allergy: Principles and Practice* (3rd ed.) St. Louis: C.V. Mosby, 1988, pp. 1176–1196.

Mrazek, D.A. "Psychiatric Complications of Pediatric Asthma." *Annals of Allergy*, 69(1992):285–290.

Mrazek, D.A., and Klinnert, M. "Asthma: Psychoneuroimmunologic Considerations." In Ader, R.; Felten, D.L.; and Cohen, N. (eds.) *Psychoneuroimmunology* (2nd ed.) Orlando, Fla.: Academic Press, 1990, pp. 1013–1035.

Mrazek, D.A.; Klinnert, M.D.; Mrazek, P.; and Macey, T. "Early Asthma Onset: Consideration of Parenting Issues." *Journal of the American Academy of Child and Adolescent Psychiatry*, 30(1991):277–282.

Strunk, R.C.; Mrazek, D.A.; Wolfson Fuhrmann, G.S.; and LaBrecque, J.F. "Physiologic and Psychological Characteristics Associated with Deaths Due to Asthma in Childhood: A Case-Controlled Study." *Journal of the American Medical Association*, 254 (1985):1193–1198,

Yellowlees, P.M., and Kalucy, R.S. "Psychobiological Aspects of Asthma and the Consequent Research Implications." *Chest*, 97(1990):628–634.

12. INFERTILITY, PREGNANCY, AND THE EMOTIONS

Groups and Organizations

RESOLVE is a national, nonprofit organization that offers information and support to infertile individuals and couples, plus education for health-care professionals. Their national office can help you find a chapter in your area:

RESOLVE
1310 Broadway
Somerville, MA 02144-1731
Business office: (617) 623-1156
HelpLine: (617) 623-0744

General References

Liebmann-Smith, Joan. *In Pursuit of Pregnancy: How Couples Discover, Cope With, and Resolve Their Fertility Problems.* New York: Newmarket Press, 1987. Reviews the medical treatments and options available, and describes the psychological and emotional aspects of infertility—with examples from interviews with infertile couples.

Professional References

Bents, H. "Psychology of Male Infertility: A Literature Survey." *International Journal of Andrology*, 8(1985):325–336.

Cook, E. "Characteristics of the Biopsychosocial Crisis of Infertility." *Journal of Counseling and Development*, 65(1987):465–470.

Domar, A.D.; Seibel, M.M.; and Benson, H. "The Mind/Body Program for Infertility: A New Behavioral Treatment Approach for Women with Infertility." *Fertility and Sterility*, 53(1990):246–249.

Homer, C.J.; James, S.A.; and Siegel, E. "Work-Related Psychosocial Stress and Risk of Preterm Low Birthweight Delivery." *American Journal of Public Health*, 80(1990):173–177.

Kennell, J.; Klaus, M.; McGrath, S.; Robertson, S.; and Hinkley, C. "Continuous Emotional Support During Labor in a U.S. Hospital." *Journal of the American Medical Association*, 265(1991):2197–2201.

Klebanoff, M.; Shiono, P.; and Rhoads, G. "Outcomes of Pregnancy in a National Sample of Resident Physicians." *New England Journal of Medicine*, 323 (1990):1040–1045.

Mahlstedt, P. "The Psychological Component of Infertility." *Fertility and Sterility*, 43(1985):335–346.

Menning, B. "The Emotional Needs of Infertile Couples." *Fertility and Sterility*, 34(1980):313–319.

Rothberg, A.D., and Lits, B. "Psychological Support for Maternal Stress During Pregnancy: Effect on Birth Weight." *American Journal of Obstetrics and Gynecology*, 165(1991):403–407.

Seibel, M.M. (ed.) *Infertility: A Comprehensive Text.* Norwalk, Conn.: Appleton & Lange, 1990.

Seibel, M.M., and Taymor, M.L. "Emotional Aspects of Infertility." *Fertility and Sterility*, 37(1982): 137–145.

Seibel, M.M. "A New Era in Reproductive Technology: In Vitro Fertilization, Gamete Intrafallopian Transfer, and Donated Gametes and Embryos." *New England Journal of Medicine*, 318(1988):828–834.

13. SOMATIZATION: WHEN PHYSICAL SYMPTOMS HAVE NO MEDICAL CAUSE

General References

Barsky, Arthur J. *Worried Sick: Our Troubled Quest for Wellness.* New York: Little, Brown, 1988. A psychiatrist who has studied the way people experience illness describes what he sees as a national obsession with sickness and health.

Professional References

Cummings, N.A. "Arguments for the Financial Efficacy of Psychological Services in Health Care Settings." In Sweet, J.J., et al. (eds.) *Handbook of Clinical Psychology in Medical Settings.* New York: Plenum, 1990, pp. 113–126.

Cummings, N.A., and Bragman, J.I. "Triaging the 'Somaticizer' Out of the Medical System Into a Psychological System." In Stern, E.M. and V.F. (eds.) *Psychotherapy and the Somatizing Patient.* Binghamton, N.Y.: Haworth Press, 1988, pp. 109–112.

Cummings, N.A., and Follette, W.T. "Psychiatric Services and Medical Utilization in a Prepaid Health Plan Setting: Part 2." *Medical Care,* 6(1968): 31–41.

Cummings, N.A., and VandenBos, G.R. "The Twenty Years Kaiser-Permanente Experience with Psychotherapy and Medical Utilization: Implications for National Health Policy and National Health Insurance." *Health Policy Quarterly,* 1(1981): 159–175.

Follette, W.T., and Cummings, N.A. "Psychiatric Services and Medical Utilization in a Prepaid Health Plan Setting." *Medical Care,* 5(1968): 25–35.

Gonik, U.; Farrow, I.; Meier, M.; Ostmand, G.; and Frolick, L. "Cost Effectiveness of Behavioral Medicine Procedures in the Treatment of Stress-Related Disorders." *American Journal of Clinical Biofeedback,* 4(1981): 16–24.

Jacobs, D.F. "Cost-Effectiveness of Specialized Psychological Programs for Reducing Hospital Stays and Outpatient Visits." *Journal of Clinical Psychology,* 43 (1987):729–735.

Rosen, J.C., and Wiens, A.N. "Changes in Medical Problems and Use of Medical Services Following Psychological Intervention." *American Psychologist,* 34 (1979):420–431.

Schlesinger, H.J.; Mumford, E.; and Glass, G.V. "Mental Health Services and Medical Utilization." In VandenBos, Gary R. (ed.) *Psychotherapy: Practice, Research, Policy.* Beverly Hills, Calif.: Sage, 1980. (Out of print.)

Yates, B.T. "How Psychology Can Improve Effectiveness and Reduce Costs of Health Services." *Psychotherapy,* 21(1984): 439–451.

14. THE RELAXATION RESPONSE

Groups, Organizations, and Clinics

Most stress management courses teach a range of self-help techniques, many of which elicit the physiological elements of the relaxation response. Many are offered by local hospitals and self-help groups throughout the United States. Your own physician, local hospital, or health maintenance organization may be able to give you relaxation training. If so, ask whether instruction is offered in techniques that elicit the relaxation response, such as progressive muscle relaxation, autogenic training, yoga, or meditation. If these elements are not an essential part of the program, consider looking for another course. (You may find one listed in the Yellow Pages under "Stress Management Programs.")

At the Division of Behavioral Medicine at the New England Deaconess Hospital, Herbert Benson and his colleagues offer groups for people dealing with hypertension, cardiac rehabilitation, cancer, AIDS, infertility, menopause, chronic pain, and insomnia. A "Healthy Lifestyles" group is also available at the Mind/Body Medical Institute for people who are currently well but interested in alleviating stress. Frequent courses are held under the aegis of Harvard Medical School's Department of Continuing Medical Education to train health-care professionals in conducting such mind/body programs. For information on any of these programs or services, contact:

The Mind/Body Medical Institute
Division of Behavioral Medicine
New England Deaconess Hospital
185 Pilgrim Rd.
Boston, MA 02215
(617) 732-9530

In addition, the first affiliate of the Mind/Body Medical Institute has been established:

The Mind/Body Medical Institute at Mercy Hospital
Stevenson Expressway at King Dr.
Chicago, IL 60616-2477
(312) 567-6700

General References

Benson, Herbert, and Klipper, Miriam. *The Relaxation Response.* New York: Avon, 1976. Describes the basic components of the relaxation response.

Benson, Herbert. *Beyond the Relaxation Response.* New York: Times Books, 1984. Examines the links between belief, spirituality, and the relaxation response.

Benson, Herbert. *Your Maximum Mind.* New York: Times Books, 1987. Explains how the relaxation response may be used to bring about other mind/body effects, maximizing performance and efficiency.

Benson, Herbert; Stuart, Eileen M.; and staff of the Mind/Body Medical Institute. *The Wellness Book: The Comprehensive Guide to Maintaining Health and Treating Stress-Related Illness.* New York: Carol, 1992. A workbook that was written for those who could not attend the clinical programs of the New England Deaconess Hospital and the Mind/Body Medical Institute.

On Audiotape
The Mind/Body Medical Institute has also developed a series of audiotapes on how to elicit the relaxation response. For information on these tapes, contact the Institute at the address above.

Professional References
Benson, H.; Beary, J.F.; and Carol, M.P. "The Relaxation Response." *Psychiatry*, 37(1974):37–46.

Benson, H.; Lehmann, J.W.; Malhotra, M.S.; Goldman, R.F.; Hopkins, J.; and Epstein, M.D. "Body Temperature Changes During the Practice of gTum-mo Yoga." *Nature*, 295(1982):234–236.

Friedman, R.; Siegel, W.C.; Jacobs, S.C.; and Benson, H. "Distress over the Non-Effect of Stress." *Journal of the American Medical Association*, 268(1992): 198.

Hoffman, J.W.; Benson, H.; Arns, P.A.; Stainbrook, G.L.; Landsberg, I.; Young, J.B.; and Gill, A. "Reduced Sympathetic Nervous System Responsivity Associated with the Relaxation Response." *Science*, 215(1982):190–192.

Wallace, R.K.; Benson, H.; and Wilson, A.F. "A Wakeful Hypometabolic Physiologic State." *American Journal of Physiology*, 221(1971):795–799.

15. MINDFULNESS MEDITATION: HEALTH BENEFITS OF AN ANCIENT BUDDHIST PRACTICE

Groups, Organizations, and Clinics

Hospital-based Mindfulness Clinics
The following hospitals and clinics now offer mindfulness training in the context of stress reduction or mind/body clinics.

Stress Reduction Clinic
University of Massachusetts Medical Center
Worcester, MA 01655
(508) 856-1616

Along with the eight-week program described in Chapter 15, which entails weekly training sessions, the Stress Reduction Clinic offers a limited number of intensive five-day residential programs to meet the needs of people who live beyond easy commuting distance to the Medical Center. Training programs in mindfulness-based stress reduction are also available for health professionals; write to the Director of Professional Education at the address above.

Awareness and Relaxation Training
Cabrillo College Stroke Center
501 Upper Park, DeLaveaga Park
Santa Cruz, CA 95065
(408) 722-9005
For correspondence:
338 Rider Rd.
Corralitos, CA 95076

Department of Psychology
The Toronto Hospital
200 Elizabeth St.
Toronto, Ontario, M5G 2C4
Canada
(416) 340-3950

Life Transition Therapy
110 Delgado Compound, Suite A
Santa Fe, NM 87501
(505) 982-4183

Mind/Body Medicine Clinic
2440 East Fifth St.
Tyler, TX 75701
(903) 592-2202

Stress Management Clinic
Rehabilitation Institute of Pittsburgh
6301 Northumberland St.
Pittsburgh, PA 15217
(412) 521-9000

Stress Reduction Clinic
LDS Hospital
Eighth Ave. and C St.
Salt Lake City, UT 84103
(801) 321-1022

Stress Reduction Group
Franklin Clinical Associates
51 Sanderson St., Suite 9
Greenfield, MA 01301
(413) 772-0211, ext. 2209
(A service of Franklin Medical Center)

Mind Body Stress Reduction Program
Arthritis-Fibrositis Center
Newton Wellesley Hospital
2014 Washington St.
Newton, MA 02162
(617) 527-7485

Stress Reduction Group
Hubbard Human Services Center
Hubbard Regional Hospital
340 Thompson Rd.
Webster, MA 01570
(508) 943-2600, ext. 285

Stress Reduction Clinic
Behavioral Associates
73 Main St.
Brattleboro, VT 05301
(802) 257-0319

Stress Reduction and Relaxation Program
4401 Wilshire Blvd.
Los Angeles, CA 90010
(310) 395-1233

Stress Reduction and Relaxation Program
Edith Nourse Rogers Memorial VA Hospital
200 Springs Rd.
Bedford, MA 01730
(617) 275-7500, ext. 560

Buddhist Groups

Most mindfulness meditation practice in this country takes place within loosely organized Buddhist networks and retreat centers where you can go for extended periods of instruction and practice. If you are not bothered by a slight Buddhist flavor and vocabulary, there are a number of mindfulness teachers and centers that offer excellent instruction and support. These centers do not take a cultish or evangelical approach toward meditation. In fact, mindfulness practice itself encourages practitioners not to get caught up in belief systems of any kind, but to inquire for themselves and chart their own paths towards understanding and clarity. The centers listed below also act as central clearinghouses for local mindfulness practice groups nationwide. Be aware that these centers do not use mindfulness as a mind/body approach to stress reduction and improving one's health, but rather in its original expression—as a path to inner development and self-understanding.

Cambridge Insight Meditation Center
331 Broadway
Cambridge, MA 02139
(617) 491-5070

Insight Meditation Society
Pleasant St.
Barre, MA 01005
(508) 355-4378

Insight Meditation West
P.O. Box 909
Woodacre, CA 94973
(415) 488-0164

General References

Goldstein, Joseph, and Kornfield, Jack. *Seeking the Heart of Wisdom: The Path of Insight Meditation.* Boston: Shambhala, 1987. Essays on mindfulness meditation and its applications by two prominent American teachers of mindfulness practice.

Kabat-Zinn, Jon. *Full Catastrophe Living: Using the Wisdom of Your Body and Mind to Face Stress, Pain and Illness.* New York: Delacorte, 1991. A detailed, step-by-step manual of mindfulness meditation and its applications for mainstream Americans.

Kabat-Zinn, Jon. *Wherever You Go, There You Are: Mindfulness Meditation in Everyday Life. Meditation for Daily Living.* New York: Hyperion, in press. Essays on integrating mindfulness into one's daily life.

Suzuki, Shunryu; ed. by Dixon, Trudy. *Zen Mind, Beginner's Mind.* New York: Weatherhill, 1970. A classic entree into Zen meditation practice.

Thich Nhat Hanh. *The Miracle of Mindfulness: A Manual on Meditation.* (2nd ed.) Boston: Beacon, 1988. A simple, elegant introduction to mindfulness practice.

On Audiotape

The following mindfulness meditation practice tapes, with the voice of Jon Kabat-Zinn, are used at the University of Massachusetts Medical Center's Stress Reduction Clinic, and can also be used in conjunction with the book *Full Catastrophe Living* (see above).

Tape 1: Guided Body Scan Meditation/Mindful Yoga 1. Side One, done lying down, is the first tape people use in the University of Massachusetts Stress Reduction Clinic. This closely guided journey through your body allows you to explore deep states of relaxation and moment-to-moment awareness. Side Two has a gentle sequence of mindful *hatha* yoga postures.

Tape 2: Guided Sitting Meditation/Mindful Yoga 2. Side One has longer stretches of silence between the instructions, allowing you to practice mindfulness on your own. Once learned, the core sitting meditation practice can be used anywhere, for any length of time. Side Two is a different sequence of mindful hatha yoga postures.

These tapes are each 45 minutes a side, and can be ordered for $10.00 *per tape* plus $1.00 per tape for postage and handling. (Massachusetts residents must add an additional $ .50 per tape for sales tax.) Checks should be made out to "Stress Reduction Tapes" and orders sent to: Stress Reduction Tapes, P.O. Box 547, Lexington, MA 02173.

Professional References

Kabat-Zinn, J. "An Out-Patient Program in Behavioral Medicine for Chronic Pain Patients Based on the Practice of Mindfulness Meditation: Theoretical Considerations and Preliminary Results." *General Hospital Psychiatry*, 4(1982):33–47.

Kabat-Zinn, J.; Lipworth, L.; and Burney, R. "The Clinical Use of Mindfulness Meditation for the Self-Regulation of Chronic Pain." *Journal of Behavioral Medicine*, 8(1985):163–190.

Kabat-Zinn, J.; Lipworth, L.; Burney, R.; and Sellers, W. "Four Year Follow-Up of a Meditation-Based Program for the Self-Regulation of Chronic Pain: Treatment Outcomes and Compliance." *Clinical Journal of Pain*, 2/3(1986):159–173.

Kabat-Zinn, J., and Chapman-Waldrop, A. "Compliance with an Outpatient Stress Reduction Program: Rates and Predictors of Program Completion." *Journal of Behavioral Medicine*, 11(1988):333–352.

Kabat-Zinn, J.; Massion, A.; Kristeller, J.; Peterson, L.; Fletcher, K.; Pbert, L.; Lenderking, W.; and Santorelli, S.F. "Effectiveness of a Meditation-Based Stress Reduction Program in the Treatment of Anxiety Disorders." *American Journal of Psychiatry*, 149 (1992):936–943.

Walsh, R.N. "The Consciousness Disciplines and the Behavioral Sciences: Questions of Comparison and Assessment." *American Journal of Psychiatry*, 137(1980):663–673.

16. HYPNOSIS: THE POWER OF ATTENTION

Groups and Organizations

Either of the professional hypnosis societies listed below can refer you to local members, all of whom have gone through rigorous screening by the societies. Both organizations recommend that their members be certified by one of the three boards of hypnosis: the American Board of Medical Hypnosis, the American Board of Dental Hypnosis, or the American Board of Psychological Hypnosis. When requesting referrals, enclose a self-addressed stamped envelope.

The American Society of Clinical Hypnosis (ASCH)
2200 East Devon Ave., Suite 291
Des Plaines, IL 60018

The Society for Clinical and Experimental Hypnosis (SCEH)
128-A Kingspark Drive
Liverpool, NY 13090
(315) 652-7299

The following organization holds clinical workshops on pediatric hypnosis:
The Society for Behavioral Pediatrics
241 East Gravers Lane
Philadelphia, PA 19118
(215) 248-9168

General References

Garfield, Charles. *Peak Performance: Mental Training Techniques of the World's Greatest Athletes.* Los Angeles: Warner Books, 1989. Describes techniques similar to self-hypnosis for improving athletic performance.

Haley, Jay. *Uncommon Therapy.* New York: W.W. Norton, 1987. Describes the therapeutic strategies used by Milton Erickson, a pioneer in hypnotherapy.

Professional References

Ament, P. "Concepts in the Use of Hypnosis for Pain Relief in Cancer," *Journal of Medicine* (NY), 13(1982):233–240.

Fromm, E., and Kahn, S. *Self-Hypnosis: The Chicago Paradigm.* New York: Guilford Press, 1990.

Olness, K., and Gardner, G.G. *Hypnosis and Hypnotherapy with Children.* (2nd ed.) Orlando, Fla.: W.B. Saunders, 1988.

Olness, K.; MacDonald, J.T.; and Uden, D.L. "Comparison of Self-Hypnosis and Propranolol in the Treatment of Juvenile Classic Migraine." *Pediatrics*, 79(1987): 593–597.

Olness, K.; Culbert, T.; and Uden, D. "Self-Regulation of Salivary Immunoglobulin A by Children." *Pediatrics*, 83(1989): 66–71.

Spiegel, H., and Spiegel, D. *Trance and Treatment: Clinical Uses of Hypnosis.* Washington, D.C.: American Psychiatric Press, 1987.

17. IMAGERY: LEARNING TO USE THE MIND'S EYE

Groups and Organizations

Imagery is easiest to learn with the assistance of an experienced professional. You can probably find one through a local hospital's wellness program, patient support group, or behavioral medicine unit. You might also query local holistic medicine practitioners or mental health professionals with an interest in health psychology. Make sure the person you choose has a professional license to practice health care or counseling; while that's not a guarantee of expertise in imagery, it does suggest some level of accountability. In addition, ask the practitioner for several references from patients he or she has treated. The following professional organizations may be able to refer you to a local qualified health-care practitioner who uses guided imagery:

The Academy for Guided Imagery
P.O. Box 2070
Mill Valley, CA 94942
(800) 726-2070

Teaches health professionals to use guided imagery through a two-and-a-half-day intensive training program and also offers a 150-hour certification program accredited by the American Psychological Association. Host of an annual November conference on imagery, the Academy has recently published its Directory of Imagery Practitioners and offers a free catalog of imagery-related books and tapes.

The Institute of Transpersonal Psychology
744 San Antonio Rd.
Palo Alto, CA 94303
(415) 493-4430

Offers training in many uses of imagery, including its applications in healing.

General References

Books generally offer more information, explanation, and theory than audiotapes, but a good audiotape will guide you through your own imagery experiences. Most self-help books and tapes teach a relatively passive approach in which the imagery is relaxing, potentially healing, or insightful. Others make an attempt to teach a more interactive approach.

Achterberg, Jeanne. *Imagery in Healing: Shamanism and Modern Medicine.* Boston: Shambhala, 1985. Explains the scientific basis of imagery techniques and the history of nonmedical healing in the Western world.

Jaffe, Dennis T. *Healing from Within: Psychological Techniques to Help the Mind Heal the Body.* New York: Simon & Schuster, 1986. Provides in-depth information about the psychological and scientific basis for imagery techniques.

Jung, Carl G. *Man and His Symbols.* New York: Doubleday, 1969. The most accessible book regarding Jung's work; illustrates how symbols relate to deeply meaningful dimensions of human life.

Rossman, Martin L. *Healing Yourself: A Step-by-Step Program for Better Health Through Imagery.* New York: Walker, 1987. An easy-to-read book with many examples of healing with imagery and scripts for nine imagery techniques for self-healing. Accompanying tapes can be ordered through Insight Publishing, P.O. Box 2070, Mill Valley, CA 94942; (800) 234-8562.

Samuels, Michael. *Healing with the Mind's Eye.* New York: Random House, 1992. An engaging book from a medical pioneer in the uses of imagery. (Out of print.)

For additional books and tapes, contact one of the following:

The Imagery Store
P.O. Box 2070
Mill Valley, CA 94942
(800) 726-2070

Offers books and tapes, for professionals and lay people, relating to imagery in medicine and healing: relaxation, pain relief, self-healing, and insight development. Also tapes of national conferences on imagery and healing. Free catalog.

The Source Cassette Learning System
Emmet Miller, M.D.
945 Evelyn St.
Menlo Park, CA 94025
(415) 328-7171

Offers tapes for relaxation, pain relief, surgery preparation, habit change, pregnancy, recovering from drug dependency, sleep disorders, and healing. Free catalog.

MindBody Health Sciences
22 Lawson Terrace
Scituate, MA 02066
(617) 545-7122

Books and tapes for medical and mental health applications. Free annual newsletter.

Professional References

Barber, T.X. "Physiologic Effects of 'Hypnotic Suggestions': A Critical Review of Recent Research (1960–64)." *Psychological Bulletin,* 63(1965): 201–222.

Sheikh, A.A. (ed.) *Imagination and Healing.* Farmingdale, N.Y.: Baywood, 1984.

Sheikh, A.A., and Shaffer, John T. (eds.) *The Potential of Fantasy and Imagination.* New York: Brandon House, 1979.

18. BIOFEEDBACK: USING THE BODY'S SIGNALS

Groups and Organizations

The Biofeedback Certification Institute of America (BCIA) offers a directory of biofeedback practitioners, their educational background and clinical experience. You can find a copy through a local biofeedback professional or a library. BCIA can also direct you by phone to professionals in your area.

Biofeedback Certification Institute of America
10200 West 44th Ave., Suite 304
Wheatridge, CO 80033
(303) 420-2902

Another resource is the Association for Applied Psychophysiology and Biofeedback, a membership organization of biofeedback practitioners which also publishes a directory. Same address as BCIA. Phone: (303) 422-8436.

Professional References

Basmajian, J.V. (ed.) *Biofeedback: Principles and Practice for Clinicians.* (3rd ed.) Baltimore: Williams and Wilkins, 1989.

Hatch, J.P.; Fisher, J.G.; and Rugh, J.D. *Biofeedback: Studies in Clinical Efficacy.* New York: Plenum, 1987.

Schwartz, M.S., et al. *Biofeedback: A Practitioner's Guide.* New York: Guilford Press, 1987.

Shellenberger, R.; Amar, P.; Schneider, C.; and Stewart, R. *Clinical Efficacy and Cost Effectiveness of Biofeedback Therapy: Guidelines for Third Party Reimbursement.* Wheat Ridge, Colo.: Association for Applied Psychophysiology and Biofeedback, 1989.

Shellenberger, R., and Green, J. A. *From the Ghost in the Box to Successful Biofeedback Training.* Greeley, Colo.: Health Psychology Publications, 1986.

19. EXERCISE FOR STRESS CONTROL

General References

American College of Sports Medicine. *ACSM Fitness Book.* Champaign, Ill.: Human Kinetics Publishers, 1992. A step-by-step guide to physical fitness by a major exercise-science organization. Helpful for people unsure of how to start an exercise program.

Gavin, James. *The Exercise Habit.* Champaign, Ill.: Leisure Press, 1992. Addresses personality and lifestyle issues and ways to make exercise a life-long habit.

Professional References

Brown, J.D. "Staying Fit and Staying Well: Physical Fitness as a Moderator of Life Stress." *Journal of Personality and Social Psychology,* 60(1991):555–561.

deVries, H.A. "Tranquilizer Effect of Exercise: A Critical Review." *Physician and Sportsmedicine,* 9 (1981):47–55.

Griest, J.H.; Klein, M.H.; Eischens. R.R.; Faris, J.; Gurman, A.S.; and Morgan, W.P. "Running as a Treatment for Depression." *Comparative Psychiatry,* 53(1979):20–41.

Kobasa, S.C.; Maddi, S.R.; and Puccetti, M.C. "Personality and Exercise as Buffers in the Stress-Illness Relationship." *Journal of Behavioral Medicine,* 5 (1982):391–404.

LaPerriere, A.; Fletcher, M.A.; Antoni, M.H.; and Klimas, N.G. "Aerobic Exercise Training in an AIDS Risk Group." *International Journal of Sports Medicine,* 12(Suppl.) (1991):S53–S57.

Sacks, M.H. (ed.) *The Psychology of Running.* Champaign, Ill.: Human Kinetics Press, 1981.

Sacks, M. "Psychological Aspects of Sports Participation." *Sports Medicine,* 8(1986):1-3.

Sacks, M. "Psychiatry and Sport." *Annals of Sports Medicine,* 5(1990):47-52.

Schwartz, G.E.; Davidson, R.J.; and Goleman, D.J. "Patterning of Cognitive and Somatic Processes in the Self-Regulation of Anxiety: Effects of Meditation Versus Exercise." *Psychosomatic Medicine,* 40(1978): 321–328.

20. SOCIAL SUPPORT: HOW FRIENDS, FAMILY, AND GROUPS CAN HELP

Groups and Organizations

Support groups for people with various illnesses are listed under chapters dealing with those illnesses. For information on other kinds of self-help groups, contact The American Self-Help Clearinghouse; call or send a self-addressed stamped envelope. (For a full description of that organization, see Chapter 25.)

The American Self-Help Clearinghouse
St. Clares-Riverside Medical Center
25 Pocono Rd.
Denville, NJ 07834
(201) 625-7101

General References

Pilisuk, Marc, and Parks, Susan H. *The Healing Web: Social Networks and Human Survival.* Hanover, N.H.: University Press of New England, 1986. Examines the role of friendships, family, the workplace, and the larger social framework in our physical and emotional well-being.

Spiegel, David. *Living Beyond Limits.* New York:

Times Books, in press. Discusses the author's research, including his ongoing studies of women with breast cancer.

Professional References
Berkman, L.F., and Syme, S.L. "Social Networks, Host Resistance, and Mortality: A Nine-Year Follow-up Study of Alameda County Residents." *American Journal of Epidemiology*, 109(1979):186–204.

Goodwin, J.S.; Hunt, W.C.; Key, C. R.; et al. "The Effect of Marital Status on Stage, Treatment, and Survival of Cancer Patients." *Journal of the American Medical Association*, 258(1987):3125–3130.

House, J.S.; Landis, K.R.; and Umberson, D. "Social Relationships and Health." *Science*, 241(1988):540–545.

Kennedy, S.; Kiecolt-Glaser, J.K.; and Glaser, R. "Immunological Consequences of Acute and Chronic Stressors: Mediating Role of Interpersonal Relationships." *British Journal of Medical Psychology*, 61(1988):77–85.

Ramirez, A.J.; Craig, T.K.; Watson, J.P.; et al. "Stress and Relapse of Breast Cancer." *British Medical Journal*, 298(1989):291–293.

Spiegel, D. "Facilitating Emotional Coping During Treatment." *Cancer*, 66(1990):1422–1426.

Spiegel, D.; Bloom, J.R.; Kraemer, H.C.; and Gottheil, E. "Effect of Psychosocial Treatment on Survival of Patients with Metastatic Breast Cancer." *Lancet*, 2(1989):888–891.

21. HEALTHY ATTITUDES: OPTIMISM, HOPE, AND CONTROL

Groups and Organizations
Cognitive therapy is a standard part of the training of many psychologists and mental health professionals. An effective treatment for depression, it can help alter pessimistic thinking. If your state psychological association cannot help, The Center for Cognitive Therapy can provide referrals to therapists trained in this technique.

The Center for Cognitive Therapy
The Science Center, Room 754
3600 Market St.
Philadelphia, PA 19104
(215) 898-4102

General References
Burns, David D. *Feeling Good: The New Mood Therapy*. New York: NAL–Dutton, 1981. An accessible introduction to cognitive therapy for depression.

Peterson, Christopher, and Bossio, Lisa M. *Health and Optimism*. New York: Macmillan, 1991. A nontechnical discussion of the recent research linking positive attitudes to good health.

Professional References
Beck, A.T. *Cognitive Therapy and Emotional Disorders*. New York: International Universities Press, 1976.

Gardner, H. *The Mind's New Science: A History of the Cognitive Revolution*. New York: Basic Books, 1987.

Peterson, C. "Explanatory Style as a Risk Factor for Illness." *Cognitive Therapy and Research*, 12(1988):119–132.

Peterson, C.; Maier, S.F.; and Seligman, M.E.P. *Learned Helplessness: A Theory for the Age of Personal Control*. New York: Oxford University Press, in press.

Peterson, C., and Seligman, M.E.P. "Explanatory Style and Illness." *Journal of Personality*, 55(1987):237–265.

Peterson, C.; Seligman, M.E.P.; and Vaillant, G.E. "Pessimistic Explanatory Style Is a Risk Factor for Physical Illness: A Thirty-Five Year Longitudinal Study." *Journal of Personality and Social Psychology*, 55(1988):23–27.

22. PSYCHOTHERAPY AND MEDICAL CONDITIONS

Groups and Organizations
The Linda Pollin Foundation for Medical Crisis Counseling
4701 Willard Ave., Suite 223
Chevy Chase, MD 20815
(301) 718-4317

Offers information on *medical crisis counseling*, a short-term approach to helping people dealing with illness.

The following organizations can refer you to local branches, which can provide information on psychological treatment and provide referrals to their members.

American Psychiatric Association
1400 K. St. NW
Washington, DC 20005
(202) 682-6000

American Psychological Association
750 First St. NE
Washington, DC 20002-4242
(202) 336-5700

National Association of Social Workers
750 First St. NE, Suite 700
Washington, DC 20002
(202) 408-8600

American Association for Marriage and Family
  Therapy
1100 17th St. NW, 10th Floor
Washington, DC 20036
(800) 374-2638

General References

Engler, Jack, and Goleman, Daniel. *The Consumer's Guide to Psychotherapy.* New York: Fireside/Simon & Schuster, 1992. A guide to making informed choices about psychotherapy—how to find the right therapist, which approaches are best for specific problems, how to tell if therapy is working.

Pennebaker, James W. *Opening Up: The Healing Power of Confiding in Others.* New York: William Morrow, 1990. Describes the physical and emotional benefits of uncovering hidden feelings, whether in psychotherapy or in a private journal.

Professional References

Climent, C.E., and Burns, B.J. *Practical Psychiatry for the Health Professional.* Manchester, N.H.: Robert B. Luce, 1984.

Fulop, G.; Strain, J.J.; Vita, J.; et al. "Impact of Psychiatric Comorbidity on Length of Hospital Stay for Medical/Surgical Patients: A Preliminary Report." *American Journal of Psychiatry,* 144(1987):878–882.

Jones, K.R., and Vischi, T.R. "Impact of Alcohol, Drug Abuse and Mental Health Treatment on Medical Care Utilization: A Review of the Research Literature." *Medical Care,* 17, Suppl. 2(1979):1–82.

Kornfeld, D.S., and Finkel, J.B. (eds.) *Psychiatric Management for Medical Practitioners.* Philadelphia: W.B. Saunders, 1982. (Out of print.)

Mumford, E.; Schlesinger, H.J.; and Glass, G.V. "Reducing Medical Costs Through Mental Health Treatment: Research Problems and Recommendations." In Broskowski, A.; Marks, E.; and Budman, S.H. (eds.) *Linking Health and Mental Health.* Beverly Hills, Calif.: Sage, 1981, pp. 257–273. (Out of print.)

Schlesinger, H.J.; Mumford, E.; Glass, G.V.; et al. "Mental Health Treatment and Medical Care Utilization in a Fee-for-Service System: Outpatient Mental Health Treatment Following the Onset of a Chronic Disease." *American Journal of Public Health,* 73(1983): 422–429.

Strain, J.J., and Grossman, S. *Psychological Care of the Medically Ill: A Primer in Liaison Psychiatry.* New York: Appleton & Lange, 1976. (Out of print.)

Strain, J.J. *Psychological Interventions in Medical Practice.* New York: Appleton & Lange, 1978. (Out of print.)

Strain, J.J.; Lyons, J.S.; Hammer, J.S.; et al. "Cost Offset from a Psychiatric Consultation-Liaison Intervention with Elderly Hip Fracture Patients." *American Journal of Psychiatry,* 148(1991):1044–1049.

Von Korff, M.; Ormel, J.; Katon, W.; and Lin, E.H. "Disability and Depression Among High Utilizers of Health Care. A Longitudinal Analysis." *Archives of General Psychiatry,* 49(1992):91–100.

23. STRESS MANAGEMENT: STRATEGIES THAT WORK

General References

McKay, Matthew; Davis, Martha; and Eshelman, Elizabeth R. (eds.) *Relaxation and Stress Workbook.* (3rd ed.) Oakland, Calif.: New Harbinger, 1988. Teaches the major stress reduction techniques available today.

Professional References

Antoni, M.H.; Baggett, L.; Ironson, G.; LaPerriere, A.; August, S.; Klimas, N.; Schneiderman, N.; and Fletcher, M.A. "Cognitive-Behavioral Stress Management Intervention Buffers Distress Responses and Immunologic Changes Following Notification of HIV-1 Seropositivity." *Journal of Consulting and Clinical Psychology,* 59(1991):906–915.

Antoni, M.H. "Psychosocial Stressors and Behavioral Interventions in Gay Men with HIV-1 Infection." *International Review of Psychiatry,* 3(1991): 383–399.

Antoni, M.H.; Schneiderman, N.; Fletcher, M.A.; Goldstein, D.; Ironson, G.; and LaPerriere, A. "Psychoneuroimmunology and HIV-1." *Journal of Consulting and Clinical Psychology,* 58(1990): 38–49.

Esterling, B.; Antoni, M.H.; Schneiderman, N.; Carver, S.; LaPerriere, A.; Ironson, G.; Klimas, N.; and Fletcher, M.A. "Psychosocial Modulation of Antibody to Epstein-Barr Viral Capsid Antigen and Human Herpesvirus Type-6 in HIV-1 Infected and At Risk Gay Men." *Psychosomatic Medicine,* 54(1992): 345–371.

Folkman, S.; Chesney, M.; McKusick, L.; Ironson, G; Johnson, D.; and Coates, T. "Translating Coping Theory into Intervention." In McKenrode, J. (ed.) *The*

Social Context of Stress. New York: Plenum, 1991, pp. 239–260

Hoffman, M.A. "Counseling the HIV-infected Client: A Psychosocial Model for Assessment and Intervention." *The Counseling Psychologist,* 19(1991): 467–542.

24. PREPARATION FOR SURGERY AND MEDICAL PROCEDURES

General References
Early in 1992, the Agency for Health Care Policy and Research, of the U.S. Department of Health and Human Services, published reports on acute pain management after surgery, medical procedures, and trauma. The reports outlined the need for better pain control and pharmacological, relaxation, and psychological approaches. The reports are available in several forms:

A patient's guide (Publication No. AHCPR92-0021)

Two quick reference guides for clinicians: one on pain management for adults (Pub. No. AHCPR 92-0019), and one on pain management in infants, children, and adolescents (Pub. No. AHCPR 92-0020).

The clinical practice guideline (Pub. No. AHCPR 92-0032).

The formal guideline report, with full backup material, is still in preparation.

To order copies of any of these materials, contact:
Center for Research Dissemination and Liaison
AHCPR Clearinghouse
P.O. Box 8547
Silver Spring, MD 20907
(800) 358-9295

Other helpful resources include:

Cohan, Carol; Pimm, June B.; and Jude, James R. *A Patient's Guide to Heart Surgery.* New York: HarperCollins, 1991.

When Your Child Needs Surgery (pamphlet). Available from the American Society of Anesthesiologists, 520 N. Northwest Highway, Park Ridge, IL 60068-2573. Send a self-addressed, stamped envelope for single copies.

On Audiotape
Linda Rodgers, C.S.W.
P.I.P. Surgical Audiotape Series, Inc.
70 Maple Ave.
Katonah, NY 10536
(914) 232-6405

Rodgers's tapes for use before, during, and after surgery include different versions for local, regional, and general anesthesia; all include suggestions and instructions with soothing synthesized music.

Steve Diamond
The Sleep Tape
P.O. Box 5032
Santa Monica, CA 90409-5032
Soothing voices and ocean sounds; no suggestions or instructions.

Music Systems for Undergoing MRI Scanning
Magnacoustics, Inc.
200 Granada St.
Atlantic Beach, NY 11509
(800) 637-2282

Professional References
Anderson, E.A. "Preoperative Preparation for Cardiac Surgery Facilitates Recovery, Reduces Postoperative Distress, and Reduces the Incidence of Acute Postoperative Hypertension." *Journal of Consulting and Clinical Psychology,* 55(1987): 513–520.

Barber, T.X. "Changing 'Unchangeable' Bodily Processes by (Hypnotic) Suggestions: A New Look at Hypnosis, Cognitions, Imagining, and the Mind-Body Problem." In Sheikh, A.A. (ed.), *Imagination and Healing.* Farmingdale, NY: Baywood Publishing, 1984, pp. 69–127.

Bennett, H.L.; Benson, D.R.; and Kuiken, D.A. "Preoperative Instructions for Decreased Bleeding During Spine Surgery." *Anesthesiology,* 65(1986): A245.

Disbrow, E.A.; Bennett, H.L.; and Owings, J.T. "Preoperative Suggestion Hastens the Return of Gastrointestinal Motility." *The Western Journal of Medicine,* in press.

Egbert, L.D.; Battit, G.E.; Welch, C.E.; and Bartlett, M.K. "Reduction of Postoperative Pain by Encouragement and Instruction of Patients." *New England Journal of Medicine,* 270(1964):825–827.

Gattuso, S.M.; Litt, M.D.; and Fitzgerald, T.E. "Coping with Gastrointestinal Endoscopy: Self-Efficacy Enhancement and Coping Style." *Journal of Consulting and Clinical Psychology,* 60(1992):133–139.

Hathaway, D. "Effect of Preoperative Instruction on Postoperative Outcomes: A Meta-Analysis." *Nursing Research,* 35(1986):269–275.

Holden-Lund, C. "Effects of Relaxation with Guided Imagery on Surgical Stress and Wound Healing." *Research in Nursing and Health,* 11(1988):235–244.

Jamison, R.N.; Parris, W.C.; and Maxson, W.S.

"Psychological Factors Influencing Recovery from Outpatient Surgery." *Behaviour Research and Therapy*, 25(1987):31–37.

Linn, B.S.; Linn, M.W.; and Klimas, N.G. "Effects of Psychophysical Stress on Surgical Outcome." *Psychosomatic Medicine*, 50(1988):230–244.

Madden, C.; Singer, G.; Peck, C.; and Nayman, J. "The Effect of EMG Biofeedback on Postoperative Pain Following Abdominal Surgery." *Anaesthesia and Intensive Care*, 6(1978):333–336.

McLintock, T.T.C.; Aitken, H.; Downie, C.F.A.; and Kenny, G.N.C. "Postoperative Analgesic Requirements in Patients Exposed to Positive Intraoperative Suggestions." *British Medical Journal*, 301(1990):788–790.

Mumford, E.; Schlesinger, H.J.; and Glass, G.V. "The Effects of Psychological Intervention on Recovery from Surgery and Heart Attacks: An Analysis of the Literature." *American Journal of Public Health*, 72(1982):141–151.

Peteet, J.R.; Stomper, P.C.; Ross, D.M.; Cotton, V.; Truesdell, P.; and Moczynski, W. "Emotional Support for Patients with Cancer Who Are Undergoing CT: Semistructured Interviews of Patients at a Cancer Institute." *Radiology*, 182(1992):99–102.

Rogers, M., and Reich, P. "Psychological Intervention with Surgical Patients: Evaluation Outcome." *Advances in Psychosomatic Medicine*, 15(1986):23–50.

25. WORKING WITH YOUR DOCTOR

General References

Stutz, David, and Feder, Bernard. *The Savvy Patient: How to Be an Active Participant in Your Medical Care.* Yonkers, N.Y.: Consumer Reports Books, 1990. Advice on communicating with your doctor and getting the best possible care in hospitals.

Ferguson, Tom. (ed.) *Medical Self-Care: Access to Health Tools.* New York: Summit Books, 1980. A large-format sourcebook for lay people and professionals interested in practicing and supporting effective self-care.

Ferguson, Tom. "How Doctors Cause Disease: An Interview with Norman Cousins," *Medical Self-Care*, Winter 1983, 12–19. Cousins focuses on the ways he believes a physician's communication of a serious diagnosis can influence the course of the illness for good or for ill.

Illich, Ivan. *Medical Nemesis: The Expropriation of Health.* New York: Pantheon, 1982. This landmark work was one of the first to describe the dark side of the health-care system and to envision a patient-centered self-help and self-care approach.

Rees, Alan M., and Hoffman, Catherine. *Consumer Health Information Source Book.* (3rd ed.) Phoenix: Oryx Press, 1990. (Available from Oryx Press, 4041 North Central Ave., Suite 700, Phoenix, AZ 85012; (800) 279–6799.) An annotated bibliography of 923 popular books and 202 pamphlets on many health topics. Also lists health-related clearinghouses, hotlines, and resource organizations.

Strasburg, Kate; Saper, Rob; Joss, Jennifer; and Lerner, Michael. *The Quest for Wholeness: An Annotated Bibliography in Patient-Centered Medicine.* Bolinas, Calif.: Commonweal, 1991. (Available from Commonweal, P.O. Box 316, Bolinas, CA 94924.) The most extensive bibliography for patient-centered medicine currently available, listing 293 books and articles. Includes two introductory essays and annotations extensive enough to be interesting and useful. The authors plan to update this bibliography regularly and welcome reader input for future editions.

White, Barbara J., and Madara, Edward J. *The Self-Help Sourcebook: Finding & Forming Mutual Aid Self-Help Groups.* (Available from the American Self-Help Clearinghouse, St. Clares Riverside Medical Center, 25 Pocono Rd., Denville, NJ 07834, (201) 625–7101.) This handbook, updated every other year (4th ed.: 1992) provides a national listing of self-help groups and guidelines for anyone interested in forming or running a self-help group.

On Audiotape

Ferguson, Tom. *Health in the Information Age.* Austin, Tex.: Self-Care Productions, 1990. (Available from Great Performance, 14964 N.W. Greenbriar Parkway, Beaverton OR 97006; (800) 433–3803.) This 90-minute cassette tape explores how the Information Age is changing our health-care system.

Newsletter

Ferguson, Tom. (ed.) *Tom Ferguson's Health in the Information Age Letter.* This quarterly publishes news and opinion about the movement toward self-care, self-help, mind/body medicine, home health care, medical consumerism, wellness, patient-centered care, and other trends. A free sample issue is available: Send a self-addressed business-size envelope with two first-class stamps to Self-Care Productions, 3805 Stevenson Ave., Austin, TX 78703; (512) 472-1333.

Professional References

Beckman, H.B., and Frankel, R.M. "The Effect of Physician Behavior on the Collection of Data." *Annals of Internal Medicine*, 101(1984):692–696.

Demers, R. Y.; Altamore, R.; Mustin, H.; Kleinman, A.; and Leonardi, D. "An Exploration of the Dimensions of Illness Behavior." *The Journal of Family Practice*, 11(1980):1085–1092.

Gartner, A., and Riessman, F. *Self-Help in the Human Services*. San Francisco: Jossey-Bass, 1977.

Greenfield, S.S.; Kaplan, S.H.; and Ware, J.E. "Expanding Involvement in Care: Effect on Patient Outcomes." *Annals of Internal Medicine*, 102(1985):520-528.

Kaplan, S.H.; Greenfield, S.S.; and Ware, J.E. "Assessing the Effects of Physician-Patient Interactions on the Outcomes of Chronic Disease." *Medical Care*, 27(Suppl. 3)(1989):S110–127.

Levin, L.S., and Idler, E.L. *The Hidden Health Care System: Mediating Structures and Medicine*. Maitland, Fla.: American Enterprise, 1981. (Out of print.)

Rost, K.M.; Flavin, K.S.; Cole, K.; and McGill, J.B. "Change in Metabolic Control and Functional Status After Hospitalization: Impact of Patient Activation Intervention in Diabetic Patients." *Diabetes Care*, 14(1991):881–889.

CONTRIBUTORS

MICHAEL H. ANTONI, PH.D., is an investigator in the Center for the Biopsychosocial Study of AIDS at the University of Miami School of Medicine. He is also a senior investigator at the Helen Dowling Institute for Biopsychosocial Medicine in Rotterdam. Antoni is an associate professor of psychology and psychiatry at the University of Miami, where he received his doctorate in clinical psychology and has won several awards for his teaching.

HENRY L. BENNETT, PH.D., is an associate clinical professor in the Department of Anesthesiology at the University of California, Davis, Medical Center, where he is also director of Intraoperative EEG and Sensory Evoked Potential Monitoring. He was trained as an experimental psychologist at UC-Davis, where he received his Ph.D. Bennett has specialized in research on the psychological aspects of surgery, and instructs medical students and residents in the operating room. He is a member of the International Anesthesia Research Society, the American Society of Anesthesiology, and the Society for Clinical and Experimental Hypnosis.

HERBERT BENSON, M.D., is the Mind/Body Medical Institute Associate Professor of Medicine, Harvard Medical School; chief of the Division of Behavioral Medicine at New England Deaconess Hospital; and founding president of the Mind/Body Medical Institute of New England Deaconess Hospital and Harvard Medical School. At Harvard, he holds the first chair in Behavioral Medicine ever endowed at any university. (Upon Benson's retirement, the chair will bear his name.) For more than two decades, Benson has been a leader in international research on the physiology of relaxation and meditation. He is also the author or coauthor of more than 100 scientific publications and five popular books on relaxation and meditation, including *The Relaxation Response*, which was a number-one national bestseller when it was published in 1975 and is still the self-help book most often prescribed by American psychologists.

LISA M. BOSSIO is a freelance writer and editor in the San Francisco Bay area whose interests include health psychology. She has edited and researched several textbooks and articles concerned with psychology and health promotion, and formerly served as a writer and editor in the U.S. Department of Education. She is the coauthor of *Health and Optimism*.

NICHOLAS A. CUMMINGS, PH.D., is president of the Foundation for Behavioral Health and of the National Academies of Practice (an interdisciplinary health policy forum made up of distinguished practitioners from nine primary health care professions). He is the chairman and C.E.O. emeritus of American Biodyne, a national treatment organization offering psychological services to five million enrollees on an HMO model. Cummings and his colleagues were responsible for designing and developing the first comprehensive mental health policy in the United States, implemented through Kaiser-Permanente. Cummings is a former president of the American Psychological Association, which has given him its highest professional award for Distinguished Contributions to Practice.

ELIZABETH A. DISBROW, M.A., is a staff research associate in the Department of Anesthesiology at the University of California, Davis, Medical Center. She wrote her master's thesis on the effects of suggestion on postoperative gastrointestinal complications, and is now working towards a Ph.D. in health psychology at UC-Davis.

TOM FERGUSON, M.D., is a graduate of the Yale University School of Medicine. He was the founding editor of the journal *Medical Self-Care* and served for many years as the medical editor of the *Whole Earth Catalog*. He currently edits *Tom Ferguson's Health in the Information Age Letter*. He has received the National Educational Press Association's Distinguished Achievement Award and the Committee for an Extended Lifetime's Lifetime Extension Award for his writings "on the rapidly expanding area of self-help and self-care." His work has been cited by John Naisbitt in his book *Megatrends* as representing "the essence of the shift from institutional help to self-help."

RONALD GLASER, PH.D., is professor and chairman of the Department of Medical Microbiology and Immunology at the Ohio State University College of Medicine. He is a fellow of the Academy for Behavioral Medicine Research and coeditor of three books on human herpes virus infections. He is also the principal investigator of two five-year research projects on stress and health, funded by the National Institute of Mental Health.

DANIEL GOLEMAN, Ph.D., received his doctorate in psychology from Harvard and served on the Harvard faculty before joining the staff of *Psychology Today* as an editor. Since 1984 he has written for *The New York Times* on health and human behavior. He is the author or editor of nine books, including, most recently, *The Consumer's Guide to Psychotherapy* (coauthored with Jack Engler). He has received the Lifetime Achievement Award of the American Psychological Association and is a fellow of the American Association for the Advancement of Science.

TED A. GROSSBART, Ph.D., is a senior associate and clinical supervisor in Beth Israel Hospital's Department of Psychiatry, and an instructor in psychology in the Department of Psychiatry at the Harvard Medical School. He has been a pioneer in the use of mind/body approaches to treat major skin, allergic, sexually transmitted, and autoimmune disorders. He is a diplomate and a fellow of the American Board of Medical Psychotherapists, and is the coauthor of *Skin Deep: A Mind/Body Program for Healthy Skin.*

JOEL GURIN is the science editor of *Consumer Reports.* A Harvard graduate in biochemistry, he has covered science and medicine as a journalist since 1975. He was a cofounder and, later, the editor in chief of *American Health*, the first health magazine ever to win the National Magazine Award for General Excellence. He has written for a score of national magazines and is the coauthor of three other books on health and medicine. He has won several national awards for his work, including the top science-writing awards of the American Association for the Advancement of Science and the National Association of Science Writers.

JIMMIE C. HOLLAND, M.D., is chief of the Psychiatry Service at New York's Memorial Sloan-Kettering Cancer Center, where she holds the Wayne C. Chapman chair in psychiatric oncology, the world's first endowed chair in this specialty. She is senior editor of the first reference text available on the psychological aspects of cancer, *Handbook of Psycho-Oncology*, and is coeditor of the international publication *Psycho-Oncology: Journal of the Psychological, Social, and Behavioral Dimensions of Cancer*. She established the International Psycho-Oncology Society, the first international network for professionals in this area; was the first president of theAmerican Society of Psychiatric Oncology/AIDS; andestablished the first training program in psychiatric aspects of cancer.

JON KABAT-ZINN, Ph.D., is director of the Stress Reduction Clinic at the University of Massachusetts Medical Center in Worcester, where he is an associate professor of medicine. He holds a doctorate in molecular biology from MIT, and has practiced mindfulness meditation since 1967. He is the author of *Full Catastrophe Living: Using the Wisdom of Your Body and Mind to Face Stress, Pain and Illness.*

JANICE K. KIECOLT-GLASER, Ph.D., is a professor of psychiatry and psychology at the Ohio State University College of Medicine. She is a fellow of the Academy of Behavioral Medicine Research and of the American Psychological Association, and has won the APA's award for Outstanding Contributions to Health Psychology. In 1990, she received the first Alumni Award for Outstanding Contributions to Scientific/Academic Psychology from the University of Miami.

SHELDON LEWIS is a senior editor of the newsletter *Health Confidential*, published by Boardroom Reports. He was director of publications at the Institute for the Advancement of Health, and editor of *Advances: The Journal of Mind-Body Health*. With his wife, Sheila Kay Lewis, he is coauthor of *The Positive Child*, a book on stress management and mind/body health for children.

JAMES A. McCARTHY, M.D., is on the staff of the Faulkner Centre for Reproductive Medicine at Faulkner Hospital in Boston. He is a fellow of the American College of Obstetrics and Gynecology and a clinical instructor at the Harvard Medical School.

DAVID A. MRAZEK, M.D., is chairman of psychiatry and chief of psychiatry and behavioral sciences at Children's National Medical Center in Washington, D.C. He is also a professor of psychiatry and pediatrics at the George Washington University School of Medicine. From 1979 to 1991, he was the director of pediatric psychiatry at the National Jewish Center for Immunology and Respiratory Medicine in Denver. He is codirector of the first major research effort, funded by the National Institute of Mental Health and the W. T. Grant Foundation, to determine the possible effect of stress on susceptibility to asthma or allergic illness in genetically vulnerable infants.

JUSTIN M. NASH, Ph.D., received his doctorate in clinical psychology from Ohio University and was a clinical research psychologist at the Pain Evaluation and Treatment Institute, University of Pittsburgh School of Medicine. He is currently on the psychology staff at the Center of Behavioral Medicine at Miriam Hospital (Providence, R.I.) and holds an appointment in the Department of Psychiatry and Human Behavior, Brown University Medical School.

KAREN OLNESS, M.D., is a professor in the Departments of Pediatrics, Family Medicine, and International Health at Case Western Reserve University. She is also director of the Division of General Academic Pediatrics in the Department of Pediatrics at Rainbow Babies and Children's Hospital in Cleveland. A pioneer in the application of mind/body techniques to children, she has served at different times as president of the Society for Behavioral Pediatrics, the American Society of Clinical Hypnosis, the Society for Clinical and Experimental Hypnosis, and the American Board of Medical Hypnosis.

KENNETH R. PELLETIER, PH.D., M.D. (hon.), is a senior clinical fellow at the Stanford Center for Research in Disease Prevention at the Stanford University School of Medicine. A leader in the development of corporate health promotion programs, he is also director of the Stanford Corporate Health Program, a collaboration between the university and 20 major corporations. Before coming to Stanford, Pelletier was an associate clinical professor of medicine at the University of California, San Francisco. He is the author of *Mind as Healer, Mind as Slayer* and other books that have been influential in bringing mind/body concepts to both professional and general audiences.

CHRISTOPHER PETERSON, PH.D., is a professor of psychology at the University of Michigan. He was formerly an associate professor of psychology at Virginia Polytechnic Institute and State University, where he did research on explanatory style and health. He is the author of several books, including texts on introductory psychology, abnormal psychology, and personality, and is coauthor of *Health and Optimism*, written for a general audience.

THEODORE PINCUS, M.D., is a professor of medicine at Vanderbilt University School of Medicine, where he was formerly chief of rheumatology and immunology. A graduate of Harvard Medical School, he served on the faculties of the Stanford University School of Medicine, The Wistar Institute, and the University of Pennsylvania School of Medicine before coming to Vanderbilt. He is a board-certified specialist in both internal medicine and rheumatology, and is a fellow of the American College of Rheumatology and the American College of Physicians.

MARTIN L. ROSSMAN, M.D., is a clinical associate in the Department of Medicine at the University of California, San Francisco. He is codirector of the Academy for Guided Imagery in Mill Valley, California, and is the author of *Healing Yourself: A Step-by-Step Program for Better Health Through Imagery*. A general practice physician for two decades, he has taught clinical guided imagery to more than four thousand health-care professionals since the early 1980s.

MICHAEL H. SACKS, M.D., is a professor of psychiatry at Cornell University Medical College, a lecturer in psychoanalysis at Columbia Psychoanalytic Center for Training and Research, and an attending psychiatrist at the Payne Whitney Psychiatric Clinic in New York City. His research interests include psychiatric education and psychiatric aspects of AIDS, as well as the psychology of sport. Sacks, editor of the book *Psychology of Running*, is a life-long runner. He began running competitively as a marathoner at age 40 and is currently taking up swimming and bicycling.

MARK S. SCHWARTZ, PH.D., joined the staff of the Mayo Clinic in Rochester, Minnesota, in 1967. He introduced behavior therapies there in 1970, and biofeedback in 1973. He served as chairman of the Biofeedback Certification Institute of America and as president of the Biofeedback Society of America (now the Association for Applied Psychophysiology and Biofeedback). In 1988, he transferred to the Mayo Clinic in Jacksonville, Florida, to develop psychological services there. He is the principal author of *Biofeedback: A Practitioner's Guide*.

NANCY M. SCHWARTZ, M.A. (formerly Nancy M. George), is a licensed mental health counselor at the Center for Psychological Services in Orange Park, Florida. She is certified by the Biofeedback Certification Institute of America in both biofeedback and stress management education, and is a member of the Association for Applied Psychophysiology and Biofeedback.

MACHELLE M. SEIBEL, M.D., is director of the Faulkner Centre for Reproductive Medicine at Faulkner Hospital in Boston. A specialist in reproductive endocrinology, he is an associate professor of obstetrics and gynecology at Harvard Medical School. His primary research interests center on the endocrinology and physiology of ovulation and encompass several other areas of infertility, including endometriosis and in vitro fertilization.

DAVID SPIEGEL, M.D., is a professor of psychiatry and behavioral sciences at Stanford University School of Medicine, where he has been a member of the faculty since 1975. He is currently director of the Psychosocial Treatment Laboratory and Faculty Psychotherapy Clinic there. Spiegel, who received his medical and psychiatric training at Harvard, is coauthor of *Trance and Treatment*, a standard textbook on the clinical uses of hypnosis. He serves on the editorial boards of the *American Journal of Psychiatry, The Journal of Psychosocial Oncology, Psycho-Oncology,* and *Health Psychology*.

JAMES J. STRAIN, M.D., is a professor of psychiatry and director of the Division of Behavioral Medicine and Consultation Psychiatry at the Mount Sinai Medical Center in New York City. He has a special interest in the psychological care of the medically ill and has 400 published communications on the subject. His research studies, funded by the National Institute of Mental Health and the National Cancer Institute, focus on the effects of psychological symptoms on medical illness. He is the mentor for the training of the Pollin International Scholar in Medical Crisis Counseling.

RICHARD S. SURWIT, PH.D., is a professor of medical psychology and associate professor of medicine at Duke University Medical Center, and research director of the Duke Neurobehavioral Diabetes Program. He is also the former director of the Psychophysiology Laboratory at Harvard Medical School. Surwit has pioneered the use of relaxation and biofeedback techniques in the treatment of Raynaud's disease, hypertension, and diabetes mellitus.

DENNIS C. TURK, PH.D., is director of the Pain Evaluation and Treatment Institute and a professor of psy-

chiatry, anesthesiology, and behavioral science at the University of Pittsburgh School of Medicine. A clinical psychologist, he has also served on the faculty of Yale University, and was a founding member of the International Association for the Study of Pain and the American Pain Society. He is a fellow of the American Psychological Association, the Academy of Behavioral Medicine Research, and the Society of Behavioral Medicine.

WILLIAM E. WHITEHEAD, PH.D., is a professor of medical psychology in the Departments of Psychiatry and Medicine at the Johns Hopkins University School of Medicine. A clinical psychologist, he has done research on the psychological and physiological aspects of gastrointestinal disorders for the past two decades. He has served on the board of directors of the Biofeedback Society of America and of the Society of Behavioral Medicine, and has recently chaired several international working groups on functional gastrointestinal disease.

REDFORD B. WILLIAMS, M.D., is director of the Behavioral Medicine Research Center and head of the Division of Behavioral Medicine at Duke University Medical Center, where he is also a professor of psychiatry and psychology and associate professor of medicine. Williams is president of the American Psychosomatic Society and past president of the Society of Behavioral Medicine. He has directed major research projects on psychology and cardiovascular disease for the National Institute of Mental Health and the National Heart, Lung, and Blood Institute. Williams received his medical training at Yale University and is board-certified in internal medicine.

INDEX